Clinical Manual for

Foundations of

Maternal-Newborn Nursing
Second Edition

Trula Myers Gorrie, M.N., R.N.,C.
Professor Emeritus
Golden West College
Huntington Beach, California

Emily Slone McKinney, M.S.N, R.N.,C.
Education Coordinator
Women's and Children's Services
Baylor Medical Center
Irving, Texas

Sharon Smith Murray, M.S.N, R.N.,C.
Professor, Health Professions
Golden West College
Huntington Beach, California

W.B. SAUNDERS COMPANY
A Division of Harcourt Brace & Company
Philadelphia London Toronto Montreal Sydney Tokyo

W.B. SAUNDERS COMPANY
A Division of Harcourt Brace & Company
The Curtis Center
Independence Square West
Philadelphia, PA 19106

NOTICE

Pharmacology is an ever-changing field. Standard safety precautions must be followed, but as new research and clinical experience broaden our knowledge, changes in treatment and drug therapy become necessary or appropriate. Readers are advised to check the product information currently provided by the manufacturer of each drug to be administered to verify the recommended dose, the method and duration of administration, and the contraindications. It is the responsibility of the treating physician, relying on experience and knowledge of the patient, to determine dosages and the best treatment for the patient. Neither the publisher nor the editor assumes any responsibility for any injury and/or damage to persons or property.

The Publisher

Clinical Manual for
Foundations of Maternal-Newborn Nursing, 2/e   ISBN 0-7216-7466-6

Copyright © 1998 by W.B. Saunders Company

All rights reserved. No part of this publication may be reproduced or transmitted in any form or by any means, electronic or mechanical, including photocopy, recording, or any information storage and retrieval system, without permission in writing from the publisher.

Printed in the United States of America.

Last digit is the print number: 9   8   7   6   5   4   3   2   1

Preface

Purpose

This Clinical Manual was written for nursing students and practicing nurses. Its handy size makes it a portable reference book that can easily be carried to the clinical area where information that relates to hands-on practice is most useful. Although the authors briefly explain essential background information and describe expected medical interventions, the focus is on nursing assessments and interventions. This Clinical Manual complements the second edition of *Foundations of Maternal-Newborn Nursing* by Gorrie, McKinney, and Murray but it can be used alone by nurses who need only a review.

Content and Organization

The manual is divided into six parts. Part I provides an overview of the antepartal period. It includes a brief review of reproductive anatomy and physiology and the hereditary and environmental factors that affect care. This section briefly covers the physiologic and psychosocial adaptations to pregnancy and the most common complications of the antepartal period.

Part II addresses the intrapartal period and briefly describes the components and processes of normal and complicated childbirth. Intrapartal nursing care, including pain management and support for the family during labor, is outlined.

Part III outlines adaptation of the normal newborn and presents necessary nursing assessments and care. In addition, this section addresses therapeutic management and nursing considerations of the most common complications of the neonatal period.

Part IV briefly describes adaptations and nursing care required during normal and complicated postpartal periods.

Major areas of concern include teaching self care and infant care, including nutrition of the infant.

Part V deals with women's health care as well as reproductive issues such as family planning and infertility. Health maintenance is emphasized, as well as the most common benign and malignant disorders of the reproductive system.

Part VI presents step-by-step guides for some of the most common procedures in maternal-newborn nursing and drug guides for specific medications.

Acknowledgments

Clinical Manual was a group effort and we sincerely thank several people at W.B. Saunders. Thomas Eoyang, vice-president and editor-in-chief, was always available and encouraging. Maura Connor-Murcar, senior editor, put the pieces together initially and kept the project moving. Elizabeth Byrd, associate developmental editor, guided the project through the early stages. Victoria Legnini, editorial assistant, calmly and patiently provided assistance with many requests. Finally, the authors relied on Marie Thomas, senior editorial assistant, to answer questions and calm frustrations before they got out of hand. We also owe a debt of gratitude to Lisa King for putting print to paper and producing the final form.

Trula Myers Gorrie, M.N., R.N.,C.
Professor Emeritus
Golden West College
Huntington Beach, California

Emily Slone McKinney, M.S.N., R.N.,C.
Education Coordinator
Women's and Children's Services
Baylor Medical Center
Irving, Texas

Sharon Smith Murray, M.S.N., R.N.,C.
Professor, Health Professions
Golden West College
Huntington Beach, California

Contents

Section One	Antepartal Period	1
Section Two	Intrapartum	91
Section Three	Normal Newborn	188
Section Four	Postpartum	281
Section Five	Women's Health Care and Reproductive Issues	349
Section Six	Procedures and Drug Guides	415
	Appendixes	469
	Bibliography	491
	Index	493

SECTION ONE

Antepartal Period

I. REPRODUCTIVE ANATOMY AND PHYSIOLOGY

A. SEXUAL DEVELOPMENT

Prenatal Development

- Genetic sex determination
  — Fertilizing spermatozoon bears an X chromosome: female results
  — Fertilizing spermatozoon bears a Y chromosome: male results
- Reproductive systems of males and females are undifferentiated during the first 6 weeks of prenatal life.
- As the prenatal female's ovaries secrete estrogen, female internal sex organs and external genitalia develop.
- As the prenatal male's testes secrete testosterone, male internal sex organs and external genitalia develop.
- After birth, the sex glands of females and males are quiet until puberty because the hypothalamus suppresses any estrogen or testosterone secreted.

Sexual Maturation

Puberty, the time when reproductive organs become fully functional, begins in late childhood and early adolescence. Puberty includes development of

- Primary sex characteristics, such as development of ova in the female's ovaries and sperm in the male's testes.
- Secondary sex characteristics, such as development of the breasts in the female and growth of facial and chest hair in the male.

Initiation of Sexual Maturation

- Hypothalamus allows increasing secretion of estrogen and testosterone; sex organs mature.
- Hypothalamus secretes more gonadotropin-releasing hormone (GnRH), which stimulates the anterior pituitary to release its hormones.
- Anterior pituitary secretes
  — Follicle-stimulating hormone (FSH).
  — Luteinizing hormone (LH).
- FSH and LH, in turn, stimulate
  — Ovaries to develop ova and secrete sex hormones, primarily estrogens and progesterone.
  — Male testes to develop sperm and secrete sex hormones, primarily testosterone.

Female Puberty

- Ovaries secrete estrogen and progesterone, causing other puberty changes.
- Breasts exhibit the earliest signs of sexual maturation.
  — Nipples enlarge and protrude.
  — Glandular tissue and milk ducts grow and develop.

- Fat deposits increase in the hips and breasts.
- Height increases at about the time of breast development.
- Bony pelvis widens.
- Pubic and axillary hair appear.
- Internal sexual organs and the external genitalia mature.
- Menarche (first menstrual period) occurs about 2–3 years after breast development begins.

Male Puberty

- Testes secrete testosterone, causing other puberty changes.
- Testes grow, followed by growth and lengthening of the penis.
- Nocturnal emissions ("wet dreams") occur.
- Pubic, axillary, facial, and chest hair appear.
- Muscle mass increases.
- Height increases. The male growth spurt begins later than the female's, but lasts longer, resulting in a greater average male height at maturity.
- Voice deepens.

Decline in Fertility

Female produces less estrogen, gradually ceases to produce ova, and has her last menstrual period (menopause) in her late 40s to early 50s. Males have a gradual decline in testosterone and sperm production, but no distinct marker such as menopause.

4 Clinical Manual for Foundations of Maternal Newborn Nursing

B. FEMALE REPRODUCTIVE ANATOMY

External Female Reproductive Organs

Figure I-1

External Female Reproductive Organs

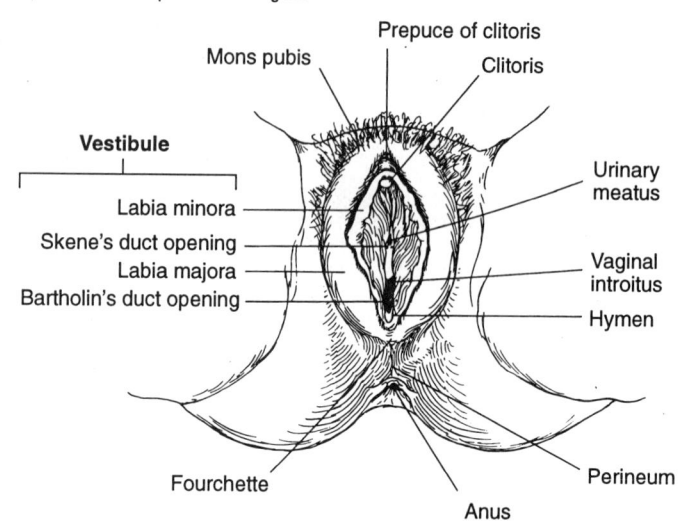

Labels: Mons pubis; Prepuce of clitoris; Clitoris; **Vestibule**; Labia minora; Skene's duct opening; Labia majora; Bartholin's duct opening; Urinary meatus; Vaginal introitus; Hymen; Fourchette; Perineum; Anus

Internal Female Reproductive Organs

Figure I-2

Internal Female Reproductive Organs, Anterior View

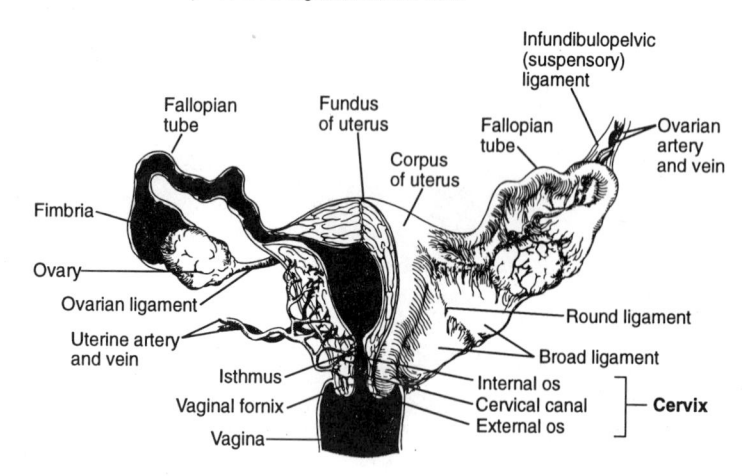

Labels: Fallopian tube; Fundus of uterus; Corpus of uterus; Infundibulopelvic (suspensory) ligament; Fallopian tube; Ovarian artery and vein; Fimbria; Ovary; Ovarian ligament; Uterine artery and vein; Isthmus; Vaginal fornix; Vagina; Round ligament; Broad ligament; Internal os; Cervical canal; External os; **Cervix**

Figure I-3

Internal Female Reproductive Organs, Mid-Sagittal View

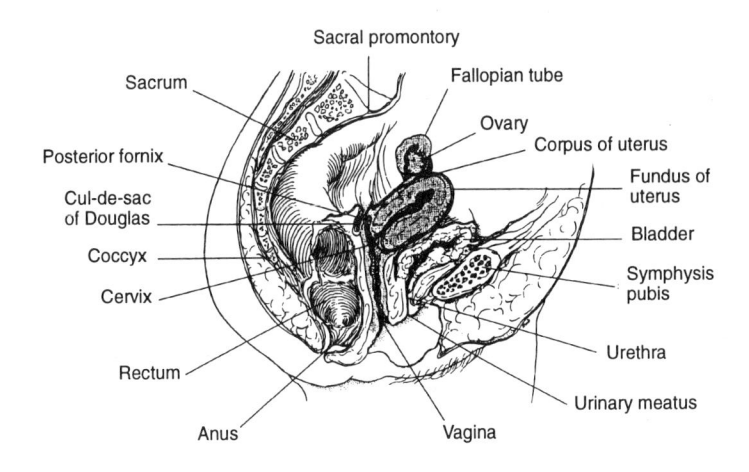

- Vagina: Tube of muscular and membranous tissue that connects the uterus with the exterior
- Uterus: Muscular organ that houses and nourishes the developing baby, then contracts to expel the fetus during labor; has three divisions and three layers
  - Divisions of the uterus
    - Corpus: Upper body of the uterus; the *fundus* is the part above where the fallopian tubes enter
    - Isthmus: Narrower zone between the corpus (above) and the cervix (below)
    - Cervix: Tubular "neck" of the uterus, about 2–3 cm long
- Layers of the uterus
  - Perimetrium: Outer layer that covers most of the uterus
  - Myometrium: Thick muscular layer containing 3 types of muscle fibers
    - *Longitudinal fibers* are found mostly in the fundus; they contract during labor to expel the fetus.

- *Interlacing fibers* in the middle layer contract around bleeding vessels after placental separation to control blood loss.
- *Circular fibers* surround the entry point of the fallopian tubes and the internal cervical os to prevent reflux of menstrual products into the tubes and to retain the fetus until the time of birth.
— Endometrium: Inner layer of the uterus that responds to cyclic variations of estrogen and progesterone during the female reproductive cycle

- Fallopian tubes: Pathway to allow the ovum released from the ovary to reach the uterus
- Ovaries: Female gonads, or sex glands
  — Produce female sex hormones
  — Mature an ovum during each female reproductive cycle

Female Support Structures

- Pelvis: Group of bones at the end of the spine, forming a "basin"; the lower pelvis (below the linea terminalis) is the most important in childbirth.

Figure I-4

Structures of the Bony Pelvis

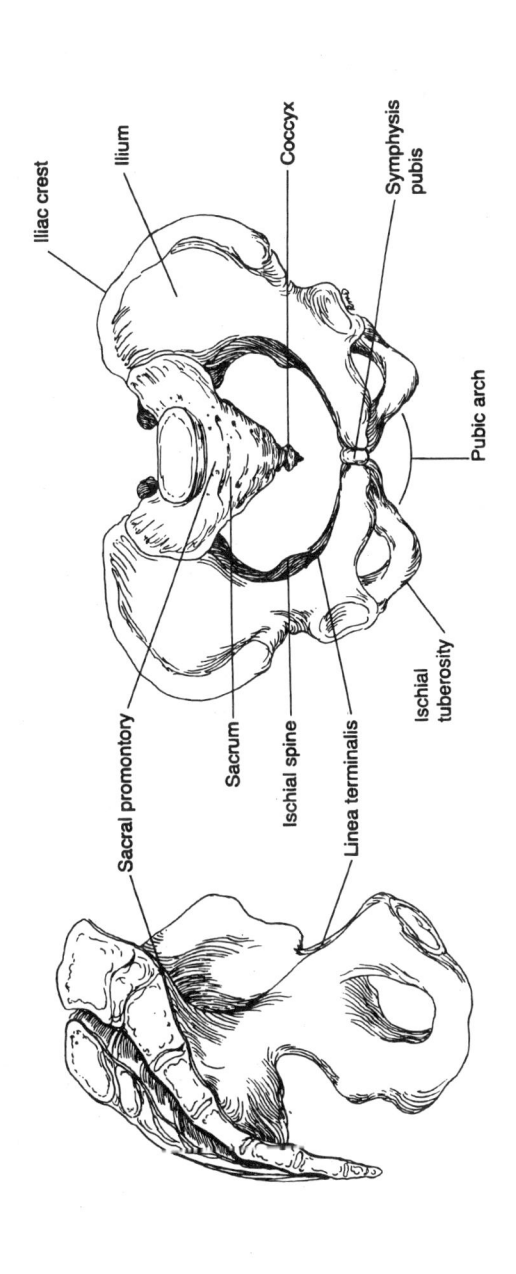

- Muscles: Paired muscles provide support for pelvic organs.
  - *Pubococcygeus*, consisting of the *pubovaginal*, *puborectal*, and *iliococcygeus* muscles, support internal pelvic structures and resist increases in intra-abdominal pressure
  - *Ischiocavernosus* muscles: Extend from the clitoris to the ischial tuberosities
  - *Transverse perineal* muscles: Extend from perineum to the ischial tuberosities

Figure I-5

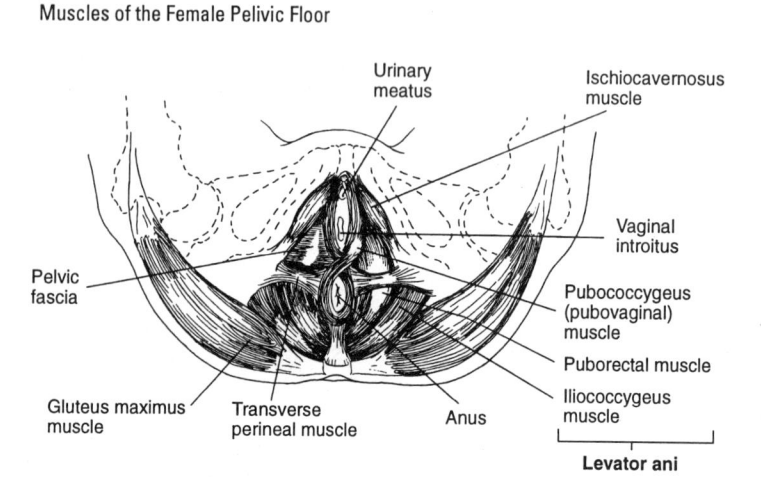

Muscles of the Female Pelivic Floor

- Ligaments: Paired ligaments stabilize the internal reproductive organs.
  - *Broad ligaments* extend from each side of the uterus to the lateral pelvic walls. Blood vessels, lymphatics, and the ovarian ligaments lie within each broad ligament.
  - *Cardinal ligaments* extend from the side walls of the cervix and vagina to the side walls of the pelvis.
  - *Ovarian ligaments* connect the ovaries to the lateral uterine walls.
  - *Infundibulopelvic (suspensory) ligaments* connect the lateral ovary and distal fallopian tubes to the pelvic side walls.

- *Round ligaments* connect the upper uterus to the connective tissue of the labia majora to maintain the uterus in the normal anteflexed position.
- *Pubocervical ligaments* connect the cervix to the interior surface of the symphysis pubis.
- *Uterosacral ligaments* support the posterior uterus by connecting it with the sacrum.

Blood Supply

- Uterus
  - Uterine arteries branch from the internal iliac artery.
  - Uterine veins drain into the internal iliac veins.
- Ovaries
  - Ovarian arteries branch from the abdominal aorta.
  - Left ovarian vein drains into the left renal vein.
  - Right ovarian vein drains into the inferior vena cava.

Nerve Supply

Functions of the reproductive system are controlled by the autonomic nervous system. Sensory and motor nerves for the reproductive organs enter the spinal cord at the T-12 through L-2 levels.

C. FEMALE REPRODUCTIVE CYCLE

The female reproductive cycle involves regular and recurrent changes in the anterior pituitary hormones which, in turn, cause cyclic changes in the ovaries, the uterine endometrium, and the cervical mucus. The cycle averages 28 days, with a range of 20 to 45 days. Significant variations from regular 28–day cycles are associated with reduced fertility.

Ovarian Cycle

- GnRH from the hypothalamus causes the woman's anterior pituitary to secrete FSH and LH, which stimulate maturation of an ovum and preparation of the uterine endometrium for implantation of a fertilized ovum.

- Follicular phase: The time during which an ovum matures, beginning with the first day of the menstrual period and ending about 12–14 days later. Several ovarian follicles begin maturation, but one outgrows the others.

- Ovulation: A surge of LH about 2 days before ovulation, accompanied by a slight decrease in estrogen, causes full maturation of one ovum within its follicle. The ovum is released from the surface of the ovary and is picked up by the fringed (fimbriated) end of the fallopian tube.

- Luteal phase: LH causes cells from the old follicle (corpus luteum) to persist for about 12 days and secrete large amounts of estrogen and progesterone to enrich the uterine lining in preparation for a fertilized ovum. If fertilization does not occur, the corpus luteum regresses and the woman has her menstrual period.

Endometrial Cycle

The endometrial cycle also consists of three phases.

- Proliferative phase: The endometrium proliferates, and endometrial glands and tiny endometrial spiral arteries and endometrial veins grow; lasts about the first 14 days of the cycle.

- Secretory phase: The endometrium further thickens, and substances are secreted to nourish a fertilized ovum; lasts about 12 days after ovulation.

- Menstrual phase: Occurs when the corpus luteum regresses because an ovum was not fertilized. Vasospasm of endometrial vessels occurs, causing the endometrium to become ischemic and necrotic, resulting in the menstrual period.

Cervical Mucus

- During most of the female reproductive cycle, the cervical mucus is thick and sticky.

- Near ovulation, it becomes clear, thin, and elastic to promote passage of sperm into the uterus and fallopian tubes to promote fertilization.

D. FEMALE BREAST

Figure I-6

Structures of the Female Breast

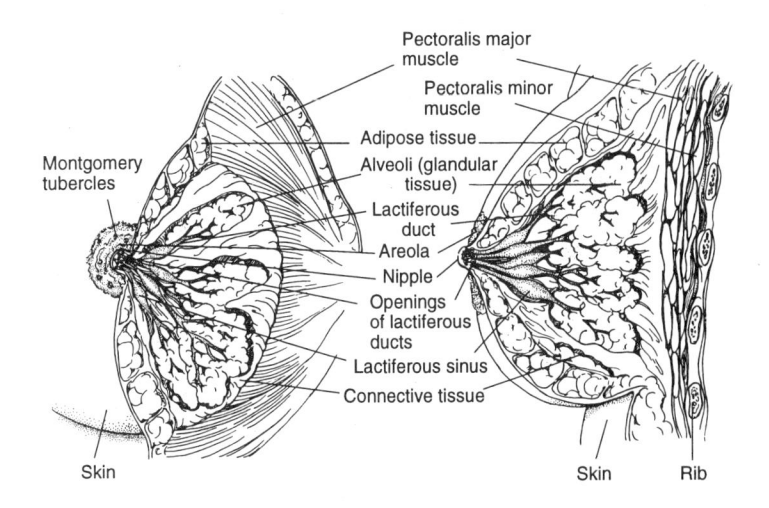

- Nipple: Sensitive erectile tissue that responds to sexual stimulation; it and the areola are more darkly pigmented than surrounding skin.
- Areola: Flattened area surrounding the nipple that contains Montgomery's tubercles, which secrete a moisturizing substance during pregnancy and lactation.
- Glandular tissue: Arranged like spokes of a wheel around a hub. Fifteen to 20 lobes comprise the glandular tissue.
- Alveoli: Small sacs that secrete the milk, which drains into the lactiferous ducts.
- Lactiferous sinuses: Widened portions of each duct that lie under the areola.

E. MALE REPRODUCTIVE ANATOMY AND PHYSIOLOGY

Figure I-7

Structures of the Male Reproductive System

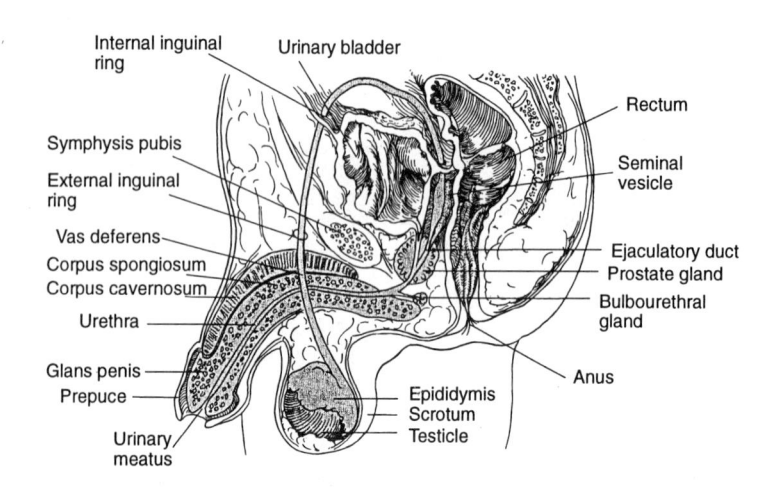

External Male Reproductive Organs

- Penis: An organ containing erectile tissue
  — Deposits sperm in the female's vagina during sexual intercourse
  — Provides passage for urine to drain from the bladder
- Scrotum: A pouch of thin skin that allows the testes to remain cooler than the core body temperature, promoting proper sperm production

Internal Male Reproductive Organs

- Testes have two functions.

— Secretion of male sex hormones, primarily testosterone, within the *Leydig cells*.

— Production and maturation of sperm within the seminiferous tubules; *Sertoli cells* nourish and support sperm during maturation.

- Accessory ducts and glands
  - Epididymis carries sperm into the vas deferens, which joins the ejaculatory duct before it then joins the urethra.
  - The seminal vesicles, prostate, and bulbourethral glands secrete seminal fluid.
    - Nourish sperm
    - Protect sperm from the acidic environment of the female's vagina
    - Enhance the motility of sperm
    - Wash all sperm out of the urethra to ensure that the maximum number are available for fertilization

II. GENETIC AND ENVIRONMENTAL INFLUENCES ON CHILDBEARING

A. CHROMOSOMES

- There are 46 paired chromosomes in the nucleus of each somatic (body) cell, other than mature erythrocytes, which do not have a nucleus.
- There are 23 single chromosomes in every germ cell (sperm or ovum).
- Studied by analyzing living cells
  - White blood cells
  - Skin fibroblasts
  - Bone marrow cells
  - Fetal cells from chorionic villi or amniotic fluid
- Care of specimens for chromosome analysis
  - No temperature extremes
  - Blood should not clot
  - Only approved preservatives

- The chromosome analysis is abbreviated by a combination of numbers and letters.
  — First number: The total number of chromosomes
  — Sex chromosomes: XY (male) or XX (female)
  — Normal male: 46, XY
  — Normal female: 46, XX
  — Additional notations describe any abnormalities; for example, Down syndrome female: 47, XX, +21 (the extra chromosome that is present in each body cell)
- Chromosome abnormalities
  — Numerical
    – Trisomy: Entire single chromosome added in each body cell; for example, trisomy 21 (Down syndrome)
    – Monosomy: Entire single chromosome missing in each body cell, for example, monosomy X (Turner's syndrome)
    – Polyploidy: One or more added full sets of chromosomes
  — Structural
    – Part of a chromosome missing or added in each body cell
    – Rearrangements of material within a chromosome
    – Two abnormally joined chromosomes

B. SINGLE GENE INHERITANCE

- Autosomal dominant traits
  — Characteristics
    – Single copy of the gene can produce the trait.
    – Males and females are equally likely to have the trait.
    – Often appear in every generation of a family, but people who have the trait may have widely varying manifestations.
    – May have multiple and seemingly unrelated effects on body structure and function.

- Transmission of trait from parent to child
    - Parent with the trait has a 50% (1 in 2) chance of passing the trait to a child.
    - Trait may arise as a new mutation from an unaffected parent.
- Autosomal recessive traits
  - Characteristics
    - Two autosomal recessive genes are required to produce the trait.
    - Males and females are equally likely to have the trait.
    - If multiple family members are affected, they are usually full siblings.
    - Consanguinity (blood relationship) of the parents increases the likelihood that the trait will appear.
    - Disorders are more likely to occur in groups isolated by geography, culture, religion, or other factors.
    - Some autosomal recessive disorders are more common in specific ethnic groups.
  - Transmission of trait from parent to child
    - Unaffected parents carry an abnormal recessive trait.
    - Each child of two carrier parents has a

      25% (1 in 4) chance of receiving both copies of the defective gene and having the disorder.

      50% (1 in 2) chance of receiving only one copy of the defective gene and being a carrier like the parents.

      25% (1 in 4) chance of receiving two normal genes and being neither a carrier nor affected.
- X-linked recessive traits
  - Characteristics
    - Gene for the trait is carried on the X chromosome.

- One copy is enough to produce the trait in a male because males have a single X chromosome, with no compensating X that does not have the trait.
- Females carry the trait, but usually are not adversely affected.
- Affected males are related to each other through carrier females.
- Affected males do not transmit the trait to their sons because they give the Y chromosome to a son.
— Transmission of trait from parent to child
- Males who have the disorder transmit the gene to 100% of their daughters.
- Sons of carrier females have a

  50% (1 in 2) chance of being affected.

  50% chance of being unaffected.
- Daughters of carrier females have a

  50% (1 in 2) chance of being carriers.

  50% of being neither affected nor carriers.
- An abnormal X-linked recessive gene may also arise by mutation.

C. MULTIFACTORIAL DISORDERS

- These disorders result from an interaction among genetic factors and environmental influence.
- Characteristics
  — Present and detectable at birth
  — Usually single, isolated defects, although the primary defect can cause other defects
- Risks of occurrence or recurrence vary. Factors that can alter the risk are
  — Number of affected close relatives.
  — Severity of the disorder in affected family members.
  — Sex of affected person(s).

- Geographic location.
- Seasonal variations.

• Infants who have several major and/or minor defects that are not directly related probably *do not* have a multifactorial defect, but have another syndrome, such as a chromosome abnormality.

D. TERATOGENS

• Environmental agents that may harm the fetus include
  - Maternal infectious agents.
  - Drugs and other substances, including therapeutic agents, illicit drugs, tobacco, and alcohol.
  - Pollutants and other substances.
  - Ionizing radiation.
  - Maternal hyperthermia.
  - Effects of maternal disorders such as diabetes mellitus or phenylketonuria.

• Avoiding fetal exposure to teratogens
  - Maternal immunization for infections such as rubella at least 3 months before pregnancy. Immunization during the immediate postpartum period is offered to nonimmune women.
  - Avoid all unnecessary drugs or using the least harmful drug that will have the desired effect.
  - Stop smoking.
  - Ingest no alcohol.
  - Avoid high-heat areas such as hot tubs or saunas.
  - Delay non-urgent radiological procedures until the first two weeks after the menstrual period begins.
  - Maintain proper diet and drug therapy for metabolic conditions such as diabetes or phenylketonuria.

III. PRENATAL DEVELOPMENT

A. PRE-EMBRYONIC PERIOD

- The first 2 days of development occur in the fallopian tube. The zygote enters the uterus about 3 days after conception.
- Implantation begins about 6 days after conception and is complete on the 10th day, usually in the uterine fundus.
- The zygote secretes human chorionic gonadotropin (hCG) to signal the woman's body that a pregnancy has begun, allowing uninterrupted estrogen and progesterone secretion from the corpus luteum to maintain the uterine endometrium.

B. EMBRYONIC PERIOD

- The embryonic period extends from the beginning of the third week through the eighth week after conception.
- The embryo is vulnerable to damage from teratogens at this time because all organ systems are developing rapidly.

C. FETAL PERIOD

- The fetal period begins 9 weeks after conception and ends with birth.
- Growth and refinement of all systems occurs.
- Teratogens may damage already formed structures, but are less likely to cause major structural damage. The central nervous system is vulnerable to damage during the entire pregnancy, however.
- During prenatal development, the relative proportions of body segments change. At 9 weeks, the head and thorax are about 7/8 of the total fetal length. At 38 weeks, the head is about 1/4 and the thorax is about 3/8 of the total fetal length.

D. TIMETABLE OF PRENATAL DEVELOPMENT

This timetable is based on *fertilization age*, about 2 weeks less than the *gestational age*, which is based on the woman's last menstrual period. CRL = crown-to-rump length

3 Weeks (1.5 mm [0.06 inches] CRL)

- Heart consists of 2 parallel tubes that begin beating.
- Three germ layers that will evolve into all body tissues develop.

4 Weeks (4.0 mm [0.16 inches] CRL)

- Neural tube (future brain and spinal cord) closes. Failure to close results in defects such as anencephaly or spina bifida.
- Eyes begin as an outgrowth of the forebrain.
- Heart tubes begin partitioning into 4 chambers.
- Upper limbs are like flippers.

6 Weeks (13 mm CRL [0.52 inches])

- Ears begin developing in the neck.
- Lung lobes (3 right and 2 left) develop.
- Most of the intestines are in the umbilical cord.
- Male and female gonads look identical.
- Fingers are webbed; feet develop slightly later.
- Primary tooth buds begin.

8 Weeks (30 mm [1.2 inches] CRL)

- Ears have their final form, but are still low-set.
- Heartbeat can be detected with ultrasound.
- Male and female genitalia begin to look different.

10 Weeks (61 mm [2.4 inches] CRL; weight 14 g [1/2 oz.])

- Intestines are now contained within the abdominal cavity.
- All parts of digestive tract are connected and patent from mouth to anus.
- Male and female genitalia more differentiated, but still easily confused.
- Fingernails begin development.
- Tooth buds for permanent teeth form below those for primary teeth.

12 Weeks (87 mm [3.5 inches] CRL; weight 45 g [1.6 oz])

- Nose and mouth are developed; palate is intact.
- Sucking reflex is present.
- Male and female genitalia can be distinguished easily.
- Lanugo hair appears.
- Heartbeat detectable with Doppler.

16 Weeks (140 mm [5.6 inches] CRL; weight 200 g [7 oz])

- Fetus swallows amniotic fluid and produces meconium in intestinal tract.
- Urine is excreted into amniotic fluid.
- Woman may begin to feel movement.
- Fingerprints are developing.

20 Weeks (160 mm [6.4 inches] CRL; weight 460 g [about 1 pound])

- Myelination of nerves begins and continues through the first year after birth.
- Heartbeat is detectable with fetoscope.
- Testes begin descent toward scrotum in males. Follicles of ovary begin developing in females.

- Mother feels fetal movements, and they may be palpable to the observer.
- Skin is covered with vernix.

24 Weeks (230 mm [9.2 inches] CRL; weight 820 g [1.8 pounds])

- Surfactant production begins in the lungs.
- Fetal activity more noticeable to woman.
- Fingerprints and footprints developed.
- Brows and lashes present.

28 Weeks (270 mm [10.8 inches] CRL; weight 1300 g [about 3 pounds])

- Erythrocyte production shifts completely to bone marrow.
- Sufficient alveoli, capillary network, and surfactant allow respiratory function, although respiratory distress syndrome is common in infants born at this time.
- Skin becomes smoother as subcutaneous fat is deposited.

32 Weeks (300 mm [12 inches] CRL; weight 2100 g [4.7 pounds])

- Testes enter the scrotum.
- Fingernails reach fingertips.
- Lanugo is disappearing.

38 Weeks (360 mm CRL [14.4 inches]; 3400 g [7.6 pounds])

- Testes are palpable in scrotum.
- Fetus has plump appearance with smooth skin.
- Vernix remains only in creases.
- Lanugo on upper back and shoulders.
- Fingernails extend beyond fingertips.
- Ear cartilage is firm.

E. AUXILIARY STRUCTURES

Placenta

- Maternal component:
  - Eighty to 100 spiral arteries arise from the uterine lining and carry oxygenated and nutrient-bearing blood into the intervillous spaces.
  - Endometrial veins drain deoxygenated blood and waste products from the placenta.
- Fetal component: Chorionic villi are tiny projections into the intervillous space that contain a fetal artery and vein to release waste products and pick up oxygen and nutrients from maternal blood.
- Theoretically, fetal and maternal blood do not mix within the placenta.

Umbilical Cord

- Two arteries carry deoxygenated blood and waste products to the placenta.
- One vein carries oxygenated blood and nutrients to the fetus.
- Wharton's jelly cushions the cord vessels.

Fetal Membranes and Amniotic Fluid

- Two membranes contain the amniotic fluid and provide some barrier against infection
  - Amnion (inner membrane)
  - Chorion (outer membrane)
- Functions of amniotic fluid are to
  - Allow symmetrical development.
  - Keep the membranes from adhering to the developing fetus.
  - Allow room and buoyancy for fetal movement.

SECTION ONE: Antepartal Period 23

F. FETAL AND POSTNATAL CIRCULATION

Figure I-8

Fetal and Postnatal Circulation

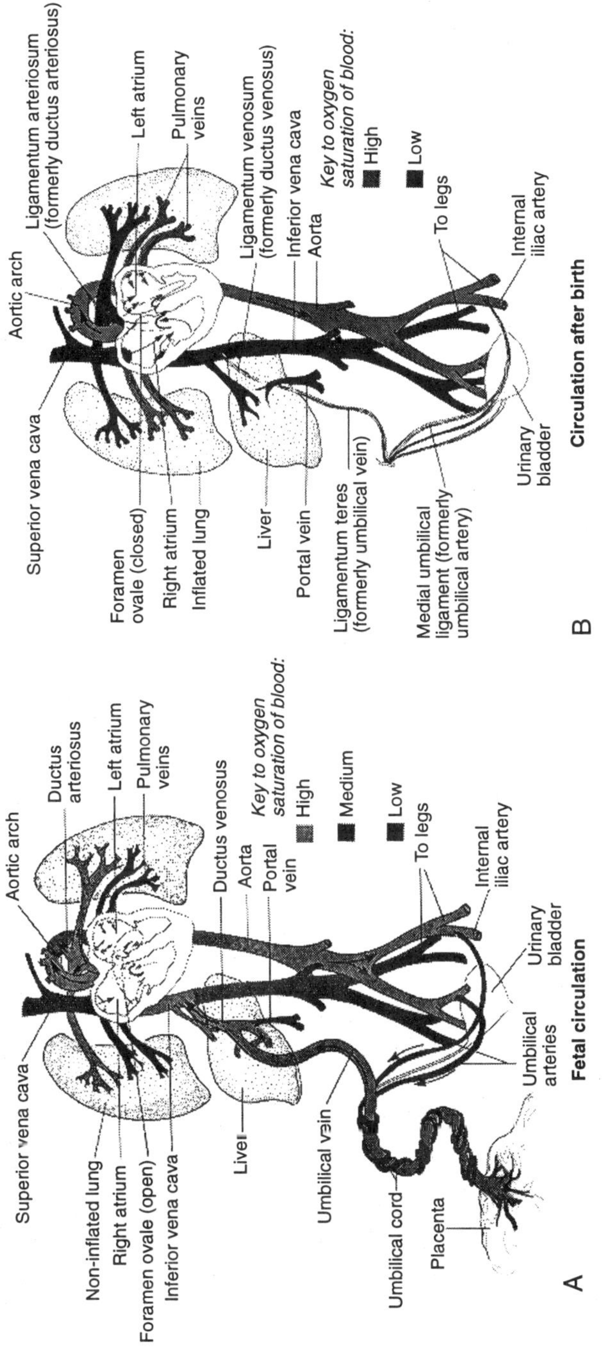

IV. ANTEPARTUM ADAPTATION

A. OVERVIEW

The average duration of pregnancy, based on the menstrual cycle, is 40 weeks or 280 days. The date on which the baby is expected, variously termed the estimated date of confinement (EDC), estimated date of delivery (EDD), or estimated date of birth (EDB), is calculated from the first day of the last menstrual period (LMP). In reality, conception occurs about 14 days later and the actual duration of pregnancy is about 266 days.

B. ESTIMATING DATE OF DELIVERY (EDD)

To compute EDD, subtract 3 months, add 7 days to the first day of the last menstrual period (LMP), and correct the year (Nagele's rule).

For example: LMP June 30, 1998
              Subtract 3 months = March 30, 1998
              Add 7 days = April 6, 1998
              Correct the year = April 6, 1999

C. TERMS TO REMEMBER

- Gravida: Any pregnancy, regardless of duration
- Multigravida: A woman who has been pregnant more than once
- Nullipara: A woman who has never completed a pregnancy beyond 20 weeks gestation
- Para: Birth after 20 weeks' gestation, regardless of whether the infant is born alive or dead
- Primigravida: A woman who is pregnant for the first time

Note: Health care providers often refer to this woman as a "primip" (short for primipara). However, she is not technically a primipara until a birth occurs.

- Primipara: A woman who has given birth after a pregnancy of at least 20 weeks
- Trimester: Division of pregnancy into time segments of about 13 weeks; typically referred to as first, second, or third trimester

D. PHYSIOLOGIC ADAPTATIONS TO PREGNANCY

Although the greatest changes occur in the reproductive system, all body systems must adapt to pregnancy. See Table I-1.

E. DIAGNOSIS OF PREGNANCY

The diagnosis of pregnancy is based on presumptive indications (subjective signs observed by the woman), probable indications (objective signs observed by examiner), and positive indications (those that can be caused only by pregnancy).

Presumptive Indications

- Amenorrhea
- Nausea and vomiting
- Fatigue
- Breast and skin changes

Probable Indications

- Abdominal enlargement
- Changes in color and consistency of cervix
- Changes in uterus (ballottement, Braxton Hicks contractions, palpation of fetal outline)
- Uterine souffle (blowing sound made by blood circulating through the placenta)
- Pregnancy tests, based on detection of human chorionic gonadotropin in blood or urine

TABLE I–1

Physiologic Adaptations to Pregnancy

SIGNIFICANT CHANGES	REASONS FOR CHANGES
Reproductive System	
Uterus	
Grows in a predictable pattern. See Fig I-9. Note that uterine height is lower at 40 weeks than at 36 weeks.	Muscle fibers stretch in all directions to accommodate the growing fetus. The fetal head drops into the pelvis near term, resulting in less pressure on the diaphragm (lightening) and easier breathing.
Cervix and Vagina	
Become softer (Goodell's sign) and bluish in color (Chadwick's sign).	Tissue is congested with blood, and connective tissue becomes swollen and loosely connected.
Mucus plug forms in cervix.	Cervical mucus increases as cervical glands proliferate.
Ovaries	
Corpus luteum secretes progesterone until the placenta is developed.	Adequate progesterone is necessary to maintain pregnancy.
Ovulation ceases.	Placenta secretes high levels of estrogen and progesterone, so gonadotropin releasing hormones are inhibited.
Breasts	
Increase in size and become highly vascular. Nipples become larger and more pigmented; tubercles of Montgomery become more prominent; colostrum is often obvious by second trimester.	Estrogen and progesterone promote growth of mammary ducts and lobes; tubercles of Montgomery secrete a substance that lubricates nipples.

SECTION ONE: Antepartal Period 27

Cardiovascular System

Blood Volume

Plasma increases by 45% over prepregnancy level.	Increased plasma is needed to transport nutrients and oxygen to the fetus and expanded maternal tissue and to compensate for blood lost at childbirth.
Red blood cells (RBCs) increase about 33%.	Extra RBCs are needed to carry oxygen; increase is less and occurs later than that in plasma volume, resulting in hemodilution and the pseudoanemia of pregnancy.
White blood cells (WBCs) increase up to 25,000/mm^3.	WBCs increase as blood volume expands during pregnancy and as a result of exertion during labor.
Blood pressure remains within normal limits.	Peripheral vascular resistance decreases due to effects of progesterone and maternal resistance to vasoconstrictors such as angiotensin II.
Clotting factors (especially fibrin and fibrinogen) increase.	Clotting factors increase to prevent postpartum hemorrhage; however, they increase the risk of thrombus formation.

Respiratory System

The ribs flare, the substernal angle widens, and the chest circumference expands. Some women experience shortness of breath in late pregnancy.	The enlarging uterus lifts the diaphragm and prevents lung expansion. Tidal volume (amount of air that is exchanged in quiet respirations) increases; mild alkalosis results.

Gastrointestinal System

Gums become hyperemic and bleed easily.	These effects are due to elevated levels of estrogen.

Gastrointestinal tone and motility decrease in the stomach and intestine, resulting in GI discomfort such as heartburn and constipation.	These effects are due to progesterone, which relaxes all smooth muscles; moreover, stomach and intestine are displaced by the enlarging uterus.
Bile becomes thicker, which predisposes to formation of gallstones.	Gallbladder hypotonic and emptying time is decreased as a result of progesterone.

Urinary System

Urinary frequency and urgency.	These effects are due to pressure of the uterus on the bladder.
Woman is at increased risk for urinary tract infection.	Stasis of urine is due to increased capacity of bladder and ureters; this is the result of decreased muscle tone due to effects of progesterone.

Musculoskeletal System

Softening of pelvic ligaments resulting in wide stance, waddling gait, and lordosis.	These changes are due to effects of the hormone relaxin and progesterone, as well as increasing uterine size that forces the woman to lean backward to maintain her balance.
Abdominal wall muscles separate (diastasis recti).	This occurs when muscles are stretched beyond their capacity in third trimester.

Integumentary System

Activity of the sweat and sebaceous glands increases; increased pigmentation such as chloasma and linea nigra.	Activity is encouraged by the increased circulation to the skin. Change is due to elevated levels of melanocyte-stimulating hormone.
Striae gravidarum ("stretch marks") may develop on breasts, buttocks, abdomen.	Due to linear tears in connective tissue; lines fade to silvery lines after childbirth.

Endocrine System

Pituitary

Follicle stimulating hormone and leutenizing hormone are suppressed.	Suppression is due to high levels of estrogen and progesterone during pregnancy.
Prolactin is released from anterior pituitary.	Prolactin prepares breasts for lactation.
Oxytocin, posterior pituitary, induces uterine contractions and the milk-ejection reflex.	This action is inhibited by high levels of progesterone during pregnancy.

Thyroid

Increase in total thyroxine produces a slight increase in size of thyroid.	This increase produces a rise in basal metabolic rate that results in an increase in cardiac output and heat intolerance.

Parathyroid

Parathyroid hormone level increases.	Higher level is needed to meet fetal demands for calcium and phosphorus.

Pancreas

Insulin production increases.	Increase is due to insulin resistance of maternal cells that begins in second trimester.

Adrenal Glands

Level of cortisol increases.	Increase is necessary for accelerated protein and carbohydrate metabolism.
Aldosterone increases.	Increase overcomes the salt-wasting effects of pregnancy and maintains expanded blood volume.

Placental Hormones

Human chorionic gonadotropin is produced.	HCGn maintains corpus luteum, which produces progesterone during the first weeks of pregnancy.
Estrogen level increases.	Estrogen stimulates uterine and breast development.
Progesterone level increases.	Progesterone maintains uterine lining, relaxes all smooth muscles, and helps prepare the breasts for lactation.
Human placental lactogen is produced.	This stimulates metabolism of glucose and converts it to fat; it is antagonistic to insulin.
Relaxin is produced.	Relaxin softens muscles and joints of pelvis.

Positive Indications

- Fetal heartbeat
- Fetal movement felt by examiner
- Visualization by ultrasound

F. PSYCHOSOCIAL ADAPTATIONS

Psychosocial adaptations to pregnancy occur gradually as the focus shifts from self to fetus as a separate, though entirely dependent, human. See Table I-2.

V. INITIAL ANTEPARTAL ASSESSMENT

A. HISTORY

- History of family, individual, and partner with particular attention to
  — Chronic diseases such as diabetes, hypertension, or heart disease

TABLE I–2

Psychosocial Adaptations to Pregnancy

FIRST TRIMESTER	SECOND TRIMESTER	THIRD TRIMESTER
Emotional Response		
Uncertainty, ambivalence, focus on self.	Fetus becomes the focus as abdomen enlarges and particularly after fetal movement is felt.	Vulnerability, increased dependence; acceptance that fetus is separate but totally dependent.
Body Image		
Little change in body contour or size; nausea and vomiting may interfere with sense of well-being.	Often proud of enlarging abdomen that indicates the fetus is growing; generally feels well as discomforts of first trimester abate.	Tends to feel negative about size, backache, waddling gait; ready for infant to be born.
Role		
Ensures "safe passage" for self and fetus by beginning prenatal care.	Seeks acceptance of fetus and her role as mother from family and significant others.	Prepares for birth; internalizes a view of how a "good" mother behaves and sets up expectations for self.
"Self" Statement		
"I am pregnant."	"I am going to have a baby."	"I am going to be a mother."

- Episodes of sexually transmissible diseases such as herpes or chemical dependency (including smoking cigarettes or use of alcohol)
- Workplace hazards, including exposure to teratogenic substances
- Religious and cultural practices and influences
• Reproductive history including
  - Gravida, para, living children, stillbirths
  - Type of births (vaginal or cesarean), hours of labor, condition and weight of infant, complications of labor or postpartum

B. PHYSICAL EXAMINATION

- Vital signs, including auscultation of maternal heart sounds
- Height, weight, and preconception weight
- Inspection and palpation of the breasts and abdomen
- Palpation of fundus. See Figure I-9, "Pattern of Uterine growth."
- Brachial and patellar reflexes for hyperreflexia, which suggests developing preeclampsia
- Pelvic examination, including external and internal genitalia, cervical cultures, and measurement of pelvic dimensions to estimate whether size seems adequate for vaginal birth
- Current pregnancy status including
  - Confirmation of pregnancy by (a) physical indications such as Chadwick's, Goodell's, and Hegar's signs; (b) use of sonography to detect a gestational sac or to visualize a viable embryo in early pregnancy; (c) fetal movement (quickening) usually felt by the mother by 20 weeks gestation (earlier for multigravidas)
  - Confirmation of gestational age by noting (a) abdominal enlargement; (b) measurement of fundal height (see Figure I-10); (c) sonography that can accurately determine fetal age early in pregnancy by measurements such the biparietal diameter of the fetal head

SECTION ONE: Antepartal Period 33

- — Fetal heartbeat that can be detected with a Doppler by 10 weeks gestation and much earlier by ultrasound examination
- — EDD based on LMP and confirmed by fundal height or sonography
- Antepartum laboratory screening (see Table I-3)
- Nutrition assessment

Figure I-9

Pattern of Uterine Growth

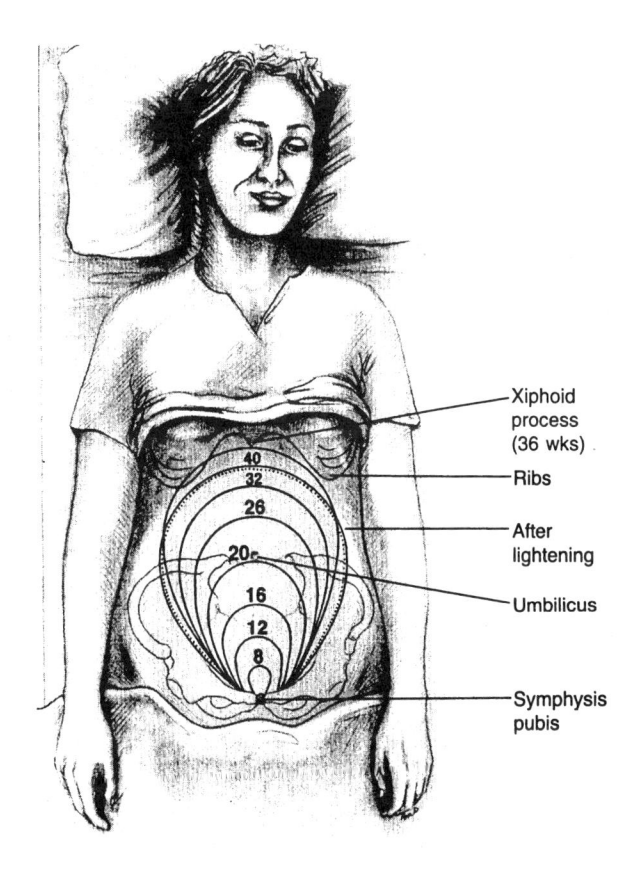

Figure I-10

Measurement of Fundal Height

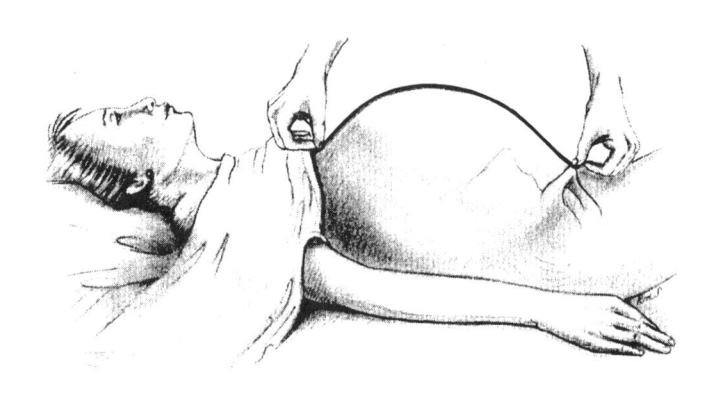

C. PSYCHOSOCIAL ASSESSMENT

Psychosocial assessment focuses on:

- Progressive acceptance of mother (and father) of pregnancy
- Availability of adequate resources and support system
- Educational needs that change over time; for instance, how to relieve nausea and vomiting is a major concern in early pregnancy, while how to care for a newborn becomes a priority during the last few weeks
- Language barriers
- Cultural beliefs or practices that may affect the pregnancy

VI. SCHEDULE OF ANTEPARTAL ASSESSMENTS

Ideally, a woman with an uncomplicated pregnancy should begin prenatal care in the first trimester and then should be evaluated every

TABLE I–3

Antepartum Tests and Procedures

TEST	PURPOSE
Initial Visit	
Blood	
Complete blood count (Hg, Hct, RBC, platelets, WBC and differential)	To screen for anemia, assess blood clotting factors, identify folic acid deficiency, and recognize infectious processes; repeat Hg and Hct at 28 and 32–36 weeks
Hemoglobin electrophoresis	For women of African, Asian, or Middle Eastern descent, to detect hemoglobinopathies such as sickle cell anemia or thalassemia
Blood type	To be prepared to intervene for hemorrhage
Rh factor	To identify possible incompatibility with fetus
Rh titers	Needed if mother is Rh-negative and father is Rh-positive; rising titer indicates danger to fetus. Repeat at 28 weeks.
Rubella antibody titer	To determine if mother is immune
Hepatitis B serology	To screen for hepatitis surface antigen, indicating that mother is a carrier of the virus
Serologic test for syphilis (RPR, VDRL)	Screen for syphilis; if positive, must confirm with FTA-ABS.
HIV antibody assay (optional)	To detect antibodies to human immunodeficiency virus

Urine

Clean voided specimen for sugar, albumin, or bacteria	Sugar suggests hyperglycemia; albumin suggests renal problems; bacteria indicate infection of bladder or kidneys.
Urine culture	To identify organisms if infection is suspected

Cervical/Vaginal Cytology

Pap smear	To screen for cervical neoplasia
Gonorrhea culture and Chlamydia test	To identify and treat sexually transmissible diseases (STDs); repeat as indicated
Examination of vaginal secretions	Foamy yellow liquid suggests *Trichomonas*; white, curd-like discharge indicates *Candida* infection
Tuberculin skin test (PPD)	To screen high-risk women for tuberculosis

Subsequent Tests

Maternal serum alpha-fetoprotein (16-18 weeks); two other markers (estriol and chorionic gonadotropin may also be examined)	Elevated levels are associated with neural tube defects; low levels suggest chromosomal defects. If abnormal, additional tests, such as amniotic fluid alpha-fetoprotein and amniocentesis, are recommended. Addition of two other markers increases sensitivity of the screening procedure.
50–gram glucose screening test (24–28 weeks)	To screen for gestational diabetes (<140 mg/dL considered normal)
3-hour glucose tolerance test	Recommended if glucose screening test levels are 140 mg/dL or greater

Culture for Group B *Streptococcus*	Colonization in late pregnancy is treated by intrapartum chemoprophylaxis.

Additional Tests for High-Risk Pregnancies

Counting fetal movements ("kick counts")	Fetal activity indicates fetal well-being. Teach mother to count movements for 20–30 minutes at specified times and to report a decrease in movements: less than 3 movements in time allotted, fewer than 10 movements in 12 hours.
Sonography (1st trimester)	To confirm pregnancy, determine fetal age, and to assess fetal growth and development.
(2nd and 3rd trimesters)	To confirm fetal presentation and position, locate the placenta, or guide other procedures, such as amniocentesis; to assess fetal movements and amount of amniotic fluid.
Nonstress test (NST)	To screen for fetal well-being by determining if the fetal heart accelerates when the fetus moves
Contraction stress test (CST)	To determine how the fetal heart responds to the stress of uterine contractions; decelerations are a nonreassuring sign.
Biophysical profile	Uses electronic fetal heart rate monitoring and ultrasonography to evaluate fetal muscle tone, fetal movements, fetal breathing movements, amniotic fluid volume, and fetal heart rate reactivity as demonstrated by NST

- 4 weeks until 28 weeks
- 2 weeks until 36 weeks
- 1 week thereafter until birth

VII. SUBSEQUENT ANTEPARTAL ASSESSMENTS

- Vital signs. Measure blood pressure while the woman is sitting with the arm supported in a horizontal position at heart level; document position, pressure, and whether Korotokoff's fourth (muffling) or fifth (disappearance of sound) was used. Vital signs, including blood pressure, should remain near prepregnancy levels, and deviations should be reported.

- Weight and pattern of weight gain (see page 48).

- Urinalysis

  Test urine for proteinuria that may indicate preeclampsia and for glycosuria that may suggest hyperglycemia.

- Fundal height

  To be accurate, this measurement must be taken when the bladder is empty. Fundal height corresponds well to weeks of gestation (particularly between 20 and 32 weeks gestation). For instance, 22 centimeters suggests 22 weeks' gestation. See Figure I-10.

- Fetal heart rate

  Normal parameters are 110 to 160 beats per minute; however, rate may be higher early in pregnancy when the fetus is very small.

- Leopold's maneuvers

  These maneuvers provide a systematic method for palpating the fetus through the abdominal wall to determine presentation and position. See Section Six, "Procedure: Leopold's Maneuver," p. 434.

VIII. HIGH-RISK FACTORS IN PREGNANCY

A *high-risk pregnancy* is defined as one in which the mother or fetus is more likely than the low-risk population to experience complications. A variety of medical, obstetrical, or social factors may increase the risk to a childbearing family. See Table I-4.

IX. COMMON NURSING DIAGNOSES

- Health-seeking behaviors: Prenatal care
- Knowledge deficit: Importance of prenatal care
- Risk for altered health maintenance related to lack of prenatal care
- Pain or backache related to muscular strain secondary to change in balance and knowledge deficit of measures to reduce strain
- Risk for altered nutrition related to nausea and anorexia
- Constipation related to lack of knowledge of preventive measures
- Family coping: Potential for growth
- Activity intolerance related to fatigue, backache, or shortness of breath

TABLE I–4

Summary of High-Risk Factors in Pregnancy

FACTORS	IMPLICATIONS
Demographic Factors	
<16 years or >35 years	Increased risk for preterm labor, pregnancy-induced hypertension, congenital anomalies
Low socioeconomic status	Increased risk for preterm labor, low-birth-weight infants
Non-Caucasian	Incidence of infant and maternal death twice that of Caucasians
Multiparity (>4 pregnancies)	Increased risk of pregnancy loss, antepartum or postpartum hemorrhage, and cesarean birth
Social-Personal Factors	
Weight <45 kg (100 lbs.)	Associated with low-birth-weight infant
Weight >90 kg (200 lbs.)	Increased risk for pregnancy-induced hypertension, gestational diabetes, difficult birth, cesarean birth
Height <154 cm (5 ft.)	Increased incidence of cesarean birth due to cephalopelvic disproportion
Smoking	Associated with preterm birth and low-birth-weight infant (<2500 grams)
Use of alcohol and other addicting drugs	Increased risk for congenital anomalies, neonatal withdrawal syndrome, and fetal alcohol syndrome

Obstetric Factors

Birth of previous infant >4000 g (8.5 lbs.)	Increased risk for birth injury, cesarean birth, neonatal hypoglycemia, and maternal gestational diabetes
Previous stillborn	Maternal psychological distress
Rh sensitization	Fetal anemia, erythroblastosis fetalis, kernicterus

Existing Medical Conditions

Diabetes mellitus	Increased risk of pregnancy-induced hypertension, fetal or neonatal death, congenital anomalies, macrosomia
Cardiac disease	Maternal risk for cardiac decompensation and maternal, fetal, or neonatal death
Renal disease	Increased risk of maternal renal failure, preterm birth, intrauterine growth restriction

Concurrent Infections

Viral or bacterial	Some, such as rubella and varicella, are preventable. Others, such as Group B *Streptococcus* infection, tuberculosis, and gonorrhea, are treatable. Without treatment there may be severe fetal or neonatal implications. See Table III-3 and pages 270-277.

X. DANGER SIGNS OF PREGNANCY

The pregnant woman and at least one other person in the family must be instructed about signs that indicate a problem that should be reported at once. See Table I-5.

XI. NURSING INTERVENTIONS

A. TEACHING HEALTH PROMOTION

- Bathing
  - Recommend daily showers or tub baths; caution the woman to take precautions to prevent falls during the third trimester when the balance has changed.
  - Suggest avoiding excessively hot water (hot tubs, jacuzzis) in early pregnancy when the fetus is developing.
- Douching
  - Emphasize that there is no hygienic need for douching, despite increased vaginal discharge.
  - Recommend that the woman follow physician or nurse-midwife's advice if douching is prescribed for medical reasons.
- Breast care
  - Instruct the woman to wash breasts and nipples with clear water and to avoid soap that removes natural lubricant.
  - Advise her to wear a good support bra with wide straps that distribute the weight evenly across the shoulders.
- Exercise
  - Recommend moderate exercise 3–4 times per week but suggest she avoid
    - Competitive exercise.
    - Vigorous exercise in hot or humid weather.
    - Strenuous exercise that exceeds 15 minutes in duration.

TABLE I–5

Danger Signs of Pregnancy

DANGER SIGN	POSSIBLE CAUSE
Vaginal bleeding	Placental abnormalities, lesions of cervix or vagina, "bloody show" (sign of labor onset)
Escape of fluid from vagina	Premature rupture of membranes
Swelling of fingers or face	Suggests development of preeclampsia (see pages 71-79)
Continuous pounding headache	Associated with chronic or pregnancy-induced hypertension
Visual disturbances (blurred vision, spots before the eyes)	Worsening preeclampsia
Persistent or severe abdominal pain	Ischemia in major abdominal vessels or abruptio placentae
Fever or chills	Infection
Painful urination	Urinary tract infection
Persistent vomiting	Hyperemesis gravidarum
Change in frequency or strength of fetal movement	Fetal compromise or death

- All exercises in supine position after 16 weeks of pregnancy.
- Any exercise that employs Valsalva maneuver.
- Emphasize the importance of taking adequate fluids before and after exercising and to stop exercises that cause undue fatigue.
- Stress the importance of checking her heart rate every 10–15 minutes and not to exceed a target heart rate that has been determined in consultation with the physician or midwife.

- Sleep and rest
  - Instruct her to use pillows to support the abdomen and back during the last trimester.
  - Recommend that she rest in a lateral position to prevent hypotension that may occur as a result of lying in a supine position.

- Employment
  - Suggest that she work out a schedule for frequent rest periods with feet elevated to prevent undue fatigue.
  - Assist her to plan ways to change positions or to walk briefly to stimulate circulation.
  - Recommend she curtail jobs that require balance during the last trimester when the center of gravity shifts and she is at greater risk to fall.

- Avoiding teratogens
  - Advise the woman to investigate her specific situation to determine possible exposure to toxic substances. Groups at risk include hairdressers, painters, printers, nurses, and laundry and dry cleaning workers.
  - Emphasize the ill effects of exposure to passive smoking.
  - Accentuate the ill effects of alcohol and illicit drugs.

- Sexual activity
  - Reassure the couple that sexual intercourse does no harm to the healthy pregnant woman.

- Suggest that they alter the position during the last trimester when supine hypotensive syndrome may result from a male-superior position.
- Advise them to curtail all sexual activity if the woman is at risk for preterm labor, if the membranes have ruptured, or if there is vaginal bleeding.

- Travel
    - Recommend that she validate that medical care is available at the destination.
    - Remind her to fasten the seat belt snugly with the lap belt under the abdomen.
    - Counsel her to stop frequently to empty her bladder and to walk around for a few minutes.
- Immunizations
    - Remind her that live virus vaccines such as those for measles, rubella, and mumps are contraindicated during pregnancy.
    - Counsel her to consult with her physician or midwife before taking any immunization during pregnancy.
- Over-the-counter drugs
    - Advise her to consult her physician, pharmacist, or midwife before taking any over-the-counter drugs.
    - Suggest that she tell the physician, nurse-midwife, and pharmacist she is pregnant if she routinely takes prescribed medications.

B. HOW TO OVERCOME THE COMMON DISCOMFORTS OF PREGNANCY

- Nausea and vomiting
    - Eat dry crackers or toast before arising in the morning, then get out of bed slowly.
    - Eat dry crackers every 2 hours to prevent an empty stomach or eat 5–6 small meals a day rather than 3 full meals.
    - Take fluids separately from meals.

- Avoid fried, greasy, or spicy foods and foods with strong odors.
- Heartburn
  - Avoid fatty foods.
  - Eat small, frequent meals; avoid overeating.
  - Sit upright after eating to reduce reflux; sleep with an extra pillow.
  - Breathe deeply and sip water to relieve burning sensation.
  - Avoid antacids that are high in sodium.
- Backache
  - Maintain correct posture with shoulders and neck straight, back flattened, and pelvis tucked under.
  - Squat, rather than bend from the waist, to pick up objects.
  - Use foot supports, arm rests, and pillows to support the back.
  - Strengthen the back by doing exercises such as the tailor position, shoulder circling, and pelvic rocking.
- Urinary frequency
  - Void when she feels the urge.
  - Maintain daytime fluid intake.
  - Decrease evening fluid intake to lessen nocturia.
- Varicosities
  - Avoid wearing constricting clothing and refrain from crossing legs at the knees because this impedes blood return from the legs.
  - Take frequent rest periods with legs elevated above the level of the hips.
  - Wear support hose or elastic stockings to prevent blood pooling in the legs.
  - Walk for a few minutes at least every 2 hours to stimulate circulation and relieve discomfort.

- Hemorrhoids
  - Establish a regular pattern of bowel elimination and avoid straining.
  - Take frequent, tepid baths; apply cool witch-hazel compresses or use anesthetic ointments to relieve existing hemorrhoids.
  - Lie on the side with the hips elevated on the pillow to promote drainage of blood from swollen hemorrhoids.
  - Push hemorrhoids back into the rectum if necessary.
  - Notify physician or midwife if there is persistent pain or bleeding.
- Constipation
  - Drink at least 8 glasses of water each day.
  - Consume foods high in fiber, such as unpeeled fresh fruit, whole grain cereals and bread, and vegetables.
  - Restrict consumption of cheese, which can cause constipation, and sweets, which increase bacterial growth in the intestine and can lead to flatulence.
  - Continue iron supplementation and consult health care provider if constipation persists. A bulk-forming or fecal-wetting agent may be prescribed.
  - Walk briskly for at least one mile to stimulate peristalsis.
- Leg cramps
  - Dorsiflex the foot and extend the leg to relieve cramp.
  - Elevate the legs frequently to improve circulation.
  - Obtain permission from physician or midwife to take aluminum hydroxide gel capsules that absorb phosphorous and raise the level of calcium in the blood.

XII. NUTRITION FOR PREGNANCY AND LACTATION

A. WEIGHT GAIN AND PATTERN OF WEIGHT GAIN

The recommended weight gain for pregnancy is 11.4–16 kg (25–35 pounds). Weight gain should follow a predictable pattern of approximately 1.6 kg (3.5 pounds) in the first trimester and a weekly gain of .44 kg (.97 pounds) in the second and third trimesters. The amount is greater for women who are under their ideal weight for height or who carry more than one fetus, and it is lower for obese women.

B. NUTRIENT NEEDS

On average, pregnant women need

- Approximately 2500 calories per day (an increase of 300 calories over nonpregnant needs).
- About 60 grams of protein (an increase of 10–15 grams).
- Additional vitamins (B_6, D, E, and folate).
- Additional minerals (iron, calcium, zinc, and magnesium).

C. FOOD SOURCES TO MEET NUTRIENT NEEDS

During pregnancy, the increased need for most nutrients may not be met unless the additional calories are selected carefully. The food pyramid can serve as a guide for healthy eating during pregnancy. The recommended daily amounts are

- Seven servings of whole-grain products (bread, cereal, pasta, rice), which form the base of the pyramid. These foods provide complex carbohydrates and fiber as well as vitamins and minerals.
- Five servings of fruits and vegetables, the next layer of the pyramid, provide vitamins, minerals, and fiber; at least one food that provides vitamin A (dark yellow vegetables and fruit, green leafy vegetables); and one that provides vita-

min C (citrus fruit, cabbage, green and red peppers, tomatoes) should be included.

- Three servings of dairy products (skim or low fat milk, cottage cheese, hard cheese) are excellent sources of protein and calcium.
- Seven ounces of protein foods (meat, fish, poultry, legumes, eggs, tofu) provide adequate protein to meet the needs of the mother and the fetus.
- Three tablespoons of unsaturated fats, represented by the tip of the pyramid, provide calories for energy but few other nutrients.

D. NUTRITIONAL RISK FACTORS

- Poverty: Carbohydrate foods are less expensive than meats, dairy products, fruits, and vegetables; therefore, low-income women may have a diet that is deficient in protein, vitamins, and minerals.
- Adolescence: The adolescent must consume enough nutrients to support her own growth and maturation as well as that of the fetus. Diets are often low in vitamins A, D, B_6, folic acid, riboflavin, calcium, and iron.
- Vegetarian diets: Vegetarian diets are often high in fiber and low in calories and may not meet the energy needs of pregnancy.
- Diets may also be low in protein unless the woman knows food combinations that provide complete proteins (whole wheat grains plus beans, rice plus peas, corn plus beans). Vegetarian diets may be particularly low in calcium and iron, and supplementation may be necessary.
- Multiparity: Women who have closely spaced pregnancies may begin a new pregnancy with inadequate nutrient stores to meet their own needs and fetal requirements. The woman with a multifetal pregnancy must provide enough calories to meet the needs of each fetus without depleting

her own stores. Suggested weight gain for a women with twins is 10–20 pounds more than for a woman with a single pregnancy.

- Lactose intolerance: Women without the enzyme lactase are unable to absorb lactose and experience nausea, bloating, flatulence, diarrhea, and cramping when they consume milk products. As a result, they may be deficient in calcium unless they eat other foods high in calcium, such as salmon or sardines with bones, dark green vegetables (broccoli, kale, collards), or tofu. They may also take lactase, which decreases their problem with milk products.

E. SUPPLEMENTATION

- Iron (30 mg per day) is prescribed for all women during the second and third trimesters because it is difficult to obtain adequate amounts through normal food intake. The dose is higher (60–120 mg per day) for women who have been diagnosed with iron-deficiency anemia. Recommend that these women
    — Take iron at different times of the day or 1–2 hours after meals to decrease nausea that some women experience.
    — Eat foods high in fiber (fresh fruits and vegetables) and drink at least 8 glasses of water a day to prevent constipation.
    — Not take iron with calcium supplements, milk products, tea, or coffee, which interfere with iron absorption.
    — Get plenty of vitamin C (in citrus fruits, tomatoes, melons, and berries) and heme iron (in meats) to increase absorption of iron.
    — Understand that iron often causes stools to be black or dark green.
- Folic acid (0.4 mg per day) is recommended for all women of childbearing age. Inadequate intake has been associated with megaloblastic anemia and neural tube defects in the fetus.

- Additional prenatal vitamins and minerals are recommended when there is reason to believe the diet is inadequate.

F. NUTRITION DURING LACTATION

The lactating woman needs additional calories, protein, magnesium, zinc, and vitamins A and C. Recommend the woman consume

- 500 kcal per day over normal needs.
- 65 grams of protein (5 grams more than needed during pregnancy).
- A diet high in fresh fruits and vegetables to meet the needs for vitamins and minerals.
- Breastfeeding mothers need reassurance that, unless they are allergic to certain foods, they can eat any food. Few foods affect the infant, and fussiness is often related to factors other than food.

XIII. EDUCATION FOR CHILDBEARING

Some of the most common educational programs offered to the childbearing family are

- Early pregnancy classes: Provide information about how the body adapts to pregnancy and how to deal with common discomforts.
- Exercise classes: Should be preceded by warm-up, should be low-impact, and should avoid excessive heart rate elevation; target heart rate is often prescribed by physician.
- Childbirth preparation classes: Describe what to expect during labor and birth and focus on self-help measures for the couple; classes include information about phases and stages of labor, pharmacologic and non-pharmacologic methods of pain relief, and supervised practice of relaxation and coping strategies.

- Selected method of childbirth education: Although most methods of childbirth education use some combination of pain management techniques, some differences exist among those listed below.
  - Dick-Read method uses education and relaxation to reduce tension (and thus pain). The method involves slow abdominal breathing in early labor and rapid chest breathing in advanced labor.
  - Bradley method was the first to include the father as a support person. Slow abdominal breathing and relaxation are used to avoid medication or other interventions.
  - Lamaze method, also called the "psychoprophylaxis" method, uses the mind to control pain. Techniques include concentration and conditioning to help the woman respond to contractions with relaxation. Class content includes preparatory exercises such as pelvic rock, tailor sitting, Kegel exercise, and stretching. Relaxation techniques include effleurage, use of a focal point, imagery, and breathing techniques.

XIV. COMPLICATIONS OF PREGNANCY

Only those complications that have a strong clinical component are presented. The reader is referred to a reference book, such as *Foundations in Maternal-Newborn Nursing*, second edition, for information about less common conditions or those that respond primarily to medical management.

A. ANEMIAS

Anemia is a condition in which there is a hemoglobin concentration of less than 10.5–11 g/dL (Laros, 1994). The most common types of anemia observed during pregnancy are iron deficiency anemia, folic acid-deficiency anemia, and sickle cell anemia.

Iron Deficiency Anemia

Most women do not have iron stores that meet the needs of pregnancy. Furthermore, it is difficult to meet pregnancy needs by diet alone, and iron supplementation with ferrous sulfate, gluconate, or fumarate is generally required. For additional information about supplementation, see page 50.

Folic Acid-Deficiency (Megaloblastic) Anemia

A deficiency in folic acid results in a reduction in the rate of DNA synthesis and mitotic activity of individual cells, resulting in large, immature erythrocytes (megaloblasts). Folate deficiency is associated with increased risk of spontaneous abortion, abruptio placentae, and fetal anomalies such as neural tube defects. As a result folate supplementation has become a standard component of care (see page 50).

Sickle Cell Anemia

Sickle cell anemia occurs when a defect in hemoglobin causes erythrocytes to be shaped like a sickle, or crescent. Pregnancy can exacerbate sickle cell anemia and bring on sickle cell crisis. This broad term may include cessation of bone marrow function, massive erythrocyte destruction resulting in hyperbilirubinemia, and severe pain caused by infarctions in the joints and major organs.

Management is based on the knowledge that dehydration, hypoxemia, extremes in temperature, exertion, and infection stimulate the sickling process. Some specific measures include

- Frequent evaluations of hemoglobin, blood count, serum iron, total iron binding capacity, and serum folate.
- Fetal surveillance studies, such as ultrasonography and biophysical profiles.
- Maintenance of adequate hydration.
- Recommendation to dress warmly in cold weather and to avoid exertion in hot weather.
- Folic acid supplementation to increase erythrocyte production.
- Rest periods throughout the day, as well as good hygienic practices and avoidance of people with infectious illnesses.
- Prompt treatment for fever or other signs of infection.
- Administration of oxygen continuously during the intrapartum period.

B. BLEEDING COMPLICATIONS OF PREGNANCY

Abortion

Abortion is the loss of pregnancy before the fetus is capable of living outside the uterus (approximately 20 weeks gestation or 500 grams). Abortion may be induced (see page 395) or spontaneous. Nurses must remember that lay people often refer to spontaneous abortion as "miscarriage."

Etiology and Predisposing Factors

The primary causes of spontaneous abortion are

- Abnormal embryonic development.
- Chromosomal defects.

- Endocrine imbalances such as insulin-dependent diabetes mellitus, hypothyroidism, or inadequate progesterone.
- Immunologic factors such as antiphospholipid antibodies.
- Infections such as bacteriuria and *Chlamydia trachomatis*.
- Systemic disorders such as lupus erythematosus.
- Anomalies of the reproductive tract, such as bicornuate uterus.

Types of Spontaneous Abortion

Spontaneous abortion is divided into six categories

- Threatened: Vaginal bleeding occurs, but the products of conception are not expelled.
- Inevitable: Abortion cannot be stopped when there is rupture of membranes and dilation of the cervix.
- Incomplete: Some, but not all, products of conception are expelled from the uterus.
- Complete: All products of conception are expelled.
- Missed: The fetus dies, but the products of conception are retained.
- Recurrent: Three or more consecutive pregnancies end in spontaneous abortion.

Signs and Symptoms

- Vaginal bleeding
- Rhythmic uterine cramping
- Backache or feeling of pelvic pressure
- Rupture of membranes
- Dilation of the cervix
- Decline in placental hormone production

Management

- Evaluation by ultrasound to determine if a fetus is present and alive
- Reassurance that bed rest does not improve the prognosis for a threatened abortion
- Analgesia as necessary
- Evacuation of the remaining products of conception if abortion is incomplete
- Administration of oxytocin, prostaglandin, or Methergine to stimulate uterine contraction and/or to control bleeding
- Intravenous fluids and blood replacement as necessary to maintain fluid and electrolyte balance
- Prophylactic Rho(D) immune globulin (RhoGAM) for all unsensitized Rh-negative mothers
- When fetal death is confirmed in a missed abortion, the usual management is to wait 3–5 weeks for spontaneous abortion to occur
- Two major complications of missed abortion: uterine infection and disseminated intravascular coagulation (DIC) (see page 64)
- Examination of the cervix and uterus to identify anatomic defects that may be the cause of recurrent abortion
- Genetic screening for factors that might increase the risk of recurrent abortion
- Suturing of the cervix (McDonald's or Shirodkar's procedure) to keep it closed and thus maintain the pregnancy if there is a history of recurrent abortion

Ectopic Pregnancy

The term *ectopic pregnancy* refers to implantation of a fertilized ovum in an area outside the uterine cavity, usually in the fallopian tube. This is a life-threatening event because of massive bleeding that can occur if the tube ruptures.

Etiology and Predisposing Factors

Ectopic pregnancy is most likely to occur when transport of the fertilized ovum through the fallopian tube is hampered. The primary predisposing factors are

- History of previous pelvic inflammatory disease.
- Previous ectopic pregnancy.
- Tubal ligation.
- Intrauterine device.

Signs and Symptoms

- Missed menstrual period and other presumptive signs of pregnancy, such as breast tenderness and nausea
- Abdominal pain and tenderness
- Pelvic mass
- Vaginal "spotting"
- Signs of internal hemorrhage such as increasing pulse, falling blood pressure, vertigo, shoulder pain due to irritation of phrenic nerve

Management

Following diagnosis, which is usually made by transvaginal ultrasound examination and assay of the beta subunit of human chorionic gonadotropin (B-hCG), management depends on whether the tube is intact or ruptured. If it is intact, initial care may include

- Administration of methotrexate, a chemotherapeutic agent to stop cell reproduction in the tube.
- An incision into the tube and removal of the products of conception (lineal salpingostomy). The goal of this procedure is to preserve the tube and to prevent hemorrhage that occurs when the tube ruptures.

If the tube is ruptured, management focuses on measures to control bleeding and to prevent hypovolemic shock. These measures include

- Administration of intravenous fluids and whole blood as necessary to maintain hemodynamic status.
- Removal of the tube (salpingectomy).
- Recognition of the family's feelings, which include grief at pregnancy loss and concern about the chances for future pregnancies.

Hydatidiform Mole

Hydatidiform mole, a form of *gestational trophoblastic neoplasia*, refers to an abnormal growth of trophoblastic cells that attach the fertilized ovum to the uterine wall. The proliferating trophoblasts fill the uterus with vesicles that resemble a cluster of grapes. The fetal part of the pregnancy fails to develop.

Types of Hydatidiform Mole

- Complete: Believed to occur when the ovum is fertilized by a sperm that duplicates its own chromosomes while the chromosomes of the ovum are inactivated.
- Partial: The maternal contribution is present but the paternal contribution is double and the karyotype is 69 XXY or 69 XYY.

Etiology and Predisposing Factors

The cause of hydatidiform mole is unknown; however, the risk factors include

- Asian or Asian descent.
- Age above 40 years.
- Age under 20 years.
- History of previous molar pregnancy.
- Stimulation of ovulation in infertility management.
- Dietary deficiency of beta-carotene and folic acid.

Signs and Symptoms

- Vaginal bleeding: may be irregular or heavy, dark brown or bright red.
- Uterine cramping may or may not be present.
- Uterus is often larger than expected based on dates of LMP.
- Fetal heart activity and fetal movement cannot be detected.
- β-hCG titers are higher than expected.
- Excessive nausea and vomiting occur.
- Vesicles may be found in the vagina.
- Signs of pregnancy-induced hypertension appear early in the pregnancy.

Management

Management includes two phases: (1) immediate evacuation after diagnosis by ultrasound examination, and (2) follow-up to detect malignant changes of the remaining trophoblastic tissue. Immediate care includes

- Specific tests such as chest X-ray to detect metastatic disease.
- Complete blood count, including assessment of clotting factors, blood typing, and crossmatching.
- Replacement of fluids and whole blood as necessary.
- General or regional anesthesia.
- Suction evacuation, followed by curettage of the uterus.
- Laboratory evaluation of tissue to identify benign or malignant cytology.
- Intravenous oxytocin to reduce blood loss.

Follow-up care protocol includes

- Evaluation of serum hCG titers for at least a year.
- Advice not to attempt pregnancy for at least a year.

- Response to feelings of sadness at loss of pregnancy and concern about the need for long-term follow-up.

Placenta Previa

In placenta previa, the placenta implants in the lower uterine segment and infringes on or covers the cervical os. Placenta previa may be marginal (extends only to the cervical os), partial (covers part of the os), or complete (extends over the entire cervical os).

Etiology and Predisposing Factors

The direct cause is unknown, but factors that have been associated with a higher incidence of placenta previa include

- Multiparity.
- Increasing maternal age.
- Prior placenta previa.
- Multiple gestation.

Signs and Symptoms

- An episode of painless uterine bleeding in the latter half of pregnancy
- Subsequent episodes of heavier bleeding
- Bleeding that occurs when labor begins (heavier and brighter than "bloody show")

Management

- Ultrasound examination to locate the position of the placenta
- Postponement of vaginal examinations that may further disrupt the placenta and cause additional bleeding
- Electronic monitoring to determine the condition of the fetus
- Evaluation of mother for signs of hypovolemia (increasing pulse, falling blood pressure, pallor, etc.)

- Laboratory examination for signs of anemia and infection (CBC, Hg, Hct) and type and crossmatch to replace whole blood as necessary
- Bedrest and careful monitoring of fetus, maternal vital signs, and vaginal bleeding if initial bleeding was scant or moderate, and if the fetus is immature and shows no signs of compromise
- Assistance for the family, who must plan for long-term bedrest, and instructions in how to monitor the mother and fetus
- Criteria for home care include
  — No evidence of active bleeding.
  — No signs or symptoms of preterm labor.
  — Home is no more than 15–20 minutes from the hospital.
  — Emergency support systems are in place for emergency transport to the hospital.
  — The presence of a responsible adult at all times.
- Preparation for cesarean delivery when fetal lungs are mature or if bleeding is excessive regardless of fetal maturity

Abruptio Placentae

Abruptio placentae, also called placental abruption or premature separation of the placenta, occurs when a normally implanted placenta separates from the uterine wall prior to the birth of the infant. The bleeding that occurs may dissect upward toward the fundus, resulting in concealed hemorrhage, or extend downward toward the cervix, resulting in external or obvious bleeding. The major dangers for the woman are hemorrhage, hypovolemic shock, and clotting disorders (DIC). The major dangers for the fetus are anoxia as placental blood flow is compromised, blood loss, or delivery before the fetus is mature.

Etiology and Predisposing Factors

- Pregnancy-induced or chronic hypertension

- Hydramnios
- Cocaine use
- Smoking
- Preterm rupture of membranes
- Short umbilical cord

Signs and Symptoms

- Abdominal pain that is severe and unremitting
- Abdominal tenderness
- Boardlike rigidity of the abdomen
- Persistent, increased uterine base tone on electronic monitor
- Vaginal bleeding
- Signs of hypovolemic shock, with or without external bleeding

Management

Management is a collaborative process that involves nurses and physicians whose major goals are to prevent hypovolemic shock and to deliver a healthy infant safely. Interventions include

- Monitor hemodynamic status of mother.
- Initiate electronic fetal monitoring to detect signs of fetal hypoxia, such as tachycardia or late decelerations.
- Insert an indwelling catheter to assess urine output accurately.
- Observe for uterine hyperactivity, such as contractions lasting longer than 90 seconds or persistent, increased uterine base tone.
- Administer intravenous fluids, whole blood, plasma, cryoprecipitate, and platelets as necessary.
- Prepare for rapid delivery to prevent fetal compromise and to control bleeding.

- Keep family informed about interventions that must often be performed quickly.
- Acknowledge the family's concern for the mother and the fetus and offer reassurance when possible.

Nursing Considerations

Vaginal bleeding is frightening for the family members, who are usually concerned about the safety of the mother as well as the fetus. Moreover, bleeding is often accompanied by pain and loss of the pregnancy. Nurses usually try to

- Confirm pregnancy and determine length of gestation according to prenatal records or history taken at initial contact.
- Evaluate vital signs, skin color and temperature, capillary return, urinary output, and level of consciousness to determine hemodynamic status.
- Evaluate the of amount of bleeding and obtain a description of the location and severity of pain.
- Monitor the condition of the fetus.
- Check laboratory values, such as hemoglobin, hematocrit, blood type, and Rh factor.
- Collaborate with physician to administer intravenous fluids and/or Rho(D) immune globulin.
- Keep the woman as comfortable as possible.
- Consider the psychological needs of the family members, who usually experience an acute sense of loss and grief when the fetus does not survive.
  — Acknowledge the parents' emotions.
  — Allow time to listen and to reflect family feelings.
  — Provide reassurance to lessen feelings of self-blame.
  — Help women express their feelings to partners and other trusted family members.
- Keep the family informed of preoperative procedures that are often performed quickly.

- Reinforce necessary follow-up care.
- Teach the family how to prevent and recognize signs of infection that may occur as a result of blood loss. Some specific measures include
  — Validating that the woman knows how to use a thermometer.
  — Instructing her to check her temperature every 8 hours for the first 3 days at home.
  — Emphasizing the importance of careful hand washing before and after changing pads.
  — Recommending that pads rather than tampons should be used until bleeding subsides.
  — Suggesting that she consult with health care provider before resuming sexual intercourse.
  — Advising her to consume foods high in iron to increase hemoglobin and hematocrit values.

C. DISSEMINATED INTRAVASCULAR COAGULATION

Disseminated intravascular coagulation (DIC) is a life-threatening complication in which anticoagulation and procoagulation factors are activated at the same time. The result is a simultaneous decrease in clotting factors and an increase in anticoagulant factors that leaves the circulating blood unable to clot.

Etiology and Predisposing Factors

Major predisposing factors include

- Missed abortion.
- Abruptio placentae.
- Pregnancy-induced hypertension.

Signs and Symptoms

- Profuse bleeding from any vulnerable area, such as intravenous sites, incisions, the gums, or nose
- Profuse bleeding from the site of placental attachment

Management

- Delivery of the fetus and placenta to stop the production of thromboplastin, which is fueling the process
- Blood replacement with whole blood, packed red blood cells, plasma, and cryoprecipitate
- Continuous monitoring of maternal vital signs to detect hypovolemia
- Documentation of location and severity of bleeding

D. DIABETES MELLITUS

Types of Diabetes Mellitus

- Diabetes mellitus that exists prior to pregnancy may be Type I (insulin dependent) or Type II (non-insulin dependent). *Oral hypoglycemic medications are teratogenic for the fetus and are not used during pregnancy.*
- Diabetes that develops during pregnancy is termed *gestational diabetes* or *pregnancy-induced glucose intolerance.*

Effects of Pregnancy on Insulin Production

Significant changes in insulin production affect all women during pregnancy. Women without diabetes adapt easily to the changes, but those with diabetes must adjust their insulin dose, diet, and exercise regimen. Changes include

- A decrease in the amount of insulin needed during the first trimester, when the expectant woman experiences anorexia, nausea, and vomiting.
- An increase in the amount of insulin needed during the second and third trimesters, when placental hormones create resistance to insulin.
- Either an increase or a decrease in insulin during the intrapartum; the amount depends on the exertion of labor and the amount of intravenous glucose administered. The amount of insulin needed is determined by frequent evaluation of blood glucose.

- A decrease in the amount of insulin needed during the postpartum period, when the hormones of pregnancy decline after the delivery of the placenta.

Effects of Diabetes on Pregnancy

Women with diabetes mellitus are at increased risk for a variety of conditions that include

- Pregnancy-induced hypertension, possibly related to previous maternal vascular damage secondary to diabetes.

- Urinary tract infections that may be due to glycosuria, which provides a nutrient-rich medium for bacterial growth.

- Hydramnios (excessive amniotic fluid) as a result of fetal hyperglycemia and consequent fetal polyuria.

- Premature rupture of membranes and preterm labor that may be related to overdistention of the uterus by hydramnios or a large fetus.

- Difficult labor, injury to birth canal, cesarean birth, and postpartal hemorrhage that are associated with fetal macrosomia.

- Ketoacidosis due to increase in ketones when fats and proteins are metabolized for energy instead of glucose.

Increased Fetal and Neonatal Risks

- Congenital anomalies, such as neural tube defects, caudal regression syndrome, and cardiac defects that are related to hyperglycemia during the period of organogenesis (first trimester)

- Perinatal death due to maternal vascular damage, pregnancy-induced hypertension, or early deterioration of the placenta

- Large infant (>4000 grams) due to fetal hyperglycemia and consequent high levels of fetal insulin (a powerful growth hormone)

- Birth injury related to macrosomia, difficult labor, and shoulder dystocia

- Intrauterine growth restriction if there is damage to maternal arterioles, resulting in poor perfusion of the placenta
- Polycythemia in response to frequent episodes of hypoxia
- Neonatal hyperbilirubinemia when excessive red blood cells are broken down, leaving large quantities of unconjugated bilirubin
- Neonatal respiratory distress syndrome due to hyperinsulinemia that retards cortisol, which is necessary for surfactant production
- Neonatal hypoglycemia following birth when serum glucose declines but neonatal insulin production remains high

Diagnosis of Gestational Diabetes Mellitus (GDM)

All women are screened for GDM during pregnancy, usually at 24–28 weeks gestation. Women at high risk to develop GDM may be screened earlier. Screening tests include

- 50-gram (1-hour) glucose challenge test (GCT); if glucose level is 140 mg/dL or greater, GTT should be performed.
- 100-gram (3-hour) glucose tolerance test (GTT); this test is positive if two or more of the following plasma levels are met or exceeded:

Fasting	105 mg/dL
1 hour	190 mg/dL
2 hour	165 mg/dL
3 hour	145 mg/dL

Predisposing Factors for Gestational Diabetes Mellitus

- Maternal age >30 years
- Prepregnancy weight >20% above ideal weight
- Family history of diabetes
- Prior birth of infant >4000 grams
- History of GDM

- Prior stillborn infant
- Prior birth of infant with congenital anomalies

Management of Gestational Diabetes Mellitus

- Dietary counseling that should emphasize:
  - Adequate calories (2200–2400 per day).
  - 50–60% of the calories should come from complex carbohydrates.
  - 10–20% should come from protein sources.
  - 25–30% should come from fat.
  - Restriction of sugars and concentrated sweets.
  - Avoidance of frozen meals, canned soups, packaged stuffing, and instant potatoes that contain excessive salt, which promotes fluid retention.
  - Small, frequent meals that include one protein source, high fiber foods, and fresh fruits and vegetables.
- Exercise regimen recommended by physician
- Instruction in self-evaluation of glucose levels
- Evaluation of fasting blood sugar and/or postprandial blood sugar
- Fetal surveillance that may include
  - Maternal assessment of fetal activity ("kick counts").
  - Nonstress tests.
  - Amniotic fluid index.
  - Biophysical profile.
- Administration of insulin if diet and exercise do not maintain normal blood glucose
- Normal prenatal care
- Opportunities for maternal decision making and control whenever possible

Assessment and Management of Preexisting Diabetes Mellitus

A team, composed of a perinatologist, obstetrician, dietitian, nurse-educator, and diabetologist, help the mother

- Maintain normal blood glucose levels.
- Give birth to a healthy baby.
- Avoid accelerated impairment of blood vessels and other organs.

Prior to pregnancy, every effort is made to achieve and maintain normal blood glucose levels. This helps prevent congenital anomalies that are strongly associated with hyperglycemia in the first trimester.

In addition, specific tests are performed to determine the effects of diabetes on maternal body systems. These tests include

- Baseline electrocardiogram.
- Evaluation for retinopathy.
- Renal function tests.
- Glycosylated hemoglobin for glucose saturation over previous 4–8 weeks.
- Maternal serum alpha-fetoprotein to screen for neural tube defects.
- Ultrasonographic evaluation of fetus, including fetal cardiac structures.
- Fetal surveillance ("kick counts", nonstress tests, contraction stress tests, biophysical profiles, amniotic fluid index) to monitor the well-being of the fetus.
- Self-monitoring of blood glucose several times each day to determine amounts of insulin needed to maintain euglycemia.
- Diet of adequate caloric intake that should be distributed among 3 meals and 2–4 snacks daily.

- Insulin therapy as necessary to maintain normal blood glucose.
- Recognition and management of hyperglycemia; signs include
  - Fatigue
  - Flushed, hot skin
  - Dry mouth; excessive thirst
  - Frequent urination
  - Rapid, deep respirations; odor of acetone on the breath
  - Drowsiness; headache
  - Depressed reflexes
- Instruction to notify the physician when signs or symptoms of hyperglycemia are noted.
- Recognition and management of hypoglycemia; signs include
  - Shakiness (tremors)
  - Sweating
  - Pallor; cold, clammy skin
  - Disorientation, irritability
  - Headache
  - Hunger
  - Blurred vision
- Treatment for hypoglycemia includes
  - Testing blood glucose when symptoms first appear.
  - If glucose is less than 60 mg/dL, boosting level by eating or drinking one of the following:
    - Eight ounces of low-fat or skim milk or 4 ounces of unsweetened fruit juice.
    - Peanut butter and crackers.
    - Glucose tablets or 1 container glucose gel.
  - Recheck blood glucose and notify health care provider if glucose level remains at 60 mg/dL or if episodes occur two or more times within a week.
- Timing of delivery as close to term as possible.

Nursing Considerations

Women respond differently to the intense medical supervision that is necessary to maintain normal blood glucose. Some fear they will be unable to control the diabetes to the degree expected. Other women may feel that they are only an "incubator" and that their feelings are unimportant as long as the fetus thrives. Nurses can facilitate communications and provide support by

- Asking broad, open-ended questions such as, "What are your major concerns?" "How do you feel about the plan of care?"

- Actively listening to concerns of the woman and her family.

- Conveying acceptance of feelings that are expressed, whether they are negative or positive.

- Allowing opportunities for control in exercise and diet whenever possible.

- Providing normal pregnancy care, which is sometimes ignored because the focus is on controlling diabetes and preventing complications.

- Providing and reinforcing information about required tests and procedures, such as nonstress tests, biophysical profile, and self-monitoring of blood glucose.

- Giving praise and encouragement for maintaining normal blood glucose and for keeping recommended appointments.

E. HYPERTENSIVE DISORDERS OF PREGNANCY

Hypertensive disease is second only to embolism as a cause of maternal death in the United States. It is also an important cause of perinatal morbidity and mortality. Despite the seriousness of the disease and the frequency with which it occurs, its origins remain unclear. What is known is that it is a multi-organ disease process that is related to vasospasm and a consequent rise in blood pressure, a decrease in cardiac output, and reduced perfusion of vital organs such as the kidneys, brain, and placenta. Figure I-11 traces the pathological processes throughout the body.

Terminology used to describe hypertension in pregnancy is not uniform, and overlapping terms are used to describe the clinical signs of the same disease process. Table I-6, "Classification of Hypertensive Disorders of Pregnancy," describes the clinical subsets accepted by the American College of Obstetricians and Gynecologists (ACOG). In clinical practice, the terms *pregnancy-induced hypertension* and *preeclampsia* are often used interchangeably. Moreover, women with chronic hypertension are at risk to develop superimposed PIH.

Predisposing Factors

- First pregnancy
- Age > 40 years
- African-American race
- Family history of PIH
- Chronic hypertension
- Chronic renal disease
- Antiphospholipid syndrome
- Diabetes mellitus
- Twin gestation
- Angiotensin gene T 235
- Low socioeconomic status and young maternal age are traditional risk factors; the actual independent contribution of these factors to the risk of PIH is questionable. (ACOG, 1996. Technical Bulletin #219. Hypertension in pregnancy).

Signs and Symptoms

The classic signs of PIH or preeclampsia are: (1) hypertension, (2) proteinuria, and (3) generalized edema. See Table I-7 for a description of mild versus severe preeclampsia. Because of potential errors, the procedure for determining blood pressure should be standardized in each institution. The woman should

Figure I-11

The Pathologic Process of Pre-Eclampsia

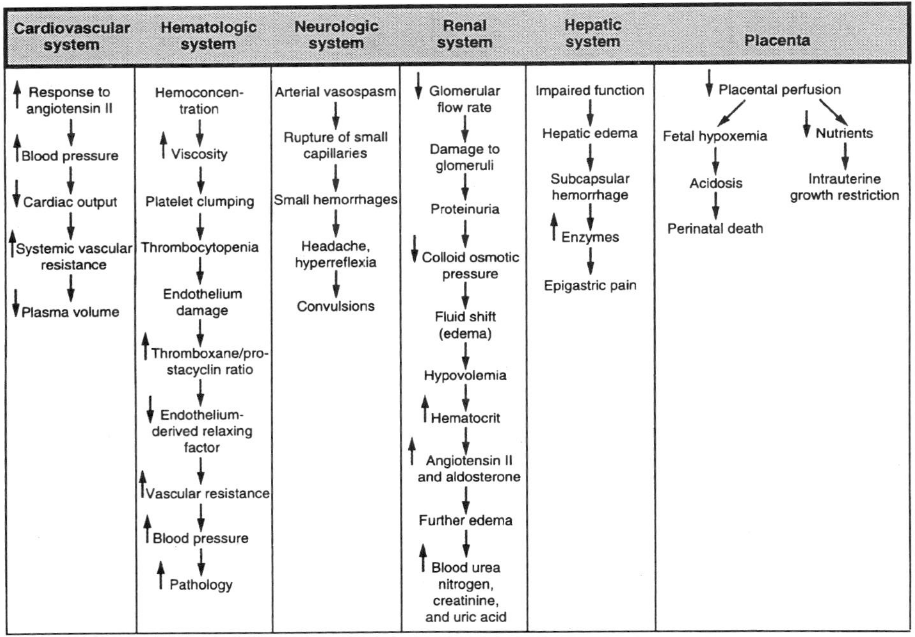

Cardiovascular system	Hematologic system	Neurologic system	Renal system	Hepatic system	Placenta
↑ Response to angiotensin II → ↑ Blood pressure → ↓ Cardiac output → ↑ Systemic vascular resistance → ↓ Plasma volume	Hemoconcentration → ↑ Viscosity → Platelet clumping → Thrombocytopenia → Endothelium damage → ↑ Thromboxane/prostacyclin ratio → ↓ Endothelium-derived relaxing factor → ↑ Vascular resistance → ↑ Blood pressure → ↑ Pathology	Arterial vasospasm → Rupture of small capillaries → Small hemorrhages → Headache, hyperreflexia → Convulsions	↓ Glomerular flow rate → Damage to glomeruli → Proteinuria → ↓ Colloid osmotic pressure → Fluid shift (edema) → Hypovolemia → ↑ Hematocrit → ↑ Angiotensin II and aldosterone → Further edema → ↑ Blood urea nitrogen, creatinine, and uric acid	Impaired function → Hepatic edema → Subcapsular hemorrhage → ↑ Enzymes → Epigastric pain	↓ Placental perfusion → ↓ Nutrients → Intrauterine growth restriction / Fetal hypoxemia → Acidosis → Perinatal death

TABLE I–6

Classification of Hypertensive Disorders of Pregnancy

Pregnancy-induced hypertension	Development of hypertension (BP >140/90 during second half of pregnancy in a previously normotensive woman
Preeclampsia	Renal involvement leads to proteinuria
Eclampsia	Central nervous system involvement leads to seizures
HELLP (hemolasis elevated liver enzymes, low platelets)	Clinical picture dominated by hematologic and hepatic signs and symptoms
Chronic hypertension	Elevation of blood pressure prior to 20 weeks gestation

Adapted from ACOG (1996). Hypertension in Pregnancy. Technical Bulletin #219.

TABLE I–7

Mild Versus Severe Preeclampsia

	MILD	SEVERE
Systolic BP	<160	>160
Diastolic BP	<100	>110
Proteinuria	Trace	> 5 g/24 hours
Creatinine	Normal	Elevated
Thrombocytopenia	Absent	Present
Oliguria	Absent	<500 mL/24 hours
Liver enzyme elevation	Minimal	Marked
Fetal growth restriction	Absent	Present
Headache, visual disturbances, abdominal pain	Absent	Present

be sitting with the arm supported in a horizontal position at heart level. The staff should agree on whether to use Korotkoff's fourth phase (muffling) or the fifth phase (disappearance). Most clinicians use the fifth phase, although it is 5–10 mm Hg lower than the fourth phase.

Management of Mild Preeclampsia

Management in the home may be possible if the woman is in stable condition with no evidence of worsening maternal or fetal status. The woman and her family must be able to adhere to a prescribed treatment plan that includes

- Bedrest with bathroom privileges only.
- Fetal movement monitoring ("kick counts").
- Blood pressure monitoring 2–4 times each day.
- Daily weights at the same time each day.
- Daily urinalysis for protein using first voided specimen.
- Uterine activity monitoring for signs of preterm labor.
- Medication administration as directed by physician.
- Documentation for home health care nurse.
- Additional fetal surveillance such as serial sonography, weekly nonstress testing, contraction stress testing, or biophysical profiles as necessary.

Management of Severe Preeclampsia

Goals of management are to prevent convulsions and to maintain the pregnancy until it is safe to deliver the fetus. Home care is not appropriate for severe preeclampsia. The woman will be hospitalized for constant assessment and management that includes

- Bedrest with reduced environmental stimuli.
- Intravenous administration of magnesium sulfate (the drug of choice in the United States to prevent convulsions). See "Drug Guide for Magnesium Sulfate" in Section Six, p. 454.

- Administration of antihypertensive medications (usually reserved for those at risk for intracranial bleeding). See "Drug Guide for Hydralazine" in Section Six, p. 451.

Nursing Considerations

Careful nursing assessment is the only way to determine whether the disease is responding to medical management or is worsening. Nursing assessments include

- Daily weights (rapid increase indicates fluid retention).
- Blood pressure to determine response to treatment.
- Respiratory rate ($MgSO_4$ causes respiratory depression; rate under 12 per minute should be reported at once).
- Breath sounds (moist breath sounds suggest pulmonary edema).
- Location and severity of edema.
- Hourly urinary output via indwelling catheter (> 30 mL/hr indicates adequate perfusion of kidneys).
- Urinalysis for proteinuria.
- Electronic monitor for changes in fetal heart rate or variability.
- Periodic monitoring for signs of labor or uterine irritability.
- Brachial and patellar reflexes plus clonus (hyperreflexia suggests increasing cerebral irritability; hyporeflexia indicates magnesium excess). See Procedure Guide in Section Six, "Assessing Deep Tendon Reflexes," p. 426.
- Level of consciousness (drowsiness, dulled sensorium indicate therapeutic effects of magnesium; non-responsive behavior or muscle weakness suggest magnesium toxicity).
- Symptoms such as headache, visual disturbances, epigastric pain (indicate increasing severity of the condition and the development of eclampsia).

- Laboratory data (elevated creatinine, elevated liver enzymes, or decreased platelets signify increasing severity of the disease; serum magnesium levels should be in therapeutic range designated by physician).

Specific Nursing Interventions

- Respond to signs of magnesium toxicity.
  - Discontinue magnesium and notify physician if respiratory rate is < 12 per minute, if deep tendon reflexes are absent, or if urinary output falls below 30 mL per hour (magnesium is excreted by the kidneys).
  - Have calcium gluconate (an antidote for magnesium sulfate) available; magnesium toxicity can be reversed by intravenous administration of 1 g (10 mL of 10%) of calcium gluconate over a 2-minute time span.
- Initiate measures to prevent eclamptic seizures.
  - Admit to private room where environmental stimuli (lights, noise, activity) can be controlled; keep the door closed.
  - Pad the door to reduce noise when it must be opened and closed.
  - Collaborate with family to reduce visitors and incoming telephone calls.
  - Group nursing assessments and care to allow long periods of quiet.
  - Move carefully and calmly around the room.
- Intervene to prevent seizure-related injury.
  - Keep the bed in the lowest position with wheels locked and side rails raised at all times.
  - Pad the side rails to prevent trauma should the woman hit them during a seizure.
  - Assemble suction and oxygen equipment in the room.

- Keep a preeclampsia tray (often called a "Tox Tray," reflecting prior time when this disease process was called "toxemia") in the room; it should contain an airway, ambu-bag with mask, ophthalmoscope, syringes, needles, tourniquet, and reflex hammer. Medications that should be readily available include magnesium sulfate, sodium bicarbonate, heparin sodium, epinephrine, phenytoin, and calcium gluconate.

- Protect the woman and fetus during a convulsion.
  - Remain with the woman and press the emergency bell for assistance.
  - Turn the woman on her side when the tonic phase begins if there is time.
  - Note the time and sequence of the convulsive activity.
  - Insert an airway following the convulsion and suction the nose and mouth to prevent aspiration.
  - Administer oxygen by mask.
  - Notify the physician as soon as possible; this is an obstetrical emergency that is associated with cerebral hemorrhage, premature separation of the placenta, fetal hypoxia, and death.
  - Administer medications and prepare for additional medical intervention as directed by the physician.

- Provide information and support for the family.
  - Explain to the family what has happened after the convulsion has ended.
  - Acknowledge that a convulsion is frightening and that it indicates worsening of the condition.
  - Respond to questions and prepare the family for future medical management that may include delivery of the infant as soon as possible.

F. HEART DISEASE

A healthy heart can adapt to the changes of pregnancy and childbirth without difficulty. If there is preexisting or underlying heart disease, however, the changes can impose a burden on an already compromised heart, resulting in cardiac decompensation and congestive heart failure. The two major categories are rheumatic heart disease and congenital heart disease. The severity of heart disease is determined by the woman's ability to endure physical activity (See Table I-8).

Signs and Symptoms

- Dyspnea, paroxysmal nocturnal dyspnea, and hemoptysis
- Syncope (fainting) with exertion
- Chest pain (angina) with exertion
- Heart murmurs
- Cardiac enlargement
- Serious arrhythmias
- Abnormal electrocardiogram or echocardiogram

TABLE I–8

Functional Classification of Heart Disease

Class I. Uncompromised, no limitation of physical activity. Asymptomatic with ordinary activity.

Class II. Slightly compromised, requiring slight limitation of physical activity. Comfortable at rest, but experience fatigue, dyspnea, palpitations, or anginal pain with ordinary activity.

Class III. Marked limitation of physical activity; comfortable at rest, but less than ordinary activity causes excessive fatigue, palpitations, dyspnea, or anginal pain; markedly compromised.

Class IV. Inability to perform any physical activity without discomfort; has symptoms of cardiac insufficiency even at rest. In general, maternal and fetal risks for Classes I and II disease are small, but risks are greatly increased for Classes III and IV.

Antepartum Management

The goal of treatment is to ensure that cardiac demand does not exceed the functional capacity of the heart. To accomplish this goal, all pregnant women with heart disease should

- Limit physical activity to remain free of symptoms of cardiac stress such as dyspnea, chest pain, or tachycardia.
- Avoid excessive weight gain that places further demands on the heart.
- Prevent anemia, which decreases the oxygen-carrying capacity of the blood and results in a compensatory increase in heart rate.
- Prevent infection; this may include the administration of prophylactic antibiotics.
- Undergo careful assessment for the development of congestive heart failure, pulmonary edema, or cardiac arrhythmias.
- Anticoagulant therapy may be necessary for those with mitral valve stenosis or septal defects.
- Antiarrhythmic therapy may be necessary for those with arrhythmias. (Digoxin, quinidine, and procainamide are not harmful to the fetus; beta-blockers are also used at times.)
- Anti-infectives may be used prophylactically.
- Diuretics are rarely used and require careful monitoring of fluid and electrolyte balance.

Intrapartum Management

Every effort is made to minimize the effects of labor on the cardiovascular system. Care includes

- Careful management of fluid administration to prevent fluid overload.
- Sims position with head and shoulders elevated.
- Oxygen administration as necessary.
- Sedation and epidural anesthesia to reduce discomfort.

- Quiet, calm environment to decrease anxiety.
- Keeping the legs level with the body during birth or lowering the legs during the third stage to minimize the risks of fluid overload when blood from the uteroplacental unit is added to central circulation.
- Using outlet forceps to shorten the second stage.
- Carefully assessing signs of circulatory overload (bounding pulse, distended neck and peripheral veins, moist rales in the lungs) during the fourth stage of labor

Postpartum Management

Women who have shown no evidence of distress during pregnancy, labor, or childbirth may decompensate during the postpartum period. They must be observed closely for signs of

- Congestive heart failure
    - Cough (frequent, productive, hemoptysis)
    - Progressive dyspnea with exertion
    - Orthopnea
    - Pitting edema of legs and feet or generalized edema of face, hands, or sacral area
    - Palpitations of the heart
    - Progressive fatigue or syncope
    - Moist rales in lower lobes
- Fluid overload.
- Infection.
- Hemorrhage.
- Thrombophlebitis.

Nursing Considerations

Nursing care focuses on teaching the woman and her family about measures that reduce the workload of the heart. These measures include

- How to avoid excessive weight gain while achieving necessary nutrients.

- How to modify activities that require energy.
  - Rest for an hour after meals.
  - Sit rather than stand whenever possible.
  - Rest whenever an activity increases heart rate.
  - Stop any activity that produces dyspnea, tachycardia, or chest pain.
- How to avoid unnecessary exposure to extreme temperatures.
- How identify and reduce emotional stress.
- How to maximize contact between the mother and newborn.

G. HYPEREMESIS GRAVIDARUM

Hyperemesis gravidarum is persistent, uncontrollable vomiting that begins in the early weeks and may continue throughout pregnancy. Consequences may include

- Severe weight loss.
- Dehydration and electrolyte imbalance.
- Loss of thiamine, retinol-binding protein, vitamin B_{12}, and chloride.
- Metabolic alkalosis (due to loss of large amounts of hydrochloric acid from the stomach).

Etiology and Predisposing Factors

The cause is unknown; however, some demographic factors have been studied. The condition is more prevalent among unmarried Caucasian women who are pregnant for the first time. Other risks may include elevated hormone levels, thyroid dysfunction, or psychologic factors.

Management

- Palliative measures such as those for "morning sickness"
- Administration of pyridoxine (vitamin B_6)

- Antiemetic medications—used with caution because of potential teratogenic effects
- Intravenous fluids and total parental nutrition

Nursing Considerations

Care usually takes place in the home, and nurses are responsible for assessing and providing care. Nursing assessments include

- Intake (oral and intravenous).
- Output (emesis, urine, bowel; 1 mL/kg/hr of urinary output suggests adequate perfusion of the kidneys).
- Drawing blood for laboratory data (elevated Hgb and Hct indicate hemoconcentration; sodium, potassium, and chloride may be depleted).
- Urinalysis for presence of ketones (suggesting starvation) or increased specific gravity (suggesting dehydration).
- Weight.

Nursing interventions focus on reducing nausea and vomiting and maintaining nutrition and fluid balance. Specific interventions include

- Offering small, frequent feedings.
- Suggesting low-fat foods and easily-digested carbohydrates (fruit, bread, rice, cereal, pasta).
- Recommending that soups and other liquids be taken between meals.
- Instructing that sitting upright after meals reduces gastric reflux.
- Providing unsolicited emotional support.

84 Clinical Manual for Foundations of Maternal Newborn Nursing

H. Rh INCOMPATIBILITY

Etiology

If blood from the Rh-positive fetus enters the bloodstream of the Rh-negative mother her body reacts by developing antibodies to the foreign antigen. Normally, fetal blood does not mingle with maternal blood. However, during labor or childbirth, small placental tears may allow a small amount of fetal blood to mix with maternal blood. The antibodies that develop as a consequence may cause problems for a subsequent pregnancy with an Rh-positive fetus. See Figure I-12.

Fetal-Neonatal Implications

Red blood cells of an Rh-positive fetus are destroyed by maternal antibodies. This destruction produces

Figure I-12

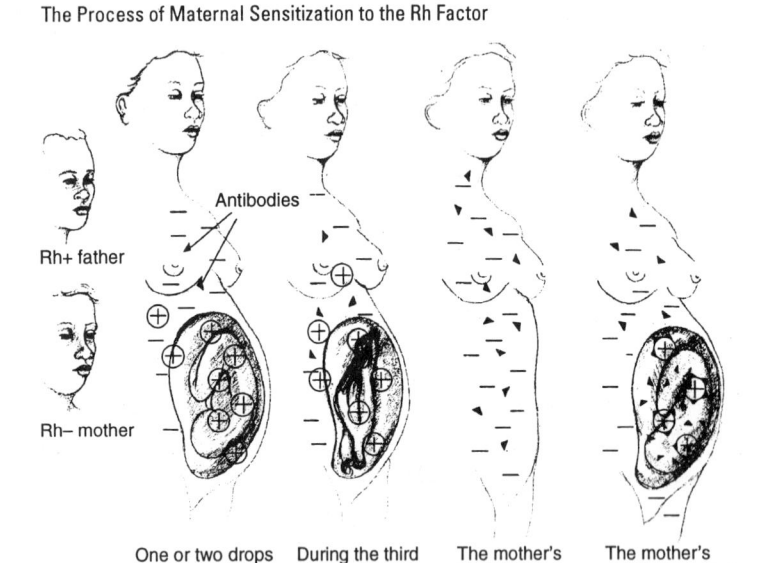

The Process of Maternal Sensitization to the Rh Factor

| One or two drops of fetal blood in the maternal circulation initiates production of antibodies | During the third stage of labor, damaged placental vessels allow exchange of maternal and fetal blood | The mother's body forms additional antibodies after birth | The mother's antibodies affect subsequent Rh+ fetuses |

- Anemia.
- Hyperbilirubinemia.
- Hypoxemia.
- Fetal death.

Management

- Prenatal screening for Rh factor for all women
- Antibody titer for all Rh-negative women
- Administration of Rho(D) immune globulin (RhoGAM, Gamulin Rh) within 72 hours to unsensitized, Rh-negative woman at 28 weeks and following amniocentesis or chorionic villus sampling, and following the birth of an Rh-positive infant (See Drug Guide, "Rho(D) Immune Globulin," Section Six, p. 462.)
- Evaluation of fetal bilirubin (by amniocentesis) if antibody titer indicates maternal sensitization
- Ultrasound examination to evaluate fetal condition

I. INFECTIONS

Infections can be mild or even asymptomatic in adults, but they are of great concern during pregnancy because they can cause catastrophic consequences for the fetus or neonate. See Table I-9 for the most common viral and nonviral infections. The most common sexually transmissible diseases and their impact on pregnancy are described in Table I-10.

TABLE I–9

Common Viral and Nonviral Infections

MATERNAL EFFECTS	FETAL-NEONATAL EFFECTS	TREATMENT
\multicolumn{3}{c}{**Viral Infections**}

Cytomegalovirus Infection

MATERNAL EFFECTS	FETAL-NEONATAL EFFECTS	TREATMENT
Mild, flu-like symptoms after exposure to body fluids such as saliva, semen, cervical mucus, and urine.	2% of all live neonates are infected with virus; 90% of this number are asymptomatic. Most serious complications are deafness, mental retardation, seizures, IUGR, blindness.	No effective therapy; antiviral agents are toxic and only temporarily suppress shedding of the virus.

Rubella

MATERNAL EFFECTS	FETAL-NEONATAL EFFECTS	TREATMENT
Fever, maculopapular rash, general malaise; maternal infection in first trimester results in multi-organ complications for the fetus.	Increase in spontaneous abortion, deafness, cataracts, mental retardation, cardiac defects, and microcephaly. Neonates shed the virus for many months.	Vaccine available for prevention; blood test of rubella titers determines maternal immunity.

Varicella Infection (Chickenpox)

MATERNAL EFFECTS	FETAL-NEONATAL EFFECTS	TREATMENT
Fever, anorexia, progressive rash (macules, papules to vesicles that crust and dry); varicella-zoster immune globulin (VZIG) administered after exposure to lessen fetal effects.	If infection occurs during first trimester, fetus is at risk for congenital varicella that includes limb hypoplasia, cutaneous scars, cataracts; exposure in later pregnancy may develop life-threatening varicella infection.	Avoid contact with infected people; report symptoms immediately; administer VZIG to infants whose mothers have chickenpox.

Genital Herpes

Virus shed from active lesions; vertical transmission from mother to infant when virus ascends after rupture of membranes, or when fetus comes into direct contact with infectious genital secretions; antiviral chemotherapy (acyclovir) is pregnancy risk category C and is used with caution during pregnancy.

Neonatal herpes infection is a major perinatal problem; symptoms are usually present within 2–3 days; mortality rate is 60% for disseminated herpes infection in newborn.

Cesarean birth if active genital lesion is present; protect infant from direct contact with lesions after birth.

Hepatitis B

Vomiting, pain, fever, jaundice, painful joints; hepatitis B vaccine available for prevention; hepatitis B immune globulin (HBIG) is administered to women who carry surface antigen (HBsAG-positive).

Prematurity, low birth-weight, neonatal death.

HBIG is administered to newborns whose mothers are HBsAG-positive; Hepatitis B vaccine is also given soon after birth.

Clinical Tip: Newborn should be bathed carefully before any injections are given to prevent infections from skin surface contamination.

Acquired Immune Deficiency Syndrome

Vertical transmission from mother to infant is between 20–40%.

No evidence of fetal embryopathy.

Encouraging results have been obtained from anti-viral medications and protease inhibitors that reduce replication of the virus and reduce vertical transmission.

Nonviral Infections

Toxoplasmosis (Protozoa Toxoplasma gondii)

Often subclinical; fatigue, muscle pains, swollen glands; transmitted through undercooked meat, contact with infected cat feces, or transplacentally.

Spontaneous abortion, low birthweight, jaundice, anemia; neurological damage may develop years later.

To prevent, cook meat thoroughly, avoid touching mouth or eyes while handling raw meat, wash hands often, avoid uncooked eggs and unpasteurized milk; avoid contact with materials contaminated with cat feces.

Group B Streptococcus Infection (Group B Streptococci)

Colonizes in the vagina, cervix, urethra, and rectum of women; usually asymptomatic, although maternal infections can occur.

Sepsis, pneumonia, meningitis of newborn; permanent neurologic sequelae are possible.

Prenatal screening cultures and intrapartum administration of penicillin to prevent neonatal infection.

Tuberculosis (Mycobacterium tuberculosis)

Transmitted by aerosolized droplets of liquid containing the bacterium that is inhaled by noninfected person; PPD is used to screen for disease during pregnancy.

Perinatal infection is rare; diagnosis made by finding bacilli in gastric aspirate of newborn.

Isoniazid (INH) plus rifampin; pyridoxine may be given with INH to prevent fetal neurotoxicity; skin-test infant and begin preventive INH therapy if necessary.

TABLE I–10

Sexually Transmissible Diseases and Vaginal Infections: Their Impact on Pregnancy

MATERNAL-FETAL-NEONATAL EFFECTS	NURSING CONSIDERATIONS

Syphilis (Causative Organism: Spirochete *Treponema pallidum*)

If untreated, the infection may pass across the placenta to the fetus and result in spontaneous abortion, a stillborn infant, premature labor and birth, or congenital syphilis. Major signs of congenital syphilis are enlarged liver and spleen, skin lesions, rashes, osteitis, pneumonia, and hepatitis.

Penicillin is the only treatment that will cure the disease without harming the fetus. Women who are allergic are desensitized and then treated. (Martens, 1994)

Gonorrhea (Causative Organism: Bacterium *Neisseria gonorrheae*)

Not transmitted via the placenta; vertical transmission from mother to newborn during birth may cause ophthalmia neonatorum. Endocervicitis and weakness of the fetal membranes increase the risk of premature rupture of membranes and preterm labor.

Ceftriaxone or cefixime with erythromycin are now recommended for penicillin-resistant organisms. The partner must also be treated to prevent reinfection. All infants are treated with an ophthalmic antibiotic at birth to prevent serious eye infections. (Lee, 1995)

Chlamydial Infection (Causative Organism: Bacterium *Chlamydia trachomatis*)

The fetus may be infected during birth and suffer neonatal conjunctivitis or pneumonitis, which manifests within 4–6 weeks. Conjunctivitis is prevented by erythromycin ophthalmic ointment. Chlamydia may also be responsible for premature rupture of membranes, premature labor, and chorioamnionitis.

Education is particularly important because Chlamydia is the most common STD in the United States, and infection is usually asymptomatic. Both partners should be treated to prevent recurrent infection. As with all STDs, the use of condoms decreases the risk of infection. Erythromycin is the recommended treatment. (Lee, 1995)

Trichomoniasis (Causative Organism: Protozoan *Trichomonas vaginalis*)

Not transmitted across the placental barrier; the organism cannot survive in the infantile, non-estrogenized vagina. Associated with premature rupture of membranes and postpartum endometritis.

Metronidazole (Flagyl) can be used safely only during the second and third trimesters because of teratogenicity. Clotrimazole may provide relief of symptoms during first trimester. (Martens, 1994)

Condylomata Acuminata (Causative Organism: Human Papillomavirus)

Transmission of condylomata acuminata, also called venereal warts, may occur during vaginal birth and is associated with the development of epithelial tumors of the mucous membranes of the larynx in children. Pregnancy can cause proliferation of lesions, which are associated with cervical dysplasia and cancer.

Podophyllin is contraindicated as treatment during pregnancy because of possible teratogenic effects. Applications of trichloracetic acid or cryotherapy are recommended instead. (Youngkin, 1995)

Vaginal Infections

Candidiasis (Causative Organism: Yeast *Candida albicans*)

Oral candidiasis (thrush) may develop in newborns if infection is present at birth. Thrush is treated with application of nystatin (Mycostatin) over the surfaces of the oral cavity four times a day for several days. Characteristic "cottage cheese" vaginal discharge with vulvar pruritus, burning, and dyspareunia. Vulva may be red, tender, and edematous.

Candidiasis (previously called *monilia*) is a persistent problem for many women during pregnancy. Effective treatment may be obtained with miconazole nitrate (Monistat) or clotrimazole (Gyne-Lotrimin), both available over the counter.

Bacterial Vaginosis (Causative Organism: *Gardnerella vaginalis**)

No known fetal effects; may be associated with postpartum endometritis. Marked by a major shift in vaginal flora from the normal predominance of lactobacilli to a predominance of anaerobic bacteria. Causes profuse, malodorous, "fishy" vaginal discharge, itching, and burning.

The causative organism is sensitive to metronidazole, which may be used during the second and third trimesters without concern about teratogenic effect. (Lee, 1995)

---

*Formerly called *nonspecific vaginitis* or *Gardnerella vaginitis*.

SECTION TWO

Intrapartum

I. NURSING CARE DURING LABOR AND BIRTH

The intrapartal period begins with the first true labor contraction and ends with the immediate recovery period after birth.

A. COMPONENTS OF CHILDBIRTH

The four major components of the birth process, often called the "four P's" of childbirth, are the powers, the passage, the passenger, and the woman's psyche.

Powers

- Two components
  - Uterine contractions: first and second stages
  - Maternal bearing-down (pushing) efforts: second stage
- Contraction cycle
  - Increment: The period of increasing strength
  - Peak (acme): The period of greatest contraction strength
  - Decrement: The period of decreasing strength
  - Interval: The period of uterine relaxation between contractions

Passage

- Bony pelvis
  - False pelvis: Above linea terminalis

- True pelvis: Below linea terminalis; the part most important to birth
- Divisions of true pelvis
  - Inlet: The upper portion, bounded by the upper border of the symphysis pubis, the sacral promontory, and the linea terminalis
  - Midpelvis (pelvic cavity): Between the boundaries for the pelvic inlet and outlet
  - Outlet: The plane of the pelvis that lies at the level of the ischial tuberosities, the lower border of the symphysis pubis, and the coccyx
- Pubic arch: Angle should be 90° or wider to allow the fetus to pass under it easily

Figure II-1

Pelvic Divisions and Measurements

Inlet

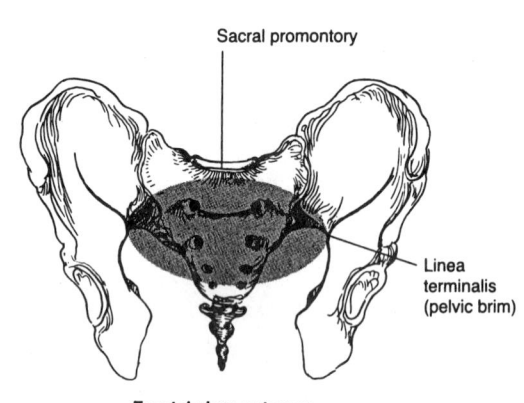

Sacral promontory

Linea terminalis (pelvic brim)

Frontal view, cutaway

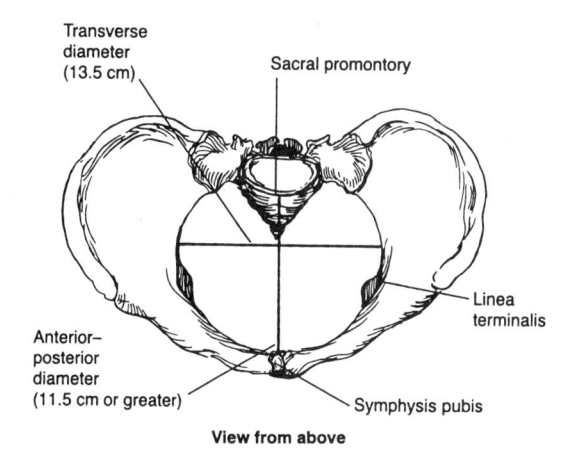

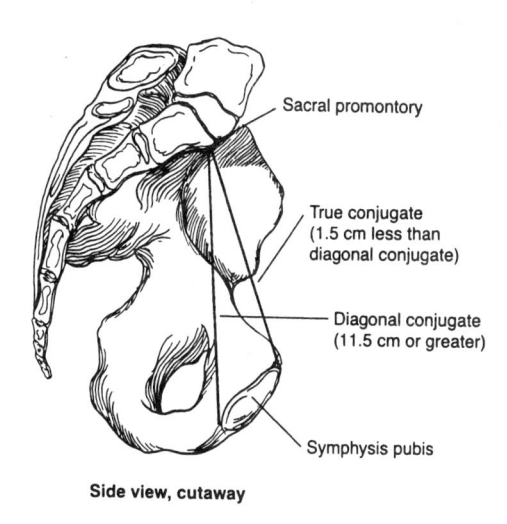

Figure II-1 *(continued)*

Pelvic Divisions and Measurements

- Transverse diameter (13.5 cm)
- Sacral promontory
- Linea terminalis
- Anterior–posterior diameter (11.5 cm or greater)
- Symphysis pubis

View from above

- Sacral promontory
- True conjugate (1.5 cm less than diagonal conjugate)
- Diagonal conjugate (11.5 cm or greater)
- Symphysis pubis

Side view, cutaway

94 Clinical Manual for Foundations of Maternal Newborn Nursing

Figure II-1 *(continued)*

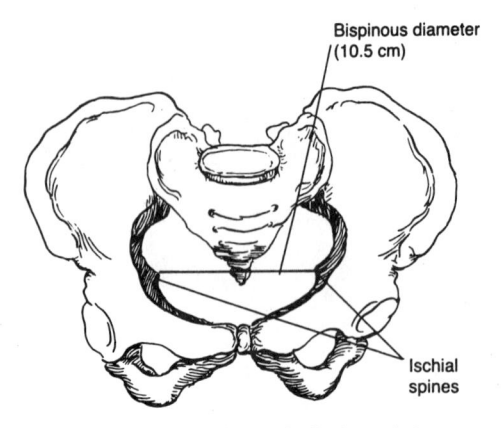

Pelvic Divisions and Measurements

View from above, with pelvis tilted anteriorly

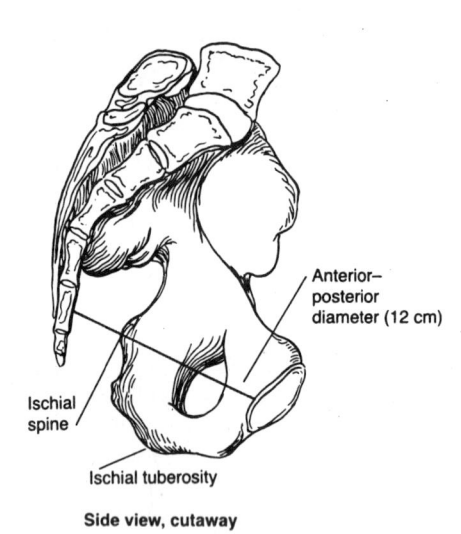

- Bispinous diameter (10.5 cm)
- Ischial spines

Side view, cutaway

- Anterior–posterior diameter (12 cm)
- Ischial spine
- Ischial tuberosity

SECTION TWO: Intrapartum 95

Figure II-1 *(continued)*

Pelvic Divisions and Measurements

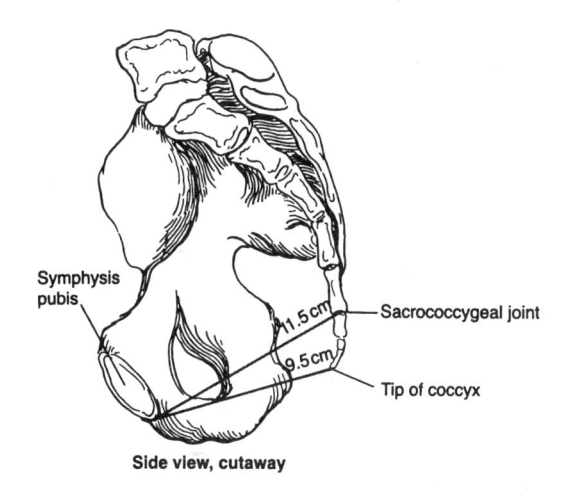

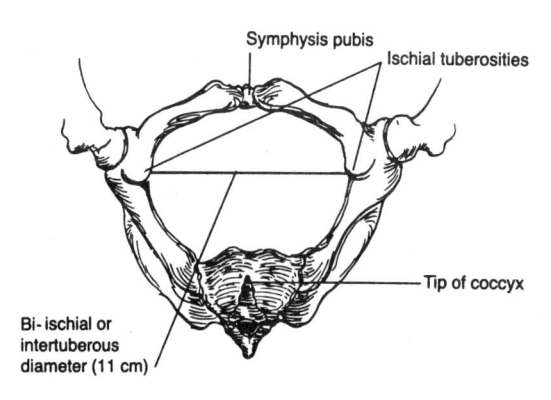

Side view, cutaway

- Symphysis pubis
- 11.5 cm — Sacrococcygeal joint
- 9.5 cm — Tip of coccyx

View from below (woman is in lithotomy position)

- Symphysis pubis
- Ischial tuberosities
- Tip of coccyx
- Bi-ischial or intertuberous diameter (11 cm)

Figure II-1 *(continued)*

Pelvic Divisions and Measurements

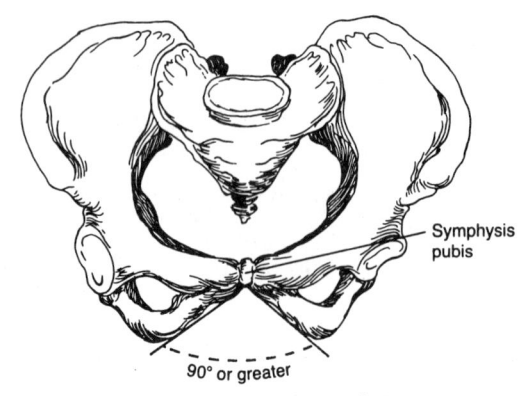

Frontal view, with pelvis tilted anteriorly

Passenger

The passenger is the fetus, plus the membranes and placenta.

- Fetal lie: Fetal orientation to the mother's vertebral column, either longitudinal, with the fetal spine parallel to the mother's spine, or transverse, with the fetus at right angles to her spine

- Fetal presentation: The fetal part that enters the pelvis, with cephalic presentations being most common (96%)
  — Cephalic presentations:
    - Vertex: Most common; fetal head is fully flexed, with the chin on the chest.
    - Military: The fetal head is in a neutral position, neither flexed nor extended.
    - Brow: The fetal head is partly extended, and may change to a vertex or face presentation as labor progresses.
    - Face: The fetal head is fully extended, with the occiput near the fetal spine.

SECTION TWO: Intrapartum 97

Figure II-2

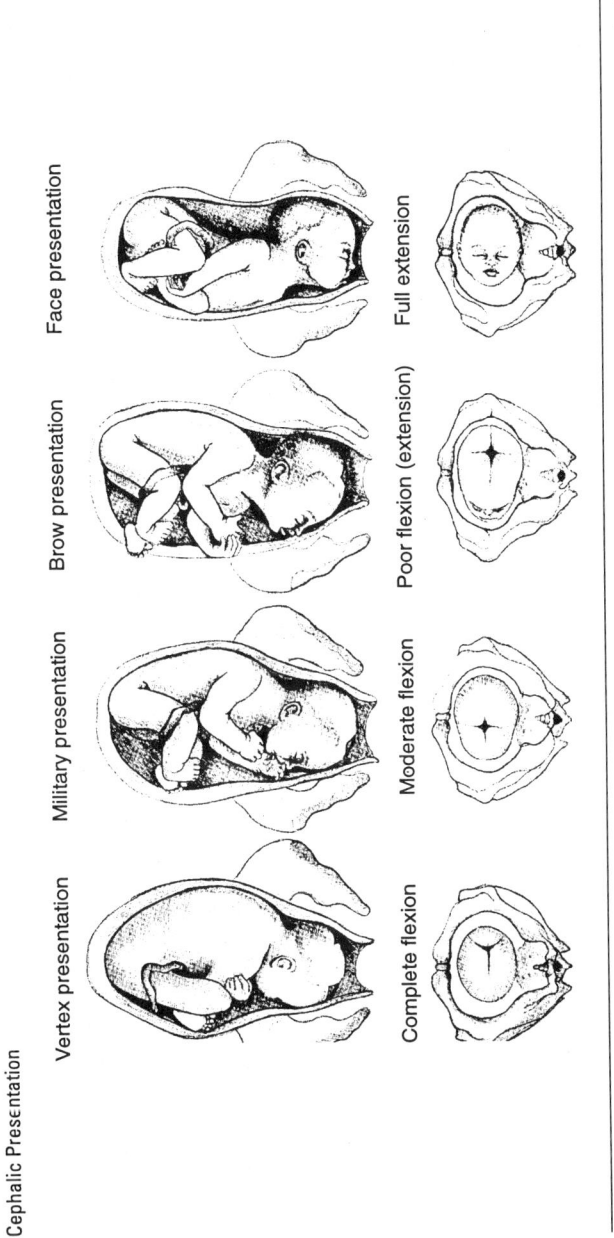

Cephalic Presentation

Four types of cephalic presentation. The vertex presentation is normal. Note positional changes of the anterior and posterior fontanelles in relation to the maternal pelvis.

- Vertex presentation — Complete flexion
- Military presentation — Moderate flexion
- Brow presentation — Poor flexion (extension)
- Face presentation — Full extension

- Breech presentations have three variations.
  - Frank breech: The fetal legs extend across the abdomen toward the shoulders, with the buttocks presenting.
  - Full (complete) breech: The fetus is flexed, with the buttocks and feet presenting.
  - Footling breech: One or both feet presenting.

- Fetal position (Abbreviations describe the relationship of a fixed fetal part in relationship to one of the four quadrants of the maternal pelvis.)
  - Right (R) or left (L) of the maternal pelvis; if the fetal part is directly anterior or posterior, this letter is omitted.
  - Occiput (O), chin (M for *mentum*), or sacrum (S) describes the fetal part used in the abbreviation. Other abbreviations may be used for less common fetal presentations.
  - Anterior (A), posterior (P), or transverse (T) describes whether the fetal point is in the mother's front or rear pelvis, or if it is between the front and back of her pelvis (transverse).

Psyche

Stress hormones called *catecholamines* can inhibit uterine contractions and placental blood flow. Excess muscle tension means that each contraction or maternal bearing down effort must work against more resistance than if the tension is less. Excess anxiety and fear consume maternal energy that she could otherwise use to cope with the demands of labor.

Cultural values affect the family's expectations of birth and satisfaction with it. Cultural values influence who the woman wants to support her during labor, how she expresses pain, and specific practices that are important to her and her family. The nurse must explore with each woman and her family what values are important to them to best determine how to make the experience as satisfying as possible.

B. CERVICAL CHANGES

- Effacement (thinning): Usually described as a percentage of its usual length or as length in centimeters; a multigravida's cervix is often thicker than a primigravida's, even during late labor
- Dilation (opening): described in centimeters

C. MECHANISMS OF LABOR

The mechanisms (or cardinal movements) of labor occur as the contractions and maternal pushing efforts propel the fetus through the pelvis.

- Descent, engagement, and flexion: The fetal head is pushed downward through the pelvis, causing the head to flex sharply on the chest.
  — Engagement occurs when the largest fetal head diameter has passed the pelvic inlet. It is described as *station*, or centimeters above or below the ischial spines, which are a 0 station.
  — Internal rotation occurs when the fetal head rotates from a transverse orientation (side-facing) within the maternal pelvis to an occiput anterior orientation (facing the mother's spine).
  — Extension occurs as the flexed fetal head descends under the symphysis pubis and meets resistance from the perineum.
  — External rotation occurs after the head is born, when it rotates passively to face one of the mother's legs. The wide diameter of the shoulders is now aligned with the anterior-posterior maternal pelvic diameter.
  — Expulsion occurs as the anterior, then posterior, fetal shoulders pass beneath the maternal symphysis pubis. The rest of the fetal body follows quickly. See Figure II-3.

Clinical Manual for Foundations of Maternal Newborn Nursing

Figure II-3

Mechanisms (Cardinal Movements) of Labor

Descent, Engagement, and Flexion

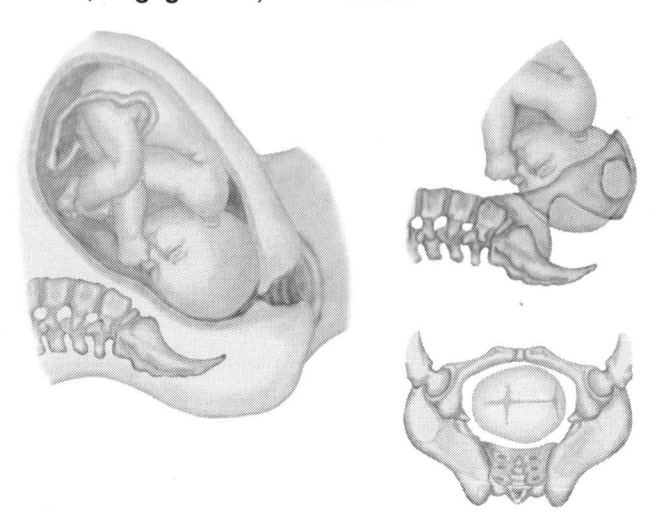

Station

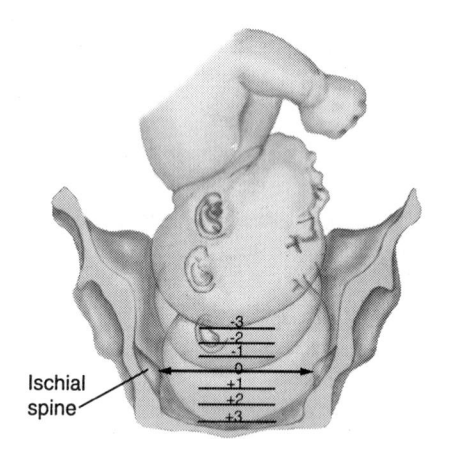

Ischial spine

Figure II-3 *(continued)*

Mechanisms (Cardinal Movements) of Labor

Internal Rotation

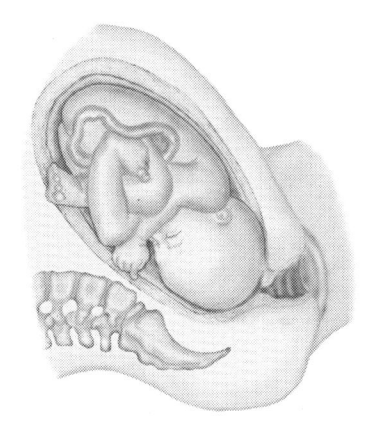

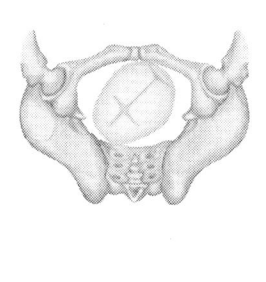

Extension

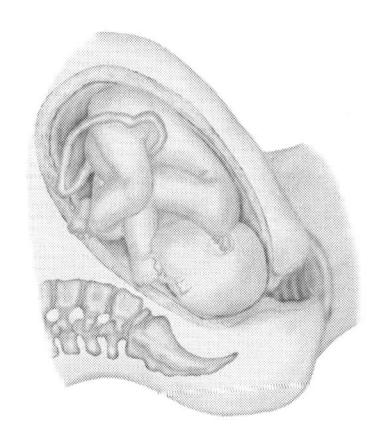

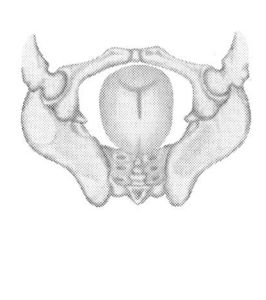

Extension beginning (internal rotation complete)

102 Clinical Manual for Foundations of Maternal Newborn Nursing

Figure II-3 *(continued)*

Mechanisms (Cardinal Movements) of Labor

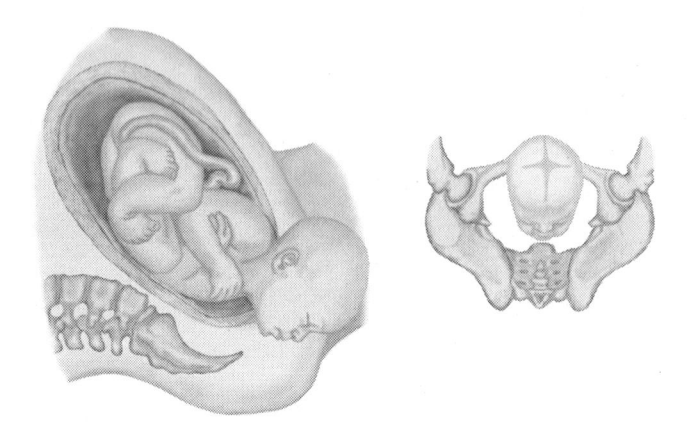

Extension complete

External Rotation

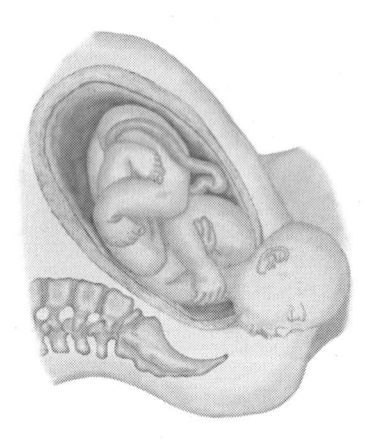

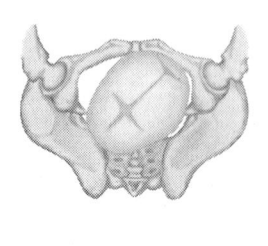

Figure II-3 *(continued)*

Mechanisms (Cardinal Movements) of Labor

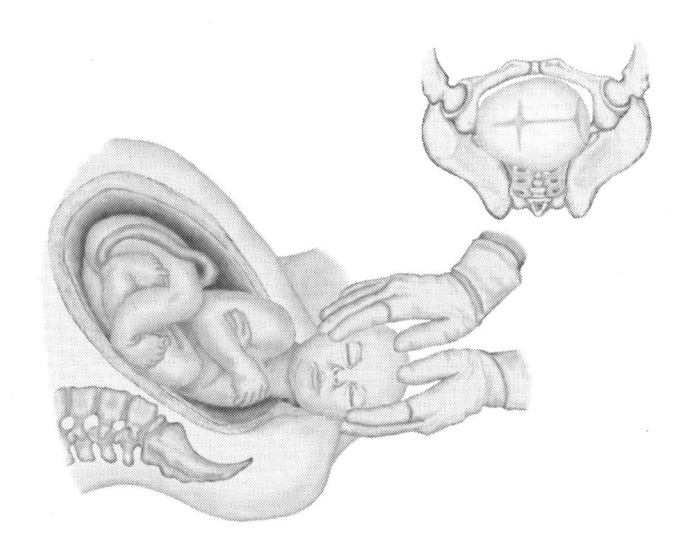

Expulsion

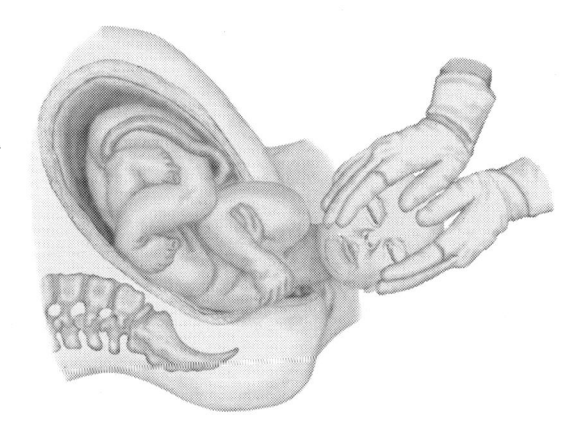

D. STAGES OF LABOR

Labor is divided into four stages.

- First stage is from onset of true labor until full effacement and dilation of the cervix; this stage has 3 phases.
  — Latent phase: 0–3 cm of cervical dilation
  — Active phase: 4–7 cm of cervical dilation
  — Transition phase: 8–10 cm (full) cervical dilation
- Second stage is from full effacement and dilation of the cervix until the birth of the infant.
- Third stage is from the birth of the infant until the birth of the placenta.
- Fourth stage is 1–4 hours after birth for physiologic stabilization and attachment within the new family.

TABLE II-1
Characteristics of Normal Labor

CHARACTERISTICS OF NORMAL LABOR

	First Stage	Second Stage	Third Stage	Fourth Stage
Duration	*Nullipara*: 8-10 hours after reaching active phase (range 6-18 hours); average rate of dilation is 1.2 cm/hour *Multipara*: 6-7 hours after reaching active phase (range 2-10 hours); average rate of dilation is 1.5 cm/hour	*Nullipara*: 50 minutes (range 30 minutes-3 hours) *Multipara*: 20 minutes (range 5-30 minutes)	5-10 minutes; up to 30 minutes; parity does not affect duration of third stage	First 1-4 hours after birth
Uterine Contractions	*Latent phase*: Mild and irregular at first, becoming more regular and longer. Frequency is about 5 minutes and duration is about 30-40 seconds by the end of latent phase	Strong, about 2-3 minutes apart; duration about 40-60 seconds. Maternal bearing-down efforts (pushing) adds to the force of contractions in propelling the fetus through the pelvis	Firmly contracted after the placenta and membranes are expelled	Uterus should be firmly contracted to control bleeding

Uterine Contractions (continued)

Active phase: Frequency is 2-5 minutes; duration 40-60 seconds. Moderate to strong intensity.		
Transition: Strong contractions, 1.5-2 minutes apart; duration 60-90 seconds		

Sensations

Often begins with a low backache or menstrual-like cramping. Gradually sweeps to the lower abdomen in a girdle-like fashion.	Urge to push or bear down with contractions. Distention of vagina and vulva may cause sensation of intense stretching or splitting.	Little discomfort; sometimes slight cramping as the placenta is passed.	Afterpains may occur, especially in multiparous women, when the uterus alternately contracts and relaxes rather than remaining continuously contracted.

Maternal Behaviors

Sociable and relaxed during early labor. Becomes more inwardly focused as labor intensifies. May temporarily lose control during transition.	Intense concentration when pushing with contractions. May seem oblivious to surroundings and doze between contractions.	Excited and relieved after baby's birth. Anxious to inspect the baby to see if he or she is normal.	Tired, but excitement may make rest difficult. Eager to become acquainted with the infant.

E. TRUE LABOR AND FALSE LABOR

Three categories help the woman and the nurse distinguish contractions that are probably false labor from those that are likely to be true labor.

TABLE II-2

How to Know Whether Labor Is "Real"

True labor differs from false labor in three categories.

FALSE LABOR	TRUE LABOR
Contractions	
Inconsistent in frequency, duration, and intensity.	A consistent pattern of increasing frequency, duration, and intensity usually develops.
A change in activity, such as walking, does not alter contractions, or activity may decrease them.	Walking tends to increase contractions.
Discomfort	
Felt in the abdomen and groin	Begins in lower back and gradually sweeps around to lower abdomen like a girdle.
May be more annoying than truly painful.	Back pain may persist in some women.
	Early labor often feels like menstrual cramps.
Cervix	
No significant change in effacement or dilation of the cervix.	Effacement and/or dilation of cervix occurs.
	Progressive effacement and dilation of cervix are most important characteristics.

F. WHEN TO GO TO THE BIRTH CENTER

When a woman should go to the birth center depends on several factors, such as the number and duration of previous labors, transportation factors, and child care needs. These are typical guidelines:

- Contractions that become progressively more regular, frequent, and have a longer duration and greater intensity
  — Nullipara: Regular contractions, about 5 minutes apart, for 1 hour
  — Multipara: Regular contractions, about 10 minutes apart, for 1 hour
- Rupture of the membranes, with or without contractions
- Bright red vaginal bleeding that is not mixed with mucus
- A substantial decrease in fetal movement
- Other concerns that do not fit these guidelines, because some women will have an atypical labor

G. ADMISSION TO THE BIRTH CENTER

If focus assessments upon admission are normal and birth is not imminent, additional nursing assessments are done.

Focus Assessments

- Fetal heart rate (FHR) and pattern: An external fetal monitor is usually applied for at least 20 minutes to obtain a baseline.
- Maternal vital signs
- Impending birth is possible if the woman says her baby is coming, if she makes grunting sounds, or is bearing down. If the woman displays signs similar to these, look at her perineum and/or perform a vaginal examination to determine her actual labor status. A vaginal examination is *not* done if the woman has bleeding other than bloody show.

Additional Assessments

TABLE II-3

Intrapartum Assessment Guide

Women who have had prenatal care have much of this information available on their prenatal record. The nurse need only verify it or update it as needed.

ASSESSMENT, METHOD (SELECTED RATIONALES)	COMMON FINDINGS	SIGNIFICANT FINDINGS, NURSING ACTION
Interview		
Purpose: To obtain information about the woman's pregnancy, labor, and conditions that may affect her care. The interview is curtailed if she seems to be in late labor.		
Introduction: Introduce yourself and ask the woman how she wants to be addressed. Ask her if she wants her partner and/or family to remain during the interview and assessment. (Shows respect for the woman and gives her control over those she wants to remain with her.)	Many women prefer to be addressed by their first names during labor.	The surname (family name) precedes the given name in some cultures. Clarify which name is used to properly address the woman and to properly identify both mother and newborn.

Culture/language: If she is from another culture, ask what her preferred language is and what language(s) she speaks, reads, or verbally understands. (Enables the most accurate data collection.)	Common non-English languages of women in the United States are Spanish or one of the Asian dialects. The most common non-English language varies with location.	Try to secure an interpreter fluent in the woman's primary language. Ask her if there are people who are not acceptable to her as interpreters (e.g., males or one from a group in conflict with her culture). Family members may not be the best interpreters because they may interpret selectively, adding or subtracting information as they see fit.
Communication: Ask the woman to tell you when she has a contraction, and pause during the interview and physical assessment. (Shows that the nurse is sensitive to her comfort and allows her to concentrate more fully on the information the nurse requests.)	Women in active labor have difficulty answering questions or cooperating with a physical examination while they are having a contraction.	If contractions are very frequent, assess the woman's labor status promptly rather than continuing the interview. Ask only the most critical questions.

Nonverbal cues: Observe the woman's behaviors and interactions with her family and the nurse. (Permits estimation of her level of anxiety. Identifies behaviors indicating that she should have a vaginal examination to determine whether birth is imminent.)

Latent phase: Sociable and mildly anxious.

Active phase: Concentrating intently with contractions; often uses prepared childbirth techniques.

The unprepared or extremely anxious woman may breathe deeply and rapidly, displaying a tense facial and body posture during and between contractions.

These behaviors suggest that birth is imminent:

1. Her statement that the baby is coming.
2. Grunting sounds (low-pitched, guttural sounds).
3. Bearing down with abdominal muscles.
4. Sitting on one buttock.

Euphoria, combativeness, or sedation suggest recent illicit drug ingestion.

Reason for *admission:* "What brings you to the hospital/birth center today?" (Open-ended question promotes more complete answer.)

Labor contractions at term are the usual reason. Observation for false labor is another common reason for admission.

Bleeding, preterm labor, pain other than labor contractions. Report these findings to the physician or nurse-midwife promptly.

Prenatal care: "Did you see a doctor or nurse-midwife during your pregnancy?" "Who is your doctor or nurse-midwife?" "How far along were you in your pregnancy when you saw the physician or nurse-midwife?" (Enables location of prenatal record.)	Early and regular prenatal care promotes maternal and fetal health.	No prenatal care or care that was irregular or begun in late pregnancy means that complications may not have been identified.
Estimated date of delivery (EDD): "When is your baby due?" (Determines if gestation is term.) "When did your last menstrual period begin?" (For estimation of EDD if woman did not have prenatal care.)	*Term gestation*: 38-42 weeks. The woman's gestation may have been confirmed or adjusted during pregnancy with an ultrasound or other clinical examination.	Gestations earlier than 38 weeks (preterm) or later than the end of the 42nd week (postterm) are associated with more fetal or neonatal problems.
Gravidity, parity, abortions: "How many times have you been pregnant?" "How many babies have you had? Were they full-term or premature?" "How many children are now living?" "Have you had any miscarriages or abortions?" "Were there any problems with your babies after they were born?" (Helps estimate probable speed of labor and anticipate neonatal problems.)	Labor may be faster for the woman who has given birth before than for the nullipara. Miscarriage is used to describe a spontaneous abortion because many lay people associate the term "abortion" with only induced abortions.	Parity of 5 or more (grand multiparity) may be associated with placenta previa (see p. 60) or postpartum hemorrhage (see p. 312). Women who have had several spontaneous abortions or who have given birth to infants with abnormalities may face a higher risk for an infant with a birth defect.

Pregnancy history (identifies problems that may affect this birth)

Present pregnancy: "Have you had any problems during this pregnancy, such as high blood pressure, diabetes, or bleeding?"	Complications are not expected.	Women having diabetes or hypertension may have poor placental blood flow, possibly resulting in fetal compromise. Some complications of past pregnancies, such as diabetes, may recur in another pregnancy. The woman who plans a VBAC may need more support and reassurance to give birth vaginally.
Past pregnancies: "Were there any problems with your other pregnancy(ies)?" "Were your other babies born vaginally or by cesarean birth?"	Women who had previous cesarean birth(s) often have a trial of labor and vaginal birth (VBAC). A woman who previously had a difficult labor may be more anxious than one who had an uncomplicated labor and birth.	
Other: "Is there anything else you think we should know so that we can better care for you?"	This open-ended question gives the woman a chance to share information that may not be elicited by other questions.	

Labor status: "When did your contractions become regular?" "What time did you begin to think you might really be in labor?" (Facilitates a more accurate estimation of the time labor began.)

Varies among women. Many women go to the birth facility when contractions first begin. Others wait until they are reasonably sure that they are really in labor.

Women who say they have been "in labor" for an unusual length of time (for example, "for two days") have probably had false labor. These women may be very tired from the annoying, nonproductive contractions.

Contractions: "How often are your contractions coming?" "How long do they last?" "Are they getting stronger?" "Tell me if you have a contraction while we are talking." (Obtains the woman's subjective evaluation of her contractions. Alerts the nurse to palpate contractions that occur during the interview.)

Varies according to her stage and phase of labor. Labor contractions are usually regular and show a pattern of increasing frequency, duration, and intensity.

Irregular contractions or those that do not increase in frequency, duration, or intensity are more likely to represent false labor. Contractions with a duration of longer than 90 seconds or intervals of full uterine relaxation shorter than 60 sec can reduce placental blood flow.

Membrane status: "Has your water broken?" "What time did it break?" "What did the fluid look like?" "About how much fluid did you lose—was it a big gush or a trickle?" (Alerts the nurse of the need to verify whether the membranes have ruptured if it is not obvious. Identifies possible prolonged rupture of membranes.)

Most women go to the birth facility for evaluation soon after their membranes rupture. If a woman is not already in labor, contractions usually begin within a few hours after the membranes rupture at term.

If the woman's membranes have ruptured and she is not in labor or if she is not at term, a vaginal examination is often deferred. Labor may be induced if she is at term with ruptured membranes.

Allergies: "Are you allergic to any foods or medicines?" "What kind of reaction do you have?" "Have you ever had a problem with anesthesia when you had dental work?" (Determines possible sensitivity to drugs that may be used.)	Record any known allergies to food and medication. As needed, describe how they affected the woman.	Allergy to seafood, iodized salt, or x-ray contrast media may indicate iodine allergy. Because iodine is used in many "prep" solutions, alternative ones should be used. Allergy to dental anesthetics may indicate possible allergy to the drugs used for local or regional anesthetics. These drugs usually end in the suffix *-caine*.
Food intake: "When was the last time you had something to eat or drink?" "What did you have?" (Helps evaluate risk for regurgitation and aspiration of stomach contents during general anesthesia.)	Record the time of the woman's last food intake and what she ate. Include both liquids and solids.	If the woman says she has not had any intake for an unusual length of time, question her more closely: "Is there any food you may have forgotten, such as a snack or a drink of water?"
Recent illness: "Have you been ill recently?" "What was the problem?" "What did you do for it?" "Have you been around anyone with a contagious illness recently?"	Most pregnant women are healthy. An occasional woman may have had a minor illness such as an upper respiratory infection.	Untreated urinary tract infections are associated with preterm labor. The woman who has had contact with someone having a communicable disease may become ill and possibly infect others in the facility.

Medications: "What drugs do you take that your doctor or nurse-midwife has prescribed?" "Are there any over-the-counter drugs that you use?" "I know this may be uncomfortable to discuss, but we need to know about any illegal substances that you use to more safely care for you and your baby." (Permits evaluation of the woman's drug intake and encourages her to disclose nonprescribed use.)

Prenatal vitamins and iron are commonly prescribed. Record all drugs the woman takes, including time and amount of last ingestion. Women who use illegal substances often conceal or diminish the extent of their use because they fear reprisals.

Drugs may interact with other medications given during labor, especially analgesics and anesthetics. Substance abuse is associated with complications for the mother and infant. If the woman discloses that she uses illegal drugs, ask her what kind and the last time she ingested them (often referred to as a "hit"). A nonjudgmental approach is more likely to result in honest information.

Tobacco or alcohol: "Do you smoke or use tobacco in any other form? About how many cigarettes a day?" "Do you use alcohol? About how many drinks do you have each day (or week)?" (Evaluates use of these legal substances.)

As in substance abuse, women may underreport the extent of their use of tobacco or alcohol.

Infants of heavy smokers are often smaller and may have reduced placental blood flow during labor. Infants of women who use alcohol may show fetal alcohol effects.

Birth plans (shows respect for the woman and her family as individuals and promotes achievement of their expectations. Enables more culturally appropriate care):

Coach or primary support person: "Who is the main person you want to be with you during labor?" Ask that person how he or she wants to be addressed, such as "Mr. Smith" or "Bob."	This is usually the woman's husband or the baby's father, but it may be her mother, sister, or a friend, especially if she is single.	The woman who has little or no support from significant others probably needs more intense nursing support during labor and after the birth. These clients are more likely to have problems with parent-infant attachment.
Other support: "Is there anyone else you would like to be present during labor?"	Women often want another support person present.	
Preparation for childbirth: "Did you attend prepared childbirth classes?" "Did someone go with you?"	Ideally, the woman and a partner have had some preparation in classes or self-study. Women who attended classes during previous pregnancies do not always repeat the classes during subsequent pregnancies.	The unprepared woman may need more support with simple relaxation and breathing techniques during labor. Her partner may need to learn techniques to assist her.

Preferences: "Are there any special plans you have for this birth?" "Is there anything you want to avoid?" "Did you plan to record the birth with pictures or video?"

Some women or couples have strong feelings regarding certain interventions. Common ones are: (1) analgesia or anesthesia; (2) intravenous lines; (3) fetal monitoring; (4) shave prep or enema; or (5) use of episiotomy or forceps.

Conflict may arise if the woman has not previously discussed her preferences with her physician or nurse-midwife or if she is unaware of what services are available where she gives birth.

Cultural needs: "Are there any special cultural practices that you plan when you have your baby?" "How can we best help you to fulfill these practices?"

Women from Asian and Hispanic cultures often subscribe to the "hot/cold" theory of illness and want specific foods after birth, such as soft-boiled eggs. They may not want their water iced.

Try to incorporate all positive or neutral cultural practices. If a practice is harmful, explain why and try to find a way to work around it if the family does not want to give it up.

Fetal Evaluation

Purpose: To determine if the fetus seems to be healthy and tolerating labor well.

Fetal heart rate (FHR): Assess by intermittent auscultation, or apply an external fetal monitor if that is the facility's policy (most common in the United States). Document FHR at least this often for the fetus at low risk for complications:

Average at term is a lower limit of 110-120 BPM and an upper limit of 150-160 BPM. Rate should increase when the fetus moves.

These signs may indicate fetal stress and should be reported to the physician or nurse-midwife:

1. Rate outside the normal limits
2. Slowing of the rate that persists after the contraction ends
3. No increase in rate when the fetus moves

1. Every hour during the latent phase
2. Every 30 min during active and transition phases
3. Every 15 min during second stage

More frequent assessments should be made of the FHR if these occur.

Labor Status

Purpose: To identify whether the woman is in labor and if birth is imminent. If she displays signs of imminent birth, this assessment is done as soon as she is admitted.

Contractions (Yields objective information about labor status): In addition to asking the woman about her contraction pattern, assess the contractions by palpation with the fingertips of one hand. A guideline is to assess:

1. Hourly during the latent phase
2. Every 30 min during the active phase
3. Every 15 min during transition and second stage

See interview section earlier in table

See interview section earlier in table. Women who have intense contractions or who are making rapid progress need to be assessed more frequently.

Vaginal examination (Determines cervical dilation and effacement; fetal presentation, position, and station; bloody show; and status of the membranes)	Varies according to the stage and phase of labor. It may not be possible to determine fetal position by vaginal examination when membranes are intact and bulging over the presenting part.	A vaginal examination is not performed if the woman reports or has evidence of active bleeding (not bloody show). Report reasons for omitting a vaginal examination to the physician or nurse-midwife.
Status of membranes: During a vaginal examination a flow of fluid suggests ruptured membranes. A Nitrazine test and/or fern test may be done. (Test needed only if it is not obvious that the membranes have ruptured.)	Amniotic fluid should be clear, possibly containing flecks of white vernix. Its odor is distinctive but not offensive. Nitrazine test with a color change to blue-green to dark blue (pH > 6.5) suggests true rupture of the membranes but is not conclusive. Fern test is more diagnostic of true rupture of membranes.	A greenish color indicates meconium staining, which may be associated with fetal compromise or postterm gestation. Thick meconium with much particulate matter ("pea soup") is most significant (see p. 244). Thick green-black meconium may be passed by the fetus in a breech presentation and is not necessarily associated with fetal compromise. Cloudy, yellowish, strong- or foul-smelling fluid suggests infection. Bloody fluid may indicate partial placental separation (p 61).

Leopold's maneuvers: Often done before assessing the FHR because they help locate the best place to assess the FHR. (Identifies fetal presentation and position. Most accurate when combined with information from vaginal examination.)

A cephalic presentation with the head well flexed (vertex) is normal.

The fetal head is often easily displaced upward ("floating") if the woman is not in labor. When the head is engaged, it cannot be displaced upward with Leopold's maneuvers.

A hard, round, freely movable object in the fundus suggests a fetal head, meaning the fetus is in a breech presentation. Less commonly, the fetus may be cross-wise in the uterus: a transverse lie.

Pain: Note discomfort during and between contractions. Note tenderness when palpating contractions. (Distinguishes between normal labor pain and abnormal pain that may be associated with a complication.)

There may be verbal or nonverbal evidence of pain with contractions, but the woman should be relatively comfortable between contractions. The skin around the umbilicus is often sensitive.

Constant pain or a tender, rigid uterus suggests a complication, such as abruptio placentae (separated placenta) (see p. 61) or, less commonly, uterine rupture (see p. 183).

Physical Examination

Purpose: To evaluate the woman's general health and identify conditions that may affect her intrapartum and postpartum care.

General appearance: Observe skin color and texture, nutritional state, and appearance of rest or fatigue. Examine the woman's face, fingers, and lower extremities for edema. Ask her if she can take her rings off and on.

Women are often fatigued if their sleep has been interrupted by Braxton Hicks contractions, fetal activity, or frequent urination.

Mild edema of the lower extremities is common in late pregnancy.

Pallor suggests anemia.

Edema of the face and fingers or extreme (pitting) edema of the lower extremities is associated with pregnancy-induced hypertension (see pp. 71-78).

Vital signs: Take the woman's temperature, pulse, respirations, and blood pressure. Reassess the temperature every 4 hrs (every 2 hrs after membranes rupture or if elevated); repeat blood pressure, pulse, and respirations every hour.

Temperature: 35.8°-37.3°C (96.4°-99.1°F)

Pulse: 60-100/min

Respirations: 12-20/min, even and unlabored.

Blood pressure near baseline levels established during pregnancy. Transient elevations of blood pressure are common when the woman is first admitted, but they return to baseline levels within about 1/2 hour.

Report abnormalities to physician or nurse-midwife. Temperature of 38°C (100.4°F) or higher suggests infection. Pulse, respirations, and FHR may also be elevated. Pulse and blood pressure may be elevated if the woman is extremely anxious or in pain. A blood pressure of 140/90 or higher is considered hypertensive. For women who did not have prenatal care, there is no baseline to compare.

Heart and lung sounds: Auscultate all areas with a stethoscope.

Heart sounds should be clear with a distinct S_1 and S_2. A physiologic murmur is common because of the increased blood volume and cardiac output. Breath sounds should be clear, with respirations even and unlabored.

The woman who is breathing rapidly and deeply may have symptoms of hyperventilation: tingling and spasm of the fingers, numbness around the lips.

SECTION TWO: Intrapartum 123

Breasts: Palpate for a dominant mass.

Breasts are full and nodular. Areola is darker, especially in dark-skinned women. Breasts may leak colostrum (clear, sticky, straw-colored fluid) during labor.

Report a dominant mass to the physician or nurse-midwife.

Abdomen: Observe for scars at the same time Leopold's maneuvers and the FHR are assessed. It is usually sufficient to assess the fundal height by observing its relation to the xiphoid process.

Striae (stretch marks) are common. If scars are noted, ask the woman what surgery she had. The fundus at term is usually slightly below the xiphoid process.

Report a previous cesarean birth to the physician or nurse-midwife. Transverse uterine scars are least likely to rupture if the woman is in labor (see p. 183). Measure the fundal height (see p. 34) if the fetus seems small or if the gestation is questionable.

Deep tendon reflexes: Assess patellar reflex. Upper extremity deep tendon reflexes should be used after epidural block analgesia.

Brisk knee jerk without spasm or sustained muscle contraction is normal. Some women normally have hypoactive reflexes.

Report absent (uncommon unless the woman is receiving magnesium sulfate) or hyperactive reflexes. Hyperactive reflexes and clonus (repeated tapping when the foot is dorsiflexed) are associated with pregnancy-induced hypertension and often precede a seizure (see pp. 71-78).

Midstream urine specimen: Assess protein and glucose levels with a dipstick. Follow instructions on the package for waiting times. Send for urinalysis if ordered.

Negative or trace of protein; negative glucose.

Proteinuria is associated with pregnancy-induced hypertension but may also be associated with urinary tract infections or a specimen that is contaminated with vaginal secretions. Glucosuria is associated with diabetes.

Laboratory tests: Women who have had prenatal care may not need additional tests. Common tests include:

1. Complete blood count (or hematocrit done on unit)	1. Hemoglobin at least 11 g/dl; hematocrit at least 33%	1. Values lower than these reduce maternal reserve for normal blood loss at birth.
2. Blood type and Rh factor	2. The woman who is Rh-negative usually has received Rh immune globulin at about 28 weeks' gestation to prevent formation of anti Rh antibodies	2. Rh-negative mothers need Rh immune globulin if their infant is Rh positive.
3. Serologic tests for syphilis	3. Negative	3. A positive test may indicate that the baby is infected and needs treatment after birth. The mother should be treated if she has not been treated already.

H. CONTINUING INTRAPARTAL CARE

Fetal Assessments

- Fetal heart rate and pattern: Assess either by intermittent auscultation or with intermittent or continuous electronic fetal monitoring (EFM). Guidelines for FHR assessment vary according to the mother's risk status and with labor events. See Table II-4, "Assessment and Documentation of Fetal Heart Rate."

TABLE II-4

Assessment and Documentation of Fetal Heart Rate

Low-Risk Patients	High-Risk Patients
First stage of labor	First stage of labor
Every 1 hr in latent phase	Every 30 min in latent phase
Every 30 min in active phase	Every 15 min in active phase
Second stage of labor	Second stage of labor
Every 15 min	Every 5 min

Labor Events

Assess fetal heart rate before:
Initiation of labor-enhancing procedures (such as artificial rupture of membranes)
Periods of ambulation
Administration of medications
Administration or initiation of analgesia or anesthesia

Assess fetal heart rate following:
Rupture of membranes
Recognition of abnormal uterine activity patterns, such as increased basal tone or tachysystole (excessive frequency)
Evaluation of oxytocin (maintenance, increase, or decrease of dosage)
Administration of medications (at time of peak action)
Expulsion of enema
Urinary catheterization
Vaginal examination
Periods of ambulation
Evaluation of analgesia and/or anesthesia (maintenance, increase, or decrease in dosage)

From NAACOG. (1990). *Fetal heart rate auscultation*. Washington, D.C.: Author.

- Amniotic fluid: Assess for color, quantity, and odor when the membranes rupture. Prepare for infant respiratory suctioning and support at birth if the fluid is meconium-stained.

Maternal Assessments

- Check vital signs every 2–4 hours.
- Labor progress: Perform vaginal exams to determine cervical effacement, dilation, and fetal descent; limit as much as possible because of possible introduction of infection.
- Monitor intake and output.
- Response to labor: Observe for the behavioral changes that are associated with labor progress. Signs that the woman may need help dealing with pain (pharmacological or nonpharmacological) include
  — Inability to use learned breathing techniques or ineffectiveness despite varying the ones used.
  — Arching her back or muscle tension that persists between contractions.
  — A tense facial expression.
  — Statements similar to "I can't take it any more."
  — Request for pain medication or other specific interventions to help her manage pain.

Common Intrapartal Nursing Diagnoses and Collaborative Problems

- Risk for altered health maintenance related to knowledge deficit regarding characteristics of false and true labor
- Anxiety or fear related to ability to meet demands of labor and labor's uncertain outcome
- Potential complication: Fetal compromise
- Pain related to uterine contractions and vaginal/perineal distention
- Risk for injury (maternal and/or fetal) related to unexpected rapid birth

Nursing Interventions

- Promoting fetal oxygenation and observing for compromise
  — Assess the fetus at appropriate intervals and labor events.
  — Encourage the woman to assume positions other than the supine, which can reduce blood flow to the placenta because of aortocaval compression.
  — Observe contractions for
    - Excessive duration (over 90 seconds)
    - Inadequate relaxation interval (less than 60 seconds).
  — Observe maternal blood pressure (hypotension and hypertension reduce placental blood flow).
  — Observe maternal temperature (increases fetal body temperature, which increases fetal oxygen demands).

Clinical Tip: Conditions Associated with Fetal Compromise

- FHR outside normal range for a term fetus: lower limit of 110–120 BPM and upper limit of 150–160 BPM
- Little or no variability in the electronically monitored FHR
- Slowing of the FHR persisting after contraction ends
- Meconium-stained (greenish) amniotic fluid
- Cloudy, yellowish, or foul odor to amniotic fluid (suggesting infection)
- Contractions lasting longer than 90 seconds
- Incomplete uterine relaxation or intervals shorter than 60 seconds between contractions
- Maternal hypotension (may divert blood flow away from the placenta to ensure adequate perfusion of the maternal brain and heart)
- Maternal hypertension (may be associated with vasospasm in spiral arteries, which supply the intervillous spaces of the placenta)
- Maternal fever (38° C [100.4° F] or higher)

- Teach the woman to avoid sustained breath-holding during pushing (the Valsalva maneuver). Prolonged breath-holding reduces placental blood flow.

- Promoting comfort
  - Reduce irritants: Dim bright lighting, especially if it shines in the woman's eyes.
  - Alter the temperature
    - Adjust the thermostat to a comfortable level.
    - Use a fan or blankets as needed.
    - Provide a cool, damp washcloth for the mother's face and neck.
    - Socks provide warmth for cold feet.
  - Change the underpad regularly. A folded terry towel absorbs more amniotic fluid than does a disposable underpad.
  - Offer hard candy, a popsicle, or ice chips to reduce mouth dryness if not contraindicated. A moist washcloth on the lips reduces a dry mouth if the woman cannot have oral intake.
  - Observe the bladder for filling that may cause discomfort or reduce the effectiveness of pharmacological pain relief methods. The woman will usually need to void every 2 hours, or more often if she has large quantities of IV fluids.
  - Have the woman change positions regularly to reduce pressure and help the fetus adapt to pelvic contours. Any position of comfort (other than supine) is usually permissible. Vertical positions work with gravity. "Back labor" may be eased by having the woman assume a position where the back of the fetal head falls away from the maternal sacral promontory, such as leaning forward or assuming a hands and knees position. During second stage, squatting enlarges the pelvic outlet slightly.
  - Water therapy in the form of a shower, tub, or whirlpool is relaxing and improves the tolerance of contractions. Nipple stimulation by the water currents

promotes natural oxytocin release from the posterior pituitary, which then stimulates contractions.

- Teaching
  - Breathing techniques
  - Usual course of labor
  - Avoiding pushing before full cervical dilation, or pushing most effectively after full dilation
  - Avoiding prolonged breath-holding (the Valsalva maneuver) during second stage
- Providing encouragement
  - Provide nursing presence with the laboring woman, which conveys respect and support.
  - Reinforce techniques the woman uses that are effective, and help her find others that may be more effective if needed.
  - Care for the woman's support person. Involve the birth partner as the couple desires. Do not expect more support of the partner than he or she can provide. Do not interfere with the woman and partner who are coping well. Encourage the partner to take a break. Food and drink can mean the difference between an effective birth partner and one who faints at birth.

Nursing Responsibilities During Birth

- Transferring the woman to a delivery room if a birthing room is not being used
- Preparing a sterile delivery table, which includes gowns, gloves, drapes, solutions, and instruments
- Performing a perineal cleansing prep
- Performing initial care and assessment of the newborn; using personal protective equipment when caring for the infant before the first bath
- Administering maternal medications, such as oxytocin, as ordered

> **Clinical Tip:** If a woman will give birth before her birth attendant arrives, get the emergency delivery tray ("precip tray"), calling for another person to bring it if it is not in the room. Put on gloves, preferably sterile, to catch the baby as it emerges. Suction the infant's mouth and nose with a bulb syringe. Dry the infant and place skin-to-skin with the mother or wrap in warmed blankets. Infant suckling at the breast stimulates maternal oxytocin release to promote placental expulsion and control of bleeding.

Nursing Responsibilities Immediately After Birth

- Care of the Infant
  - Observe and support respiratory function.
    - Perform an Apgar at 1 and 5 minutes. See Table II-5.
    - Suction excess secretions with a bulb syringe or suction catheter; teach parents the use of the bulb syringe at the first opportunity.
  - Support temperature regulation.
    - Dry the infant thoroughly, including the hair, and wrap in warm blankets.
    - A hat reduces heat loss from the large surface area of the head.
  - Methods to add heat
    - Place the infant in skin-to-skin contact with a parent.
    - Place the infant in a radiant warmer without hat and blankets; a skin probe allows the warmer heat to rise and fall according to the infant's needs.
- Care of the mother
  - Observe for hemorrhage
    - Check vital signs every 15 minutes during the first hour, every 30 minutes during the second hour, and hourly until discharge from the recovery area.

TABLE II-5
Apgar Score*

Assessment	0	1	2
Heart rate	Absent	Below 100/min	100/min or higher
Respiratory effort	No spontaneous respirations	Slow respirations or weak cry	Spontaneous respirations with a strong, lusty cry
Muscle tone	Limp	Minimal flexion of extremities; sluggish movement	Flexed body posture; spontaneous and vigorous movement
Reflex response	No response to suction or gentle slap on soles	Minimal response (grimace) to suction or gentle slap on soles	Responds promptly to suction or a gentle slap to the sole with cry or active movement
Color	Pallor or cyanosis	Bluish hands and feet	Pink (light-skinned) or absence of cyanosis (dark-skinned)

*The Apgar score is a method of rapid evaluation of the infant's cardiorespiratory adaptation after birth. The nurse scores the infant at 1 minute and 5 minutes in each of five areas. The assessments are arranged from most important (heart rate) to least important (color). The infant is assigned a score of 0 to 2 in each of the five areas and the scores are totaled. General guidelines for the infant's care are based on three ranges of 1 minute scores:

0 1 2 3 4	5 6 7	8 9 10
Infant needs resuscitation.	Gently stimulate by rubbing the infant's back while administering oxygen. Determine whether mother received narcotics, which may have depressed infant's respirations. Have naloxone (Narcan) available for administration.	Provide no action other than support of the infant's spontaneous efforts and continued observation.

SECTION TWO: Intrapartum

> **Clinical Tip:** A rising pulse is the first sign of hypovolemic shock; the blood pressure usually falls later.

- Observe uterine fundus for firmness, height, and position. The uterus should be firm, midline, and about halfway between the symphysis and umbilicus. Actual height varies with the woman's parity and the size of her infant. If the uterus is soft, it should be massaged until firm.
- Observe bladder with fundal checks. A high uterine fundus that may be displaced to one side suggests a full bladder, which interferes with uterine contraction. Measure the first two voidings; each should be about 300–400 mL. Expect more rapid bladder filling and possible difficulty voiding if the woman received epidural anesthesia for birth.
- Observe lochia with each vital sign and fundal check.

    Watch for excess lochia pooling under the woman's buttocks and back.

    More than one saturated standard pad (not those having cold packs in them) per hour is excessive.

    Report large clots (small ones are common) or a continuous bright red trickle of blood when the fundus remains firm (suggests a bleeding laceration in the birth canal).

— Promote comfort
   - Provide warmth in the form of a warm blanket and/or a portable radiant warmer. Warm drinks may be comforting.
   - Apply cold packs to the perineal area in the form of a glove filled with shaved ice or a chemical cold pack. Wrap the glove in a washcloth or similar wrap to avoid placing the latex next to the woman's perineal skin.

- Provide analgesia: Oral analgesic drugs such as hydrocodone with acetaminophen are common.
- Early care of the new family
  - Provide time for the parents and newborn to get acquainted with as little interruption as possible. Do infant assessments and care while parents hold the baby, if possible.
  - Initiate breastfeeding. The infant is often alert at this time, and stimulating the woman's nipples also causes oxytocin secretion from her pituitary, aiding in control of bleeding.
  - Observe for expected behaviors in early parent-infant interactions
    - Use of high-pitched, affectionate tones
    - Seeking eye contact with the infant
    - Gradually progressing from tentative fingertip touching of the infant, to palm touch, to enfolding the infant

II. INTRAPARTAL FETAL ASSESSMENT

A. FACTORS THAT IMPACT FETAL OXYGENATION

- Maternal blood flow to the placenta
- Maternal blood oxygen saturation
- Exchange of oxygen and carbon dioxide in the placenta
- Blood flow from the placenta, through the umbilical vessels, to the fetus
- Fetal circulatory and oxygen-carrying functions

TABLE II-6

Conditions Associated with Decreased Fetal Oxygenation

Antepartum Period
Maternal history
  Prior stillbirth
  Prior cesarean birth
  Chronic diseases, such as cardiac disease, hpertension, and diabetes
  Drug abuse
Problems identified during pregnancy
  Fetal growth restriction
  Gestation >42 weeks
  Marked decrease in fetal movement
  Multifetal gestation
  Pregnancy-induced hypertension
  Gestational diabetes
  Placenta previa
  Maternal severe anemia
  Maternal infection

Intrapartum Period
Maternal problems
  Hypotension
  Hypertonic uterine contractions
  Abnormal labor: preterm or dysfunctional
  Prolonged ruptured membranes
  Chorioamnionitis
  Fever
Fetal or placental problems
  Abnormal fetal heart rate
  Meconium-stained amniotic fluid
  Abnormal presentation or position
  Prolapsed cord
  Abruptio placentae

B. TYPES OF INTRAPARTAL FETAL ASSESSMENT

Intrapartal fetal assessment primarily involves observation of the fetal heart rate and uterine contractions. Other factors that relate to fetal well-being include maternal vital signs and character of amniotic fluid.

Low-Tech Approach

- Involves intermittent auscultation of fetal heart rate with Doppler or fetoscope (see "Procedure: Auscultating the Fetal Heart Rate," p. 430.) plus intermittent palpation of uterine contractions for frequency, duration, intensity, and resting interval. See "Procedure: Palpating Contractions," p. 432.
- Provides a more natural birthing environment.
- Assesses the fetus and uterine activity for a small percentage of the total labor.

Electronic Fetal Monitoring (EFM)

- Variations
  — Continuous, with only occasional interruptions (such as toileting)
  — Intermittent, assessed at regular intervals during labor
- EFM provides more total information and allows identification of subtle trends in the fetal response to labor.
- EFM lends a more technical atmosphere to the birthing room.

C. ELECTRONIC FETAL MONITORING EQUIPMENT

- External equipment is non-invasive, but less accurate than internal. See "Procedure: External Fetal Heart Rate and Contraction Monitoring," p. 421.
- Internal equipment has greater accuracy, but is invasive and requires ruptured membranes and some cervical dilation. See "Procedure: Internal Fetal Heart Rate and Contraction Monitoring," p. 423.

136 Clinical Manual for Foundations of Maternal Newborn Nursing

D. EVALUATING ELECTRONIC FETAL MONITORING STRIPS

- The fetal heart rate is recorded in the upper grid of the paper strip; uterine activity is recorded in the lower grid.
- Fetal heart rate and uterine activity patterns must be evaluated together.

Fetal Heart Rate

- Baseline rate
  - Normal: For the term fetus, a lower limit of 110–120 BPM, and an upper limit of 150–160 BPM (some sources say that 120 BPM is the lower limit of normal); preterm fetus generally has a higher rate
  - Bradycardia: Less than 110–120 BPM, persisting at least 10 minutes
  - Tachycardia: Greater than 150–160 BPM, persisting at least 10 minutes
- Variability: fluctuations in the baseline FHR. Two types are
  - Short-term variability (STV): Changes in the fetal heart rate from one beat to the next (beat-to-beat); most accurately assessed with an internal spiral electrode
  - Long-term variability (LTV): Broader fluctuations that are apparent over 1-minute intervals (about 3–6 cycles/min)
- Presence of periodic changes
  - Accelerations: Increase in the FHR of at least 15 BPM above the baseline, lasting at least 15 seconds; reassuring pattern
  - Decelerations
    - Early: Usually caused by fetal head compression
      Begin after the contraction begins
      End before contraction ends
      Reassuring pattern
    - Late: Associated with uteroplacental insufficiency

Begin after the contraction begins (often after it peaks)

End after the contraction is over

Nonreassuring pattern

- Variable: Associated with umbilical cord compression

    Variable in appearance

    Often have no consistent relation to contractions

    Sharp in onset and sharp in offset

    No uniform agreement about classification; ACOG guideline (1995) states that variable decelerations are significant when the FHR repeatedly decreases to less than 70 BPM and persists at that level for at least 60 seconds before returning to the baseline.

TABLE II-7

Reassuring and Nonreassuring Fetal Heart Rate Patterns

Reassuring Patterns

Baseline rate: Stable, with a lower limit of 110-120 BPM and an upper limit of 150-160 BPM at term

Variability of 6-25 BPM

Accelerations with fetal movement: At least 15 BPM above the baseline for at least 15 sec

Uterine activity:

   Contraction frequency: no more frequent than every 2 min

   Contraction duration: no longer than 90 sec

   Interval between contractions at least 60 sec

   Uterine resting tone: uterus relaxed between contractions (with external monitor); uterine resting tone <20 mmHg (with intrauterine pressure catheter)

Nonreassuring Patterns

Tachycardia

Baseline FHR > 160 BPM for at least 10 min
   Mild: 161-180 BPM
   Severe > 181 BPM

Maternal fever (fetal tachycardia may be the first sign of an intrauterine infection)
Maternal dehydration
Maternal or fetal hypoxia
Fetal acidosis
Maternal or fetal hypovolemia
Fetal cardiac arrhythmias
Maternal severe anemia
Maternal hyperthyroidism
Drugs administered to mother (such as terbutaline)

Bradycardia

Baseline FHR < 110 BPM for at least 10 min
   Baseline rates between 100 and 110 BPM are usually not associated with fetal compromise if there are no nonreassuring patterns

Fetal head compression
Fetal hypoxia
Fetal acidosis
Fetal heart block
Umbilical cord compression
Second-stage labor with maternal pushing

Decreased or Absent Variability

FHR baseline has a smooth, flat appearance

Fetal sleep (usually lasts no longer than 30 min at a time)
Fetal hypoxia with acidosis
Drug effects:
   CNS depressants
   Local anesthetic agents

Late Decelerations

Recurrent decelerations with a uniform appearance and a consistent relation to the contraction; begin after the contraction starts (usually at the peak) and do not return to baseline until after the contraction ends	Uteroplacental insufficiency, which may be secondary to: Maternal hypotension Excess uterine activity Placental interruption, such as abruptio placentae or placenta previa Pregnancy-induced or chronic hypertension Maternal diabetes Maternal severe anemia Maternal cardiac disease

Variable Decelerations

Sharp in onset and offset Appearance and relationship to contractions is not consistent, may occur as a non-periodic pattern (randomly)	Umbilical cord compression, which may be secondary to: Prolapsed cord Nuchal cord (around fetal neck) Oligohydramnios (abnormally small amount of amniotic fluid) Cord between fetus and mother's uterus or pelvis, without obvious prolapse Cord between fetal body parts Knot in cord

Abbreviations: BPM, beats per minute; FHR, fetal heart rate

Clarifying Questionable EFM Data

- Fetal scalp stimulation
  — Apply pressure to the fetal scalp with the gloved finger and sweep the fingers in a circular motion.
  — Acceleration of the FHR (which may not be immediate) of at least 15 BPM for at least 15 seconds is reassuring.
  — Stimulation should not be done if a vaginal examination is contraindicated.

- Vibroacoustic stimulation
  - Apply an artificial larynx to the mother's lower abdomen and turn it on for up to 3 seconds.
  - Acceleration as in fetal scalp stimulation is reassuring.
- Fetal scalp blood sampling: The physician obtains a sample of fetal blood to determine the fetal blood pH.
  - Normal fetal scalp pH: 7.25–7.35
  - Acidosis: less than 7.20 (birth may be hastened by forceps or cesarean delivery)
  - Borderline: 7.20–7.24 (sample may be repeated)
- Umbilical cord blood analysis: Sampling after birth to determine pH, PCO_2, PO_2, bicarbonate, and base deficit. Analysis helps identify whether acidosis exists and whether it is respiratory (short-term), metabolic (prolonged), or mixed.
  - Draw blood into heparinized syringes from an umbilical cord artery or a fetal artery on the placenta surface.
  - Cap syringes promptly to prevent altering values.
  - Samples are reliable for 30–60 minutes at room temperature. Ice the samples if testing will be later than this time.

E. INTERVENING FOR NONREASSURING EFM PATTERNS

Identifying the Cause

- Assess maternal vital signs to identify hypotension, hypertension, or elevated temperature.
- Review maternal medications.
- Perform vaginal examination to identify palpable prolapsed cord.

Interventions for Nonreassuring Patterns

The specific intervention(s) chosen depend on the probable cause that was identified. Common interventions are listed here.

- Increase placental perfusion.
  - Position on side, or other than the supine, to avoid aortocaval compression.
  - Observe for excess uterine activity.
    - Stop oxytocin if that is causing excess activity.
    - A tocolytic drug, such as terbutaline (0.125–0.25 mg intravenously or 0.25 mg subcutaneously), may be given.
  - Increase nonadditive IV solution to expand maternal blood volume.
- Increase maternal blood oxygen saturation by giving oxygen at 8–10 L/min with a snug face mask.
- Reduce cord compression.
  - Reposition woman.
    - Turn side to side.
    - Elevate hips.
  - Perform amnioinfusion if ordered.
- Initiate internal EFM if no contraindication.
- Notify birth attendant of
  - Pattern that was identified.
  - Nursing interventions to correct the problem.
  - Fetal response.

III. PAIN MANAGEMENT DURING CHILDBIRTH

The intrapartal nurse usually employs both nonpharmacological and pharmacological pain management to assist women during labor.

A. NONPHARMACOLOGICAL TECHNIQUES

Assist Relaxation

- Control the environment.
  — Reduce bright lights.
  — Mask outside noise with music or even television.
- Increase personal comfort.
  — Keep reasonably clean and dry.
  — Offer ice chips to reduce dry mouth.
- Reduce anxiety and fear.
  — Provide explanations.
  — Call her a "mother" or a "woman," not a "patient."

Cutaneous Stimulation

- Self-massage
  — Effleurage
  — Tracing circles or figure-8s on the bed
- Massage by others
  — Palm or sole stimulation
  — Temples or shoulders
  — Sacral pressure
    - Pressure should be continuous and firm.
    - A hand over the woman's hip helps steady her during sacral pressure.
    - Slight movement of the hand may increase effectiveness.
    - Two tennis balls in a sock may be used.

Thermal Stimulation

- Cool cloths to the face
- Ice in a glove (covered with washcloth) applied to lower back
- Warm whirlpool or shower
- Alternating heat with cold to reduce habituation

Mental Stimulation

Teach woman to use

- A focal point.
- Imagery, usually of a pleasant scene or experience. The woman imagines herself in that setting. As she breathes, she can picture oxygen entering her body to nourish her baby and tension leaving as she exhales.
- Music or peaceful sounds. Headphones help mask outside noise. The music's rhythm can help her pace her breathing.

Breathing Techniques

- First stage: Cleansing breath (like a sigh) at beginning and end of contraction
  - Slow paced breathing: Use of slow, deep breathing to promote relaxation and sufficient oxygenation
  - Modified paced breathing: More rapid rate, but more shallow and rapid breathing during the peak of a contraction
  - Patterned paced breathing: Pant-blow in various types of patterns
  - Avoiding pushing: Blowing repeatedly using short puffs when the urge to push occurs before complete cervical dilation
- Second stage
  - Cleansing breaths as usual
  - Pushing: Using either as near continuous pushing as possible, or pushing for 5–6 second intervals

B. PHARMACOLOGICAL TECHNIQUES FOR LABOR

Systemic Drugs

TABLE II-8
Drugs Commonly Used for Intrapartum Pain Management

Drug/Dose	Comments
Opioid Analgesics	
Meperidine (Demerol) 12.5–50 mg every 2–4 hr IV	Respiratory depression (primarily in the neonate) is the main side effect
Butorphanol (Stadol) 1 mg every 3–4 hr; range 0.5–2 mg IV	Has some narcotic antagonist effects; should not be given to the opiate-dependent woman (may precipitate withdrawal) or after other narcotics such as meperidine (may reverse their analgesic effects); also a respiratory depressant
Nalbuphine (Nubain) 10 mg every 3–6 hours IV	Same as butorphanol
Adjunctive Drugs	
Promethazine (Phenergan) 12.5–25 mg every 4–6 hr IV	Duration of action is longer than most narcotics; enhances respiratory depressant effects of narcotics Given to relieve pruritus from epidural narcotics
Diphenhydramine (Benadryl) 10–50 mg every 4–6 hr IV	
Hydroxyzine (Atarax, Vistaril) 25–100 mg IM Z-track only	See promethazine.
Narcotic Antagonists	
Naloxone (Narcan) Adult: 0.4–2 mg IV To reverse pruritus from epidural opioids: 0.04–0.2 mg IV or IV infusion 5–10 µg/kg/hr Neonate: 0.1 mg/kg IV (umbilical vein) or intratracheal	Action shorter than most narcotics it reverses; must observe for recurrent respiratory depression and be prepared to give additional doses For neonatal resuscitation
Naltrexone (Trexan): 3–6 mg p.o. × 1 dose	Long-acting drug to relieve pruritus from epidural narcotics (investigational when used for this purpose)

IV = intravenously; p.o. = orally; IM = intramuscularly.

Regional Techniques for Labor Pain Management

Epidural Block

- Injection of anesthetic into the epidural space, between the dura and the spinal canal
- Local anesthetic (often with a small dose of an opioid analgesic) injected intermittently or continuously during labor

> **Clinical Tip:** All drugs injected into the epidural or subarachnoid spaces are preservative-free.

- A small (3 mL) test dose is injected before giving the full dose to distinguish the epidural space from the subarachnoid space; 3 mL does not provide anesthetic effect if catheter is in the epidural space.
- Adverse effects or complications
  — Maternal hypotension
    - Rapid infusion of warmed intravenous solution offsets the vasodilation effects of the epidural.
    - Ephedrine 10–15 mg IV (in 5 mg increments) may be given to raise the blood pressure.
  — Bladder distention
  — Prolonged second stage because of the reduced maternal urge to push
  — Epidural catheter migration, possibly resulting in an intense, absent, too-high, or unilateral block
  — Nausea and vomiting, primarily when opioids are given
  — Pruritus, or itching of the face and neck, with epidural narcotic use
  — Delayed maternal respiratory depression for up to 24 hours, depending on the epidural opioid used (usually post-cesarean birth)
  — Dural puncture, leading to cerebrospinal fluid leakage and spinal headache

— Contraindicated if woman has allergy to anesthetic, coagulation defects, hypovolemia, or infection in area of insertion

Intrathecal Opioid Analgesics

- Injection of a preservative-free opioid analgesic into the subarachnoid space; reinjection may be required.
- Advantages
  - Allows smaller dose of opioid for pain relief
  - Reduces pain without sedation
  - No motor block
  - No hypotensive effects
- Disadvantages
  - Limited duration of action
  - Inadequate relief for late labor and birth
- Adverse effects or complications
  - Nausea and vomiting
  - Pruritus

Local Infiltration

- Infiltration of the perineal area just before performing an episiotomy or suturing a laceration
- Few adverse effects

Pudendal Block

- Injection of local anesthetic in the area of the pudendal nerves, near the ischial spines; the perineum is also infiltrated.
- Few adverse effects

Subarachnoid (Spinal) Block

- Injection of a single dose of local anesthetic into the subarachnoid space

- Can be done quicker than epidural, if emergency cesarean birth is required
- Contraindications, adverse effects, and precautions similar to those for epidural block

Management of Post-Spinal Headache

- Headache may occur after either epidural or subarachnoid block.
- Medical treatment and nursing care
  — Bedrest, with flat head of bed
  — Oral or intravenous hydration
  — Blood patch: Injection of 10–15 mL of the woman's blood (obtained by sterile technique) into the epidural space to form a patch over the leaking area.

General Anesthesia

- Infrequently used, but may be required for some women having cesarean birth
  — Refusal or a poor candidates for epidural or subarachnoid block
  — When rapid cesarean birth is required and there is not time to establish either epidural or subarachnoid block
- Primary risks and prevention measures
  — Maternal aspiration of acidic gastric contents
    - Restrict intake to clear fluids or nothing by mouth if surgery is anticipated
    - Drugs to reduce gastric acidity, such as
      Sodium citrate and citric acid (Bicitra)
      Ranitidine (Zantac)
      Cimetidine (Tagamet)
      Famotidine (Pepcid)
    - Drugs to reduce secretions, such as glycopyrrolate (Robinul)
    - Drugs to speed gastric emptying, such as metoclopramide (Reglan)

- Use cricoid pressure (Sellick's maneuver) to block the esophagus by pressing the trachea downward toward the cervical spine
— Newborn respiratory depression
  - Reduce the time from induction of anesthesia to cord clamping
  - Keep anesthesia level light until cord is clamped.
— Uterine relaxation: Observe the uterine fundus for firmness, quantity of lochia, and urine output during recovery.

IV. OBSTETRICAL PROCEDURES

A. AMNIOTOMY

Amniotomy is the artificial rupture of the membranes, typically abbreviated AROM.

Indications

- Induce or stimulate labor
- Allow internal electronic fetal monitoring and fetal scalp blood sampling

Contraindications or Precautions

- High fetal presenting part
- Fetal presentation other than cephalic
- Placenta previa
- Any contraindication to labor or vaginal examination

Risks

- Prolapse of the umbilical cord
- Infection
- Abruptio placentae (premature separation of the placenta)

Technique

- Sterile technique is used.
- Physician or nurse-midwife does vaginal examination.
- Membrane perforator is passed through the cervix, and the membranes are snagged with the hook to create a hole.

Nursing Considerations

- Document baseline FHR for 20–30 minutes.
- Assist with the procedure.

- Place several underpads under the woman's buttocks.
- Open the package containing the hook using sterile technique.
- Drop sterile lubricant on the birth attendant's sterile gloved fingers.

- Document quantity, color, odor of amniotic fluid; FHR.
- Promote comfort by changing underpads regularly.
- Observe for complications.
  - Assess the fetal heart rate for at least one minute after amniotomy. Prolapse of the umbilical cord usually causes slowing of the FHR, with variable decelerations.
  - Check the woman's temperature every 2 hours (or according to facility policy). Report a temperature above 38°C (100.4°F). Monitor FHR for a rate above 160 BPM, which may precede maternal temperature elevation. Observe for foul-smelling or yellowish fluid.

B. INDUCTION AND AUGMENTATION OF LABOR

Induction is the initiation of labor. *Augmentation* is stimulation of labor contractions that have already begun. Techniques are similar for both.

Indications

- Pregnancy-induced hypertension
- Premature rupture of the membranes without onset of labor
- Chorioamnionitis
- Maternal conditions, such as diabetes or renal or pulmonary disease
- Conditions suggesting fetal compromise, such as intrauterine growth restriction, post-term gestation, maternal-fetal blood incompatibility
- Fetal death

- Mother having a history of rapid labors who lives a long distance from the birth center
- Arranging the birth of a baby expected to have problems at a specialized center
- Labor that began spontaneously slows or stops because of poor contractions

Contraindications or Precautions

- Placenta previa
- Umbilical cord prolapse
- Abnormal fetal presentation
- High fetal presenting part
- Active genital herpes infection
- Maternal pelvic structural abnormalities
- Previous classic (vertical) uterine incision

Risks

- Hypertonic uterine activity, manifested by contractions that
  — Are too close (less than 2 minutes apart)
  — Are too long (over 90 seconds)
  — Are too strong (higher than 90 mmHg with intrauterine pressure catheter)
  — Have too short a resting interval (less than 60 seconds relaxation) or incomplete relaxation (resting tone higher than 20 mmHg with intrauterine pressure catheter)
- Uterine rupture
- Maternal water intoxication (more likely if a dextrose and water IV solution is used or if infusion rate is higher than 20 mµ/min)

Technique

- Cervical ripening may be done to soften the cervix before the induction.
  - Prostaglandin E_2
  - Hydrophilic inserts such as Dilapan, Lamicel, or laminaria tents
- Oxytocin
  - Administer intravenously.
  - Oxytocin line is inserted into the primary line as close as possible to the venipuncture site.
  - Start slowly, increase gradually, and regulate with an infusion pump.
  - Infusion rate may be reduced when the woman is in the active phase of labor.
  - May be used for serial induction, with oxytocin solution given over a 2–3 day period for 8–10 hours each day.
  - A lower rate of oxytocin infusion is usually required for augmentation than for induction of labor.

Nursing Considerations

- Observe for hypertonic contractions as described earlier.
- Observe fetal heart rate and patterns that suggest reduced placental exchange:
  - Bradycardia
  - Tachycardia
  - Late decelerations
- Nursing actions for excessive contractions or nonreassuring FHR patterns
  - Reduce or stop the oxytocin infusion.
  - Increase the rate of the primary (nonadditive) IV solution.
  - Do not allow the woman to assume a supine position.
  - Give 100% oxygen by snug face mask at 8–10 L/min.

— Give ordered tocolytic drug, such as terbutaline or magnesium sulfate.
— Notify birth attendant.
- Check blood pressure and pulse every 30–60 minutes or with each oxytocin rate increase. Check temperature every 2–4 hours, depending on previous readings and membrane status.
- Record intake and output to identify fluid retention.
- After birth, observe for uterine atony, especially if the woman receives oxytocin for a long time.

C. EXTERNAL CEPHALIC VERSION

Version involves changing the fetal presentation, usually from breech to cephalic. External version is the more common, although an internal version is sometimes done in a twin birth.

Contraindications or Precautions

- Vaginal birth is unlikely
- Maternal uterine malformations
- Previous cesarean birth with a vertical uterine incision
- Fetopelvic disproportion
- Placenta previa
- Multifetal gestation
- Oligohydramnios
- Ruptured membranes
- Cord around the fetal body or neck
- Uteroplacental insufficiency
- Engagement of the fetal presenting part into the pelvis

Risks

- Entanglement and compression of the umbilical cord
- Abruptio placentae

Technique

- Perform nonstress test to evaluate fetal health and placental function.

- Perform ultrasound examination to determine fetal gestational age and fetal presentation and to identify the adequacy of amniotic fluid; ultrasound also guides the fetal manipulations.

- Administer a tocolytic drug to relax the uterus during the version.

- Physician pushes the fetal breech out of the pelvis in a forward or backward roll, guiding the fetal head downward into the pelvis.

Nursing Considerations

- Maintain NPO until after procedure and return of maternal and fetal status to baseline levels.

- Assess maternal vital signs before and every 5 minutes during the procedure.

- Perform nonstress test.

- Explain side effects of the planned tocolytic drug, emphasizing that these abate soon after the drug is stopped.

- Administer the drug as ordered.

- Monitor FHR with Doppler or real-time ultrasound during procedure. Fetal bradycardia may occur during the procedure, but the rate usually returns to normal when manipulations stop.

- Monitor maternal vital signs and FHR; monitor for regular contractions or ruptured membranes after the procedure.

- Give Rh immune globulin (RhoGAM) to the Rh-negative woman, as indicated.

- Review signs and symptoms of true labor and teach guidelines for returning to the birth center.

D. FORCEPS AND VACUUM EXTRACTION

These procedures assist fetal expulsion by allowing the physician to apply traction to the fetal head. Forceps may assist fetal head rotation as well as descent.

Indications

- Maternal
  - Exhaustion
  - Poor pushing effectiveness
  - Cardiac or pulmonary disease
  - Intrapartum infection demanding prompt birth
- Fetal
  - Prolapsed umbilical cord (if birth can be accomplished quickly with the procedure; otherwise cesarean birth is done)
  - Premature separation of the placenta
  - Nonreassuring FHR patterns

Contraindications or Precautions

- Severe fetal compromise
- High fetal station
- Acute maternal conditions, such as congestive heart failure or pulmonary edema
- Fetopelvic disproportion

Risks

- Maternal: laceration or hematoma of the vagina
- Fetal/neonatal
  - Ecchymoses
  - Facial or scalp lacerations or abrasions
  - Facial nerve injury
  - Cephalhematoma
  - Subgaleal or intracranial hemorrhage

Technique

- Complete cervical dilation is required.
- Catheterization provides more room in the pelvis.
- Anesthesia is a regional block such as pudendal or epidural.
- Episiotomy is common.
- Classifications of forceps are based on station of the fetal head when forceps are applied:
  — Outlet: The fetal head is on the perineum, with the scalp visible at the vaginal opening without separating the labia.
  — Low: The leading edge of the fetal skull is at station +2 (about 2 cm below the level of the mother's ischial spines) or lower.
  — Mid-forceps: The leading edge of the fetal skull is between a 0 (at the level of the ischial spines) and a +2 station.

Nursing Considerations

- Add a catheter to the delivery instrument set.
- Continue FHR observations and notify the physician if the rate is lower than 100 BPM.
- Observe mother and infant for forceps-related trauma.
- Apply cold to the woman's perineum for 12 hours.
- Reassure parents that the reddening and bruising of the infant's skin where forceps were applied is temporary. Cold is not applied to the infant's skin because it would cause hypothermia.
- Observe infant for infection that may gain entry via skin breaks and for facial asymmetry that suggests facial nerve injury.

E. EPISIOTOMY

Indications

- Fetal
  - Similar to those for forceps or vacuum extraction
  - Reduction of pressure on the head of a small preterm fetus
- Maternal
  - Control of the direction and extent to which the vaginal opening is enlarged (controversial)
  - A straight, clean-edged incision that can be simpler to repair than a large perineal laceration

Contraindications or Precautions

There are no real contraindications, although routine performance of an episiotomy remains controversial. The physician or nurse-midwife must make the decision just before birth.

Risks

- Infection
- Perineal pain that may last longer than pain associated with spontaneous tears

Technique

- Done when fetal presenting part has crowned to a diameter of about 3–4 cm
- Two types
  - Median: Cut along a line from the vaginal fourchette toward the anus
    - Less blood loss, scarring, and postpartum pain
    - More likely to extend into the anal sphincter because of limited room to enlarge vaginal opening
  - Mediolateral: Cut at an angle from the vaginal fourchette toward the left or right

- More enlargement of vaginal opening and less risk of tearing into the anal sphincter
- More blood loss, pain, and scarring; longer painful intercourse

Nursing Considerations

- Actions to reduce need for episiotomy
  — Help woman push in an upright position.
  — Apply warm perineal compresses.
  — Perform perineal massage.
- Post delivery
  — Observe the perineum for hematoma and edema.
  — Apply cold compresses for first 12 hours; apply perineal heat after 12 hours.

F. CESAREAN BIRTH

Indications

- Maternal or fetal compromise
- Dystocia
- Fetopelvic disproportion
- Pregnancy-induced hypertension, if prompt delivery is needed
- Maternal diseases such as diabetes, heart disease, or cervical cancer, if labor is not advisable
  — Active genital herpes
  — Some previous uterine surgical procedures, such as a classic cesarean incision
  — Persistent nonreassuring fetal heart rate patterns
  — Prolapsed umbilical cord
  — Fetal malpresentations, such as breech or transverse lie
  — Hemorrhagic conditions, such as abruptio placentae or placenta previa

Contraindications or Precautions

- Fetal death
- Fetus that is not expected to survive
- Maternal coagulation defects

Risks

- Maternal
  - Infection
  - Hemorrhage
  - Urinary tract trauma
  - Thrombophlebitis
  - Paralytic ileus
  - Atelectasis
  - Anesthesia complications
- Neonatal
  - Inadvertent preterm birth
  - Transient tachypnea of the newborn
  - Persistent fetal circulation
  - Injury, such as laceration, bruising, or other trauma

Technique

The reason for the cesarean (planned or unplanned) and time pressure will modify some of these steps.

- Test for fetal lung maturity before planned cesarean birth (lecithin/sphingomyelin [L/S] ratio and assessment for presence of phosphatidylglycerol [PG] and phosphatidylinositol [PI]).
- Initiate fetal monitoring for 20–30 minutes before a scheduled cesarean birth.
- Administer drugs to reduce gastric acidity or control respiratory secretions. Other than ordered oral medications, the woman remains NPO.

- Laboratory tests vary with the maternal and fetal conditions.
  - Complete blood count
  - Clotting studies
  - Blood typing and screening; crossmatching may be done if the woman is anemic or if she has an increased risk for hemorrhage.
- Anesthesia
  - Epidural or subarachnoid block is preferred
  - General may be required if regional is not possible or refused
- Incisions
  - Skin
    - Pfannenstiel (transverse, or "bikini")
    - Vertical
  - Uterine
    - Low transverse (preferred)
    - Low vertical
    - Classic (high vertical)

Nursing Considerations

- Provide emotional support; need varies according to the reason for the cesarean birth.
  - Identify concerns and misunderstandings about the current or prior cesarean births. Teach the woman and her support person to reduce their fear of the unknown.
  - Use a calm and confident manner, even if the cesarean is done in an emergency situation.
  - Visit the woman and her partner after birth to answer questions they may have or fill in gaps in their understanding.

> **Clinical Tip:** A woman's support person may be anxious and physically exhausted after hours of supporting her in labor. Do not expect more support from this person than he or she can provide.

Preoperative

- Teach the woman and her partner about cesarean birth.
  - Preoperative procedures and their purposes
  - Intravenous line and catheter, which are usually removed within 24 hours after birth
  - Reassurance that pressure and pulling sensations are normal and that the anesthesia clinician will regularly assess her pain management needs.
  - If general anesthesia is planned, reassure her that she will be asleep before the incision is made even though all preparations are done before anesthesia is begun.
  - Appearance of the operating room and explanations of who will be present
    - Cool room
    - Narrow surgery table
    - When her partner can come in (Preoperative preparations may take 30–45 minutes in a non-emergency cesarean birth.)
  - Recovery room
    - Equipment, such as a pulse oximeter and automatic blood pressure cuff
    - Routine assessments and interventions
      Vital signs
      Fundus and lochia checks
      Coughing and deep breathing
    - Exercises to promote circulation in her legs
    - Comfort interventions, such as medication and positioning
  - Maintaining NPO status, other than for ordered drugs to control gastric secretions.
- Preoperative preparation
  - Abdominal shave depends on the expected skin incision.
    - For Pfannenstiel skin incision, shave from about 3 inches above the pubic hairline to the mons pubis (about where her legs come together).

- For vertical skin incision, shave from just above the umbilicus to the mons pubis.
— An indwelling catheter, often inserted after a regional anesthetic takes effect, reduces the chance for bladder injury during the procedure. If a general anesthetic is planned, the catheter is inserted before induction of anesthesia to reduce fetal exposure to the anesthetic.
— Intravenous infusion
- Prophylactic intravenous antibiotic

Intraoperative

- Transfer and position to prevent injury
  — Pad bony prominences.
  — Secure the woman's position with a safety strap across her thighs.
  — Place a wedge under one hip or tilt the operating table to reduce aortocaval compression.
  — Route the indwelling catheter drain tube under her leg and place bag near the head of the table so the anesthesia clinician can monitor urine output.
- Verify proper function of machines such as suction, monitors, electrocautery.
- Apply leads for cardiac monitoring and pulse oximetry readings.
- Apply a grounding pad for electrocautery use.
- Cleanse the incision with sterile water or saline and apply a sterile dressing.
- Clean blood and amniotic fluid from the woman's abdomen, buttocks, and back before transferring her to a bed after surgery.
- Transfer the woman smoothly to reduce pain and prevent hypotension.
- Care for the infant, as in vaginal birth.

Postoperative

- Assessments are typically done every 15 minutes during the first 1–2 hours, then every 30–60 minutes until transfer to her postpartum room.
  - Check blood pressure, pulse, and respirations at the intervals noted; check temperature at recovery room admission and according to protocol thereafter.
  - Monitor pulse oximetry (continuous). Have the woman take several deep breaths if oxygen saturation falls below 95%.
  - Assess for return of motion and sensation (if a regional block was given).
  - Assess level of consciousness (particularly if general anesthesia or sedating drugs were given).
  - Check abdominal dressing, including character and amount of drainage.
  - Assess uterine firmness and position (midline or deviated).
  - Note lochia quantity and presence of any clots.
  - Assess urine output (quantity, color, other characteristics).
  - Monitor intravenous infusion (solution, rate of flow, condition of site, secondary infusions).
  - Pain relief needs
    - PCA (patient-controlled analgesia) pump
    - Intermittent injections
    - Epidural narcotics provide long-lasting analgesia.

Clinical Tip: To relax her abdominal muscles during fundal checks, have the woman flex her knees and take slow deep breaths. Gently "walk" the fingers toward her fundus to determine uterine firmness.

V. INTRAPARTAL COMPLICATIONS

A. DYSFUNCTIONAL LABOR

Dysfunctional labor has many causes. Maternal and fetal risks vary with the specific labor dysfunction, but often include

- Infection.
- Fetal hypoxia.
- Maternal or fetal injury.

Problems of the Powers

Ineffective Contractions

- Causes
  - Maternal fatigue
  - Maternal inactivity
  - Fluid and electrolyte imbalance
  - Hypoglycemia
  - Excessive analgesia or anesthesia
  - Maternal catecholamines secreted in response to stress or pain
  - Disproportion between the maternal pelvis and the fetal presenting part
  - Uterine overdistention, such as with multiple gestation or hydramnios
- Characteristics
  - Ineffective contraction patterns are classified as hypotonic or hypertonic.
  - The characteristics and therapeutic management differ.
- Nursing considerations
  - Hypotonic dysfunction
    - Encourage position changes.
    - An abdominal binder may help if the woman's abdominal wall is very lax (usually multiparas).

- Hypertonic dysfunction
  - Promote uterine blood flow by avoiding the supine position.
  - Provide pain relief.
  - Promote general comfort.
- Provide emotional support and reassurance to the woman and her family.

Ineffective Maternal Pushing

- Causes
  - Use of incorrect pushing techniques or inappropriate pushing positions
  - Fear of injury because of pain and tearing sensations felt by the mother when she pushes
  - Decreased or absent urge to push
  - Maternal exhaustion
  - Analgesia or anesthesia that suppresses the woman's urge to push
  - Psychological unreadiness to "let go" of her baby
- Therapeutic management: Forceps or cesarean birth may be required if the woman continues to be unable to push her baby out.
- Nursing considerations
  - Observe maternal and fetal vital signs for signs that either is not tolerating the prolonged second stage.
    - Maternal fever (over 38°C [100.4°F])
    - Fetal tachycardia (often the first sign of infection)
    - Any other nonreassuring fetal heart rate pattern
    - Amniotic fluid having a foul or strong odor, a yellow color, or a cloudy appearance
  - Encourage upright positions while pushing, such as squatting, semi-sitting, side-lying, or pushing while sitting on the toilet.

- Teach the woman how her tissues gradually stretch to accommodate the baby. Warm perineal compresses or perineal massage may increase perineal distensibility.
- Coach the woman to push if she cannot feel the urge because of regional block analgesia.
- Have the exhausted woman push only when she feels the urge, or with every other contraction.
- Provide oral and/or intravenous fluids, as ordered.
- Reassure the woman that there is no arbitrary time limit for the duration of second stage labor.

Problems with the Passenger

Fetal Size

Macrosomia

Birth weight is greater than 4000 g (8.8 pounds). Size is relative, however, and a woman with a large pelvis may easily give birth to an infant larger than this, while a woman with a small or abnormally-shaped pelvis may be unable to deliver a smaller infant. Also, a woman with a small pelvis may be able to deliver a large infant if all other factors (fetal position, uterine contractions, etc.) are favorable.

Shoulder Dystocia

The fetal shoulders are trapped behind the woman's symphysis after the fetal head is born. The "turtle sign" is characteristic of shoulder dystocia: the fetal head retracts against the perineum as soon as it emerges. Shoulder dystocia is more likely to occur if the fetus is large.

> **Clinical Tip:** A shoulder dystocia is an urgent situation because the umbilical cord is deep in the pelvis, subject to compression. Yet the infant cannot breathe because the thorax is compressed.

- Therapeutic management involves the birth attendant and the nurse.
  - McRobert's maneuver: The woman flexes her thighs sharply against her abdomen to straighten the pelvic curve.
  - A supported squat has an effect similar to that of McRobert's maneuver and adds gravity to the forces of maternal pushing.
  - Suprapubic pressure toward the maternal sacrum displaces the fetal shoulder from above the maternal symphysis.
  - *Fundal pressure should not be used* because it can further impact the fetal shoulders above the maternal symphysis.
- Nursing considerations
  - Assist the birth attendant in the listed methods to relieve shoulder dystocia.
  - Check the newborn's clavicles for crepitus, deformity, or bruising that suggests fracture.

Abnormal Fetal Presentation or Position

Rotation Abnormalities

The fetus in a vertex presentation does not complete rotation into the occiput anterior position. The fetal head may remain in an occiput posterior or occiput transverse position. Some women may be able to deliver their infants in an occiput posterior position, but most cannot.

- Causes
  - Large fetus
  - Poor fetal head flexion, which increases the diameters presented to the maternal pelvis
  - Small or abnormally-shaped maternal pelvis
  - Inadequate contractions or maternal pushing to assist fetal rotation

- Characteristics
  - Prolonged labor
  - The woman usually feels intense back and/or leg pain ("back labor") that is poorly relieved with analgesia.
- Therapeutic management
  - Forceps to assist rotation and descent of the fetal head
  - Cesarean birth if the rotation abnormality persists
- Nursing considerations
  - Encourage position changes to favor fetal head rotation
    - Hands and knees; rocking the pelvis back and forth while on hands and knees encourages rotation.
    - Side-lying (on her left side if the fetus is in a right occiput posterior [ROP] position and on her right side for a left occiput posterior [LOP] position)
    - The lunge, in which the mother places one foot on a chair with her foot and knee pointed to that side. She lunges sideways repeatedly during a contraction for 5 seconds at a time. It can also be done in a kneeling position. The nurse or her partner must secure the chair and help her balance.
    - Squatting (for second-stage labor)
    - Sitting, kneeling, or standing while leaning forward.
  - Pain management techniques
  - Check for maternal and newborn injuries after birth
    - Vaginal hematoma
    - Newborn cephalhematoma or forceps marks

Breech Presentation

External version may be attempted if the fetus remains in a breech presentation near term. If the fetus remains breech, cesarean birth is common. Vaginal breech birth may be recommended if

- The maternal pelvis is of normal size and shape.
- The estimated fetal weight is under 3600 g (8 pounds).

- Other complications, such as placenta previa or prolapsed cord, are not present.

Multifetal Gestation

- Intrapartal risks include
  - Dysfunctional labor caused by uterine overdistention (hypotonic dysfunction).
  - Abnormal presentation of one or both fetuses.
  - Greater risk for fetal hypoxia.
  - Maternal postpartum hemorrhage caused by uterine atony.
- Vaginal birth considerations include
  - Fetal presentations.
  - Maternal pelvic size.
  - Presence of other complications.
- Nursing considerations
  - Monitor each twin's FHR separately. Continue monitoring the second twin after the first twin's birth.
  - Observe for hypotonic labor dysfunction.
  - Duplicate equipment and staff to care for each infant.
  - One nurse remains free to care for the woman.
  - Observe fundal height and firmness, lochia, and maternal vital signs after birth to detect uterine atony.

Problems of the Passage

Pelvis

Women may have any of four types of pelvis, and most women have characteristics of more than one type. The different pelvic types have different prognoses for vaginal birth. Those other than the gynecoid are likely to cause dysfunctional labor. Therapeutic management and nursing considerations are similar to those listed for dysfunctional labor.

- Gynecoid (50% of women)
  - Round, cylindric shape with a wide pubic arch

- Good prognosis for vaginal birth
- Anthropoid (25% of white women, 50% of nonwhite women)
  - Long, narrow oval shape with a narrow pubic arch
  - Fetus is more likely to be born in an occiput posterior (face up) position
- Android (30% of women)
  - Heart or triangular shape with narrow diameters and a narrow pubic arch
  - Poor prognosis for vaginal birth
- Platypelloid (3% of women)
  - Flat shape with a wide, short oval and a wide pubic arch
  - Poor prognosis for vaginal birth

Maternal Soft Tissue

The most common soft tissue obstruction of labor is a full bladder. The woman often has pain that remains after epidural analgesia. Assess for bladder filling and encourage the woman to void every 1–2 hours, or more often if she has received large amounts of intravenous fluids. Catheterize her if she cannot void.

Problems of the Psyche

Nursing care of the woman's psyche is directed toward helping her relax and work with the forces of labor.

- Establish a trusting relationship with the woman and her family.
- Make the environment comfortable by adjusting temperature and light.
- Promote physical comfort, such as cleanliness.
- Provide accurate information.
- Implement nonpharmacological and pharmacological pain management.

- Implement appropriate nursing care for any other type of labor dysfunction.

Abnormal Labor Duration

Prolonged Labor

- Parameters for normal labor progress
  — Cervical dilation rate of at least 1.2 cm/hour in the nullipara and 1.5 cm/hour in the parous woman
  — Fetal descent rate of at least 1 cm/hour in the nullipara and 2 cm/hour in the parous woman
- Causes and characteristics: Any of the previously discussed problems of the powers, passenger, passage, or psyche usually cause a prolonged labor. If the cause can be identified, specific therapeutic management and nursing care is directed toward that cause.
- Risks
  — Maternal infection, intrapartum or postpartum, particularly with prolonged membrane rupture
  — Neonatal infection, which may be severe or fatal
  — Maternal exhaustion
  — Higher levels of anxiety and fear during a subsequent labor
- Nursing considerations
  — Limit vaginal examinations as much as possible. Use behavioral cues to help determine when a vaginal examination is truly necessary.
  — Observe maternal vital signs every 2–4 hours and FHR with fetal monitoring. Note particularly fetal or maternal tachycardia, or elevated maternal temperature. Report a temperature of 38°C (100.4°F) or higher.
  — Observe amniotic fluid for a cloudy or yellow color and a strong or foul odor. Change underpads regularly to keep the woman relatively dry.
  — Observe for signs associated with fetal hypoxia, such as bradycardia, tachycardia, loss of variability, and/or late decelerations. See p. 138.

- Use appropriate position changes to foster labor progress.
- Promote comfort and conservation of maternal energy.
- Observe intake and output. Provide ordered IV fluids. If oral fluids are allowed, juice, lollipops, popsicles, or other clear liquids help moisten the woman's mouth and maintain her hydration and energy stores.
- Provide emotional support. Encourage and praise her use of coping skills. Tell her when she makes progress. Reassure her of fetal well-being, if true.
- Observe the newborn for signs of sepsis. See p. 270.
- Obtain cultures of maternal (uterine cavity or placenta) and newborn (multiple cultures) secretions as ordered. Use correct specimen containers for aerobic and anaerobic organisms. Transport to the lab promptly.
- Administer prophylactic antibiotics to mother and infant as ordered.

Precipitate Labor

- Causes
  - Unusually strong labor contractions (natural or oxytocin-stimulated)
  - Large maternal pelvis relative to the fetal size
- Characteristics: Birth occurs within 3 hours of labor onset.
- Risks
  - Maternal trauma: Uterine rupture, cervical lacerations, or vaginal or vulvar hematoma.
  - Fetal trauma: Fetal hypoxia, intracranial hemorrhage, or nerve damage
- Therapeutic management
  - No specific interventions if contractions are not so strong that they impair fetal oxygenation
  - Tocolytic drugs to reduce contractions that are too intense
  - Supplemental oxygen

- Nursing considerations
  - Promote fetal oxygenation.
    - Maintain a side-lying position.
    - Administer oxygen at 8–10 L/min by face mask.
    - Maintain adequate blood volume by titrating the nonadditive IV flow rate.
  - Stop any oxytocin infusion.
  - Give ordered tocolytic drugs.
  - Help woman use nonpharmacologic pain management measures because progress may be too fast to allow medications such as opioid analgesia or regional block. Focus on helping the woman cope with one contraction at a time.
  - Be prepared to assist with birth if it occurs before the birth attendant arrives.

B. PREMATURE RUPTURE OF THE MEMBRANES

- Definitions
  - *Premature rupture of the membranes* (PROM): Rupture of the amniotic sac before true labor, regardless of gestational age.
  - *Preterm premature rupture of the membranes* (PPROM): Rupture of the amniotic sac earlier than the end of the 37th week of gestation, with or without contractions.
- Causes
  - Infections of the vagina or cervix, such as gonorrhea, group B *Streptococcus*, and *Gardnerella vaginalis*
  - Chorioamnionitis
  - Incompetent cervix
  - Fetal abnormalities or malpresentation
  - Hydramnios
  - Amniotic sac with a weak structure
  - Recent sexual intercourse
  - Nutritional deficiencies

- Risks
  - Infection, maternal and newborn, either before or after birth; infection can be both a cause and a result of prematurely ruptured membranes.
  - Newborn complications of prematurity, particularly if birth occurs before 34 weeks of gestation
  - Umbilical cord compression
  - Fetal/neonatal complications of reduced amniotic fluid volume: reduced lung volume with respiratory distress, deformities secondary to compression.
- Therapeutic management
  - Determining if membranes are truly ruptured with a Nitrazine and/or fern test
  - Assessment of fetal lung maturity
  - Culture of secretions to identify infection
- If gestation is at or near term, management may include
  - Walking to stimulate contractions.
  - Oxytocin induction of labor.
- If gestation is preterm, management may include observation in the hospital for a few days to rule out infection.
- Nursing considerations
  - Specific care depends on whether the gestation is term or preterm, whether labor will be induced, or whether the woman will be discharged to await labor.
  - Client teaching before discharge (undelivered)
    - Avoid sexual intercourse, orgasm, or insertion of anything into vagina, which increases the risk for infection caused by ascending organisms and can stimulate contractions.
    - Avoid breast stimulation if the gestation is preterm; breast stimulation can cause release of oxytocin from the posterior pituitary and thus stimulate contractions.
    - Check temperature at least four times a day, reporting any temperature over 37.8°C (100°F).

C. PRETERM LABOR

Labor is preterm if it begins after the 20th week but before the end of the 37th week of gestation.

- Risks

TABLE II-9

Maternal Risk Factors for Preterm Labor

Medical History	Obstetric History
Uterine or cervical anomalies	Previous preterm birth
Diethylstilbestrol (DES) exposure as a fetus	Previous preterm labor
History of cone biopsy	Previous first trimester abortions (>2)
Low weight for height	Previous second trimester abortion
Chronic illness (such as cardiac, renal, hypertension)	History of previous pregnancy losses (2 or more)
	Incompetent cervix

Present Pregnancy	Lifestyle and Demographics
Uterine distention (such as multifetal pregnancy or hydramnios)	Little or no prenatal care
Abdominal surgery during pregnancy	Poor nutrition
Uterine irritability	Age under 18 or over 40
Uterine bleeding	Low education level
Dehydration	Low socioeconomic status
Infection	Smoking >10 cigarettes daily
Anemia	Nonwhite
Incompetent cervix	Chronic physical or psychological stress
Pre-eclampsia	Substance abuse
Preterm premature rupture of membranes (PPROM)	
Fetal or placental abnormalities	

- Characteristics
  - Uterine contractions that may or may not be painful; the woman may not feel contractions at all
  - A sensation that the baby is frequently "balling up"
  - Cramps similar to menstrual cramps
  - Constant low backache
  - Sensation of pelvic pressure or a feeling that the baby is pushing down
  - Pain, discomfort, or pressure in the vulva or thighs
  - Change or increase in vaginal discharge (increased, watery, bloody)
  - Abdominal cramps with or without diarrhea
  - A sense of "just feeling bad" or "coming down with something"
- Therapeutic management
  - More frequent prenatal visits for women at increased risk for preterm labor
  - Fetal fibronectin determination to help the health care provider decide on the best course of action: watchful observation, or more aggressive treatment with tocolytic drugs and drugs to accelerate fetal lung maturity
  - Identifying conditions that contraindicate continuing the pregnancy, such as pregnancy-induced hypertension, maternal hypovolemia, chorioamnionitis, or fetal compromise
  - Treating conditions associated with preterm labor, such as urinary tract infection
  - Transport of a woman who is likely to deliver preterm to a facility with neonatal intensive care facilities
  - Home uterine activity monitoring, which includes transmission of uterine activity data over the phone and 24-hour availability of perinatal nurses
  - Measures to stop preterm labor before it reaches the point of no return, usually after 3 cm of cervical dilation; measures chosen depend on the probable cause of preterm labor, but may include the following:

- Restricting activity, although the usefulness of this measure has been questioned
- Hydration with oral and/or intravenous fluids
- Tocolytic drugs
- Corticosteroids to accelerate fetal lung maturation

TABLE II-10

Drugs Used in Preterm Labor

DRUG/ PURPOSE	COMMON DOSES*	SIDE OR ADVERSE EFFECTS
β-Adrenergics (tocolysis) Ritodrine	IV: Start at 0.05 mg/min (50 µg/min). Increase by 0.05 mg/min until labor stops or significant side effects develop. Maximum dose is 0.35 mg/min (350 µg/min). Hold rate for 60 min after contractions stop, then decrease by 0.05 mg/min (50 µg/min) increments until lowest effective dose is reached. Hold this dose for 12 hr. *Oral:* Give first oral dose before discontinuing IV ritodrine. 10 mg q 2 hr or 20 mg q 4 hr for 24-48 hr. Maximum daily oral dose: 120 mg/day.	Side effects are dose-related and more prominent during increases in the infusion rate than during maintenance therapy. Cardiovascular: maternal and fetal tachycardia. Wide pulse pressure Pulmonary: Shortness of breath, chest pain Gastrointestinal: Nausea, vomiting, diarrhea, ileus Tremors, jitteriness, restlessness, feeling of apprehension Metabolic alterations: hyperglycemia; hypokalemia Pulmonary edema (more likely if the woman receives corticosteroids at the same time)

Terbutaline	See Drug Guide: Terbutaline (p. 464)	Cardiovascular: Maternal and fetal tachycardia, palpitations, cardiac arrhythmias, chest pain, wide pulse pressure

See Drug Guide: Terbutaline (p. 464)

IV: Begin at 0.0025 mg/min (2.5 µg/min). Increase by 0.0025 mg/min (2.5 µg/min) at 20-min intervals until contractions stop (maximum of 0.02 mg/min [20 µg/min]) or significant side effects develop. Maintain dose for at least 1 hr; then reduce rate at 20-min intervals to reach lowest effective dose. Continue maintenance dose for 12 hr after contractions stop before changing route of administration.

Subcutaneous (SC) (most common parenteral route): 0.25 mg (250 µg) every 1-3 hr. Continuous pump may be used for SC administration.

Oral: 2.5-5 mg every 2-4 hr.

Cardiovascular: Maternal and fetal tachycardia, palpitations, cardiac arrhythmias, chest pain, wide pulse pressure

Respiratory: Dyspnea, chest discomfort

Central nervous system: Tremors, restlessness, weakness, dizziness, headache

Metabolic: Hyper-glycemia, hypokalemia

Gastrointestinal: Nausea, vomiting, reduced bowel motility

Skin: Flushing, diaphoresis

Infection at injection site (subcutaneous terbutaline pump)

Magnesium sulfate (tocolysis)	IV loading dose: 4-6 g; continue at 2-4 g/hr Higher doses can usually be given than for pre-eclampsia because these women usually have normal renal function.	Side and adverse effects are dose-related, occurring at higher serum levels. Depression of deep tendon reflexes Respiratory depression Cardiac arrest (usually at serum levels above 12/mg/dl) Less serious side effects include: Lethargy, weakness, visual blurring, headache, sensation of heat, nausea, vomiting, constipation Fetal-neonatal effects: Reduced FHR variability. Hypotonia
Indomethacin (tocolysis)	*Oral or rectal*: 25-50 mg every 6 hr for 48 hr. Discontinue if birth is imminent or likely to occur within 24 hr. 48 hr is a common maximum time for administration.	Gastrointestinal Epigastric pain, gastrointestinal bleeding Fetus: May have constriction of the ductus arteriosus and decreased urine output. Decreased urine output is associated with oligohydramnios, which may result in cord compression. Adverse fetal effects usually resolve within a day after treatment is stopped.

Nifedipine (tocolysis)	Oral: 30 mg initially; 20 mg 4 hr later	Maternal flushing Transient maternal tachycardia Maternal hypotension
Corticosteroids (accelerating fetal lung maturation) * Betamethasone * Dexamethasone	Betamethasone: 12 mg IM for two doses, 24 hr apart Dexamethasone: 6 mg IM q 12 hr for four doses Greatest fetal benefits if at least 24 hr elapse between first dose and birth	Concurrent administration with beta-adrenergics and corticosteroids has been associated with development of pulmonary edema. May worsen conditions such as diabetes and hypertension and may delay wound healing.

---

*Doses and frequency of administration are common, but protocols do vary.

- Nursing considerations
  — Teach pregnant women the signs of early preterm labor. Reinforce these and inquire about them at each office visit, particularly for women at increased risk.
  — Help the woman change risk factors that can be changed, such as nutritional deficiencies or smoking.
  — Refer for assistance, such as to food supplement programs (WIC).
  — Teach woman and her partner to promptly report signs or symptoms associated with preterm birth. Teach her how to be assertive in seeking prompt care so measures to prevent preterm birth are likely to be more effective.
  — Observe for conditions that may contraindicate continuing the pregnancy.
    – Assess the blood pressure to identify hypotension or hypertension.

- Assess temperature and pulse to detect elevations associated with infection.
- Monitor the FHR for patterns associated with compromise, such as abnormal rates, loss of variability, and late or severe variable decelerations. Significant reduction of fetal movement also suggests compromise.
— Observe for treatable conditions that increase the likelihood of preterm birth, such as urinary or reproductive tract infections.
— Observe for preterm premature ruptured membranes.
— Help woman cope with activity restrictions.
— Provide oral and/or intravenous hydration as ordered. Observe for signs of dehydration if the woman has had a febrile illness or has vomiting and/or diarrhea (dry skin and mucous membranes, elevated temperature, scant and concentrated urine).
— Administer ordered tocolytic drugs and drugs to speed fetal lung maturation. Teach the woman correct use and precautions if she will be self-administering these drugs.

D. INTRAPARTAL EMERGENCIES

Medical and nursing management often overlap when caring for a woman and her fetus during an intrapartum emergency. Written standard protocols often provide direction for nursing actions in an emergency.

Prolapsed Umbilical Cord

- Characteristics
  — Umbilical cord slips into a position to be compressed between the maternal pelvis and the fetal body.
  — Cord compression is more severe during contractions.
- Risks
  — A fetus that remains at a high station
  — A very small fetus

- Breech presentations, especially a footling breech
- Transverse lie
- Hydramnios

- Signs
  - Complete: Cord is visible at vaginal opening.
  - Partial: Cord is not visible externally, but is palpated during vaginal examination.
  - Occult: Cord is neither visible nor palpable, but FHR patterns, such as severe variable decelerations or bradycardia, suggest cord compression.

- Management
  - Relieve pressure on the cord.
    - Position the woman's hips higher than her head

      Knee-chest position

      Trendelenburg position

      Elevate hips with pillows while maintaining a side-lying position
    - With a gloved hand, push the fetal presenting part upward. Maintain this position until the physician orders it stopped, which may not be until a cesarean incision is made.
  - Give oxygen at 8–10 L/min by face mask.
  - Give a tocolytic drug, such as terbutaline, to inhibit contractions.
  - If cord protrudes, do not attempt to replace it. Towels moistened with warm saline retard cooling and drying if there will be any delay in delivery.
  - Delivery will be as rapid as possible, usually by cesarean.
  - Provide emotional support. Explain what is happening simply and calmly. Encourage the woman and her partner to ventilate their feelings after birth.

Uterine Rupture

- Characteristics
  - The uterine wall is torn to a varying degree. Classifications of uterine rupture
    - Complete: Having a direct communication between the uterine and peritoneal cavities
    - Incomplete: Rupture into the peritoneum covering the uterus or into the broad ligament but not into the peritoneal cavity
    - Dehiscence: A partial separation of an old uterine scar
  - Signs and symptoms vary with the degree of rupture. Dehiscence may have no signs or symptoms.
    - Abdominal pain and tenderness, which may or may not be severe
    - Chest pain, pain between the scapulae, or pain on inspiration
    - Hypovolemic shock
    - FHR patterns associated with impaired fetal oxygenation, such as late decelerations, reduced variability, tachycardia, or bradycardia
    - Absent fetal heart tones
    - Cessation of uterine contractions
    - Palpation of the fetus outside the uterus
- Causes and risks
  - Previous uterine incision; the woman who has had a classic cesarean incision has a greater risk than does the woman who has had a low transverse incision.
  - High parity, with a thin uterine wall
  - Blunt trauma
  - Intense labor contractions, particularly if there is fetopelvic disproportion
- Management
  - Identify women who have increased risk for rupture and remain alert for its signs and symptoms.

- Give ordered tocolytic drugs for hypertonic contractions.
- Give oxygen at 8–10 L/min.
- Expedite birth, usually by cesarean.
- Provide blood and fluid replacement.
- Observe for excessive postpartum bleeding and hypovolemic shock that may occur if a rupture was not detected earlier.

Uterine Inversion

- Characteristics
  - The uterus turns inside out, either partially or completely.
  - Signs and symptoms
    - Absence of the uterus from the lower abdomen
    - Depression in the fundus of the uterus, felt with palpation
    - Interior of the uterus visible through the cervix or protruding into the vagina
    - Hemorrhage, shock
    - Severe pelvic pain
- Causes and risks
  - Pulling on the umbilical cord before the placenta detaches from the uterine wall
  - Fundal pressure during birth
  - Increased intra-abdominal pressure
  - An abnormally adherent placenta
  - Congenital weakness of the uterine wall
  - Fundal placenta implantation
  - Fundal pressure on an incompletely contracted uterus after birth
- Management
  - Establish two IV lines for fluid and blood replacement.

- Give tocolytic drugs to stop uterine contractions. General anesthesia may be needed.
- Give oxytocin after the uterus is replaced. Oxytocin is not given until the uterus is repositioned to avoid trapping the inverted fundus in the cervix.
- Observe for signs of hypovolemia after birth (tachycardia, falling blood pressure, inadequate [less than 30 mL/hour] or absent urine output with an indwelling catheter in place). Cardiac monitoring to identify dysrhythmias and invasive hemodynamic monitoring may be ordered.
- Observe the uterus for firmness, height, and deviation from the midline.

Amniotic Fluid Embolism

Amniotic fluid embolism occurs when amniotic fluid is drawn into the maternal circulation and carried to the woman's lungs. It is most likely to occur if labor contractions are very intense. Embolism of meconium-stained amniotic fluid is often fatal.

- Characteristics: Amniotic fluid embolism usually becomes apparent after birth.
  - Abrupt respiratory distress
  - Heart failure
  - Circulatory collapse
  - Disseminated intravascular coagulation (see p. 64)
- Management
  - Cardiopulmonary resuscitation
  - Oxygen with mechanical ventilation
  - Blood transfusion
  - Correction of coagulation deficits with platelets or fibrinogen

Trauma

- Causes
  - Accidents

- Assault
- Suicide
- Types of trauma
  - Blunt (automobile accidents, battering)
  - Penetrating (knife or gunshot wounds)
  - Burns
  - Electrical injuries
- Fetal/neonatal complications
  - Direct injury due to skull fracture, intracranial hemorrhage
  - Indirect injury due to abruptio placentae, maternal hypovolemia, or uterine rupture
  - Death of the mother (most common cause of fetal death)
  - Neurologic deficits sometimes found in survivors
- Management
  - Stabilization and care of maternal life-threatening injuries, then stabilization of the fetus
  - Delivery if the maternal condition warrants and the fetus is likely to survive
  - Delivery of the dead or extremely immature fetus if that will improve the maternal outcome
- Nursing considerations
  - Place a wedge under one hip to prevent supine hypotension and improve placental blood flow.
  - Observe vital signs (frequency depends on maternal condition). Monitor FHR if the fetus has reached a viable gestational age.
  - Observe urine output for quantity (at least 30 mL/hour), and for presence of blood.
  - Observe for and report signs of abruptio placentae (vaginal bleeding with uterine pain and tenderness; increase in uterine height).

- Palpate for contractions because pain from injury or impairment of consciousness may mask labor symptoms. Contractions may not be evident on a fetal monitoring strip.
- Prepare for birth of an infant who may be immature and/or need resuscitation.
- Provide emotional support. Explain what is occurring simply and honestly. Support the partner. Give the woman and her family an opportunity to ventilate their feelings after the emergency has passed.

> **Clinical Tip:** Although the nurse is usually anxious in an emergency situation, it is important to keep a calm attitude. The woman and her family quickly pick up on the staff's anxiety, and theirs will escalate. Remain with the woman to reduce fears of abandonment. If possible, hold her hand. Speak in a low, calm voice.

SECTION THREE

Normal Newborn

I. THE PROCESSES OF ADAPTATION

A. RESPIRATORY SYSTEM ADAPTATION

- Initiation of respirations occurs by stimulation of the respiratory center in the brain
  — Chemical factors: Decreased blood oxygen (PO_2) and pH and increased blood carbon dioxide (PCO_2) levels
  — Thermal factors: Change in temperature from the uterus to the colder air environment
  — Tactile stimuli: Handling at birth
  — Mechanical factors: Compression and release of the chest during birth
- Surfactant production
  — Reduces surface tension within the alveoli and prevents collapse of alveoli with exhalation
  — Produced in adequate amounts by 34–36 weeks of gestation
- Fetal lung fluid is absorbed by the circulatory and lymphatic systems. Absorption is accelerated by labor and may be delayed by cesarean birth.

B. CARDIOVASCULAR ADAPTATION

- Closure of the ductus arteriosus causes blood to flow to the lungs for oxygenation.
- Closure of the foramen ovale directs blood from the right atrium to the right ventricle.

- Closure of the ductus venosus causes blood to pass through the liver for filtration.
- Dilation of the pulmonary vessels allows blood flow into lungs.
- Closure is functional at first and not permanent for weeks after birth. It can be reversed in the early days.

C. NEUROLOGICAL ADAPTATION

Thermoregulation

- Neonates lose heat by four methods.
  - Evaporation from exposure of wet surfaces to air and from insensible water loss from the skin and respiratory tract; examples include amniotic fluid on the skin at birth, bathing.
  - Conduction from direct contact with objects cooler than the infant's skin (cold hands, circumcision restraint boards, etc.); heat can be gained by conduction too (warm blankets, the mother's skin).
  - Convection: heat transfers to air surrounding the infant (air conditioning, people moving).
  - Radiation: heat transfers to cooler objects that are not in direct contact with the infant (cold windows, outside walls, walls of incubators).
- Effects of cold stress
  - Increased metabolism (with increased use of glucose and oxygen)
  - Decreased surfactant production
  - Respiratory distress
  - Hypoglycemia
  - Metabolic acidosis
  - Jaundice
- Cold stress may lead to nonshivering *thermogenesis*, the oxidation of brown fat to produce heat.

- It begins before there is a change in core (rectal) temperature.
- It produces fatty acids that interfere with bilirubin transport and increase risk for jaundice.

- Neutral thermal environment is a temperature at which infants maintain a stable body temperature without an increase in oxygen or metabolic rate. The range of neutral thermal environmental temperatures is 32–34°C (89.6–93.2°F) for healthy, unclothed, full-term newborns.

- Hyperthermia
  - Caused by overheating from poorly regulated heating equipment (radiant warmers, warming lights, or incubators)
  - Increases metabolic rate and need for oxygen and glucose
  - Vasodilation causes insensible fluid losses

D. HEMATOLOGICAL ADAPTATION

- Normal breakdown of unneeded erythrocytes may cause physiologic jaundice (see Hyperbilirubinemia, p. 234).
- Polycythemia increases the risk of jaundice and may damage the brain or other organs from stasis.
- High leukocyte levels do not necessarily indicate infection. Increased numbers of immature leukocytes or decreased platelets are signs of infection.
- Newborns cannot synthesize vitamin K, which is necessary for normal clotting, until normal flora are established in the intestines.
- Maternal intake of drugs such as phenytoin, phenobarbital, or aspirin during pregnancy interferes with clotting ability in the newborn.
- See Laboratory Values in the Newborn, Appendix B.

E. GASTROINTESTINAL SYSTEM

- The stomach capacity is about 6 mL/kg at birth but expands to about 90 mL within the first few days of life.
- The stomach empties within 2–4 hours of feedings.
- Regurgitation often occurs due to the relaxed cardiac sphincter.
- Normal intestinal flora are established within a few days of birth.
- The stools pass through three stages.
  - Meconium stools are thick, sticky, tar-like, greenish-black in color, and are usually passed within 24 hours of birth. Suspect obstruction if meconium is not passed within 36–48 hours.
  - Transitional stools are greenish–brown and looser in consistency.
  - Milk stools are characteristic of the type of feeding the infant receives.
    - Breast milk stools are seedy, mustard color, very soft, with a sweet-sour smell. Newborn should have at least three stools a day, but may have ten or more.
    - Formula stools are pale yellow to light brown, firm, and have the odor of feces. Newborn may have one or several daily.

F. HEPATIC SYSTEM

- A blood glucose level below 40 mg/dL in the term infant indicates hypoglycemia. See "Hypoglycemia," pp. 240, and "Procedure: Blood Glucose Screening for Newborns," p. 424.
- The liver conjugates bilirubin by the following steps.
  - Unconjugated bilirubin travels on plasma albumin binding sites to the liver.
  - It is changed to the conjugated form by glucuronyl transferase passed into the bile and the duodenum.

- The conjugated bilirubin is reduced to urobilinogen by normal intestinal flora and is excreted in the stool.
- A small percentage of conjugated bilirubin is deconjugated by the intestinal enzyme β-glucuronidase, reabsorbed into the bloodstream and carried back to the liver, where it must be conjugated again for excretion.

G. URINARY SYSTEM

- The first voiding is usually within 24 hours of birth. Suspect hypovolemia due to inadequate intake or kidney abnormalities if there is no void within 48 hours. Normal voiding pattern is 2–6 per day during first days, then 5–25 daily.
- Normal urine output is 1–3 mL/kg/hr.
- Normal specific gravity is 1.001–1.020. Large increases in fluids (such as excess intravenous fluid) cause fluid overload.
- Seventy-eight percent of the newborn's body is water, with much of it in the extracellular spaces where it can be easily lost.
- Insensible water loss occurs due to the large body surface area, rapid respiratory rate, and radiant heaters.
- Daily fluid need is 65 mL/kg (30 mL/pound) during the first 2 days of life, then 100–150 mL/kg (45–68 mL/pound).
- Maintenance of acid-base and electrolyte balance may be precarious.
- Ability to filter waste products from the blood is decreased.
- Urate crystals may leave a pink stain on the diaper, but this is normal.

H. IMMUNE SYSTEM

- The hypothalamus and inflammatory responses are immature. Leukocytes may be slow to respond and inefficient. Fever and leukocytosis are often not present in the newborn with infection.

- Immunoglobulins (serum globulins with antibody activity) help protect newborns from infection.
  - IgG from the mother provides temporary immunity to bacteria and viruses to which the mother has developed immunity. Preterm infants may have much less IgG. Most passive immunity lasts about 3 months.
  - IgM is produced by the infant and helps protect against gram-negative bacteria. High IgM levels indicate exposure to infection in utero because it does not cross the placenta.
  - IgA is not produced in adequate amounts until 6–12 weeks after birth. It helps protect the gastrointestinal and respiratory systems. A form of IgA is present in colostrum and breast milk.

I. PSYCHOSOCIAL ADAPTATION

Periods of Reactivity

In the early hours after birth, the infant goes through changes called the periods of reactivity.

- First period of reactivity
  - Infants are active, alert, and often interested in breastfeeding.
  - Respirations are as high as 80 breaths/minute. There may be crackles, retractions, nasal flaring, and increased mucus secretions.
  - The heart rate may be as high as 180 beats/minute.
  - After about 30 minutes, the infant becomes sleepy.
- Period of sleep
  - This period lasts about 2–4 hours.
  - Pulse and respirations are normal, temperature may be low.
- Second period of reactivity
  - This period lasts about 4–6 hours.

- Infants are alert, interested in feeding, and may pass meconium.
- Infants may have increased pulse and respirations, cyanosis, or apnea.
- Infants may gag or regurgitate and have increased mucus secretions.

Behavioral States

There are six different behavior states in the newborn.

- Quiet sleep state
  - Deep sleep without eye movements
  - Quiet, regular respirations
  - Little or no response to noise or stimuli
- Active sleep state
  - Movement, startles from disturbances, brief fussing
  - Rapid, irregular respirations
  - Rapid eye movements (REM)
  - May return to sleep or awaken
- Drowsy state
  - Eyes closed or glazed and unfocused
  - Startling, slow movement
  - May progress to sleep or awake states
- Quiet alert state
  - Intense gazing at objects or people
  - Excellent time for bonding
- Active alert state
  - Fussy, restless, seems aware of discomfort
  - Respirations faster and irregular
- Crying state
  - Continuous, lusty crying

II. NURSING ASSESSMENTS

A. INITIAL ASSESSMENTS

- Examine the infant immediately after birth for respiratory problems and obvious anomalies. Intervene appropriately.
- When infant is stable, perform a more thorough assessment. See Table III-1, "Summary of Newborn Assessments."
- Assess vital signs every 30 minutes until stable for 2 hours. See "Procedure: Vital Sign Assessments," p. 428.

B. DOCUMENTATION

Record all marks, bruises, rashes, or other abnormalities.

- Describe location, size, color, elevation, and texture of each mark.
- Record subsequent changes in appearance.

C. ASSESSMENT OF GESTATIONAL AGE

- This assessment determines the number of weeks from conception to birth based on physical and neurological characteristics. The New Ballard Score (Fig. III-1) is frequently used.
- Neuromuscular characteristics
  - Posture and degree of flexion: Observe the position of the infant at rest.
  - Square window sign: Measure the angle between the palm and the forearm when the hand is bent at the wrist as far as possible.
  - Arm recoil: Measure the degree of flexion after the infant's arms are fully flexed at the elbows for 5 seconds, pulled straight down to the sides, and released.
  - Popliteal angle: Measure the angle at the popliteal space when the thigh is flexed against the abdomen and the lower leg is straightened.

TABLE III-1

Summary of Newborn Assessment

NORMAL AND NORMAL VARIATIONS	ABNORMAL (COMMON CAUSES)	NURSING ACTIONS

Initial Assessment

Assess for obvious problems first. If infant is stable and has no problems that require immediate attention, continue with complete assessment.

Vital Signs

See "Procedure: Vital Sign Assessments," p. 428.

Temperature

36.5–37.5° C (97.7–99.5° F) axillary, 36.5–37.6° C (97.7–99.7° F) rectal. Axillary is the preferred site.	*Decreased* (infection, hypoglycemia, CNS problem, cold environment). *Increased* (infection, environment too warm).	*Decreased*: Institute warming measures and check in 30 minutes. Check blood glucose. *Increased*: Remove excessive clothing. Check for dehydration. *Decreased or increased*: Look for signs of infection. Check radiant warmer temperature setting. Check thermometer for accuracy. Report abnormals to physician.

SECTION THREE: Normal Newborn 197

Pulses

Heart rate at 120–160/minute (100 sleeping, 180 crying). Rhythm regular. Point of maximum impulse (PMI) at the 3rd to 4th intercostal space, slightly to the left of the midclavicular line, may be visible. Brachial, femoral, and pedal pulses present and equal bilaterally.	Tachycardia (respiratory problems, anemia, infection, cardiac conditions). Bradycardia (asphyxia, increased intracranial pressure). PMI to the right (dextrocardia, pneumothorax). Absent or unequal pulses (coarctation of the aorta). Murmurs (functional or congenital heart defects) and arrhythmias should be assessed by skilled practitioners.	Note the location of murmurs. Report abnormal rates, rhythms, sounds, pulses.

Respirations

Rate 30–60 (average 30–40) per minute. Respirations irregular, shallow, unlabored. Chest movements symmetric. Breath sounds present and clear bilaterally.	Tachypnea, especially after the first hour. Slow respirations (maternal medications). Nasal flaring. Grunting (respiratory distress syndrome). Gasping (respiratory depression). Periods of apnea more than 20 seconds or with change in heart rate or color (respiratory depression, sepsis, cold stress). Asymmetry or decreased chest expansion (pneumothorax). Intercostal, xiphoid, subcostal, or supraclavicular retractions	Mild variations: continued monitoring. Expect to clear in early hours after birth. Persistent or severe: suction, give oxygen, call physician, and initiate more intensive care.

or seesaw respirations (respiratory distress). Coarse, rales, crackles, rhonchi (fluid in the lungs). Bowel sounds in the chest (diaphragmatic hernia).

Blood Pressure

Average 70 mm Hg systolic and 45 mm Hg diastolic. Varies with activity and gestational age.	Hypotension (hypovolemia, shock, sepsis). Difference of 20 mm Hg between the arms and the legs (coarctation of the aorta).	Report abnormal blood pressures. Prepare for intensive care if very low.

Measurements

See "Procedure: Weighing and Measuring the Newborn," p. 445.

Weight

Weight: 2500–4000 grams (5 pounds, 8 ounces–8 pounds, 13 ounces). Weight loss up to 10% in the early days.	*Above normal range* (LGA, maternal diabetes). *Below normal range* (SGA, preterm, multifetal pregnancy, medical conditions in mother that affect intrauterine growth). Weight loss above 10% (dehydration, feeding problems).	Determine cause. Monitor for complications common to cause.

Length

48–53 cm (19–21 inches).	*Below normal range* (SGA, congenital dwarf). *Above normal range* (LGA, maternal diabetes).	Determine cause. Monitor for complications common to the cause.

Head Circumference

33–35.5 cm (13–14 inches). Head approximately 1/4 of the infant's length.	*Small* (SGA, microcephaly, anencephaly). *Large* (LGA, hydrocephalus, increased intracranial pressure).	Determine cause. Monitor for complications common to the cause.

Chest Circumference

30.5–33 cm (12–13 inches). Generally 2–3 cm less than the head circumference.	Large (LGA). Small (SGA).	Determine cause. Monitor for complications common to the cause.

Posture

Flexed extremities resist extension, return quickly to flexed state. Hands usually clenched. Movements symmetrical. Slight tremors on crying. Breech—extended, stiff legs. "Molds" body to caretaker's when held, responds by quieting when needs met.	Limp, flaccid, "floppy," or rigid extremities (preterm, hypoxia, medications, CNS trauma). Hypertonic (fetal abstinence syndrome, CNS damage). Jitteriness or tremors (low glucose or calcium levels). Opisthotonos, seizures, stiff when held (CNS damage).	Seek cause, report abnormalities.

Cry

Lusty, strong.	High-pitched (increased intracranial pressure). Weak, absent, irritable, cat-like mewing (neurologic problems). Hoarse or crowing (laryngeal irritation).	Observe for changes, report abnormalities.

Skin

Color pink or tan (according to race) with acrocyanosis. Vernix caseosa in creases. Small amounts of lanugo over the shoulders, sides of the face, forehead, upper back. Skin turgor good with quick recoil. Some cracking and peeling of the skin.
Normal variations: Milia. Erythema toxicum (flea bite rash). Puncture on the scalp (from electrode). Mongolian spots. Telangiectatic nevi (nevus simplex or "stork bites").

Color: Cyanosis of the mouth and central areas (hypoxia). Pallor (anemia, hypoxia). Gray (hypoxia, hypotension). Red, sticky, transparent skin (very preterm). Ruddy (polycythemia). Greenish-brown discoloration of the skin, nails, cord (possible fetal compromise, postterm). Yellow vernix (blood incompatibilities). Jaundice (pathologic in the first 24 hours). Thick vernix (preterm).

Delivery marks: Bruises on the body (pressure), scalp (vacuum extractor) or face (cord around neck). Petechiae (pressure, low platelets, infection). Forceps marks. Birthmarks: Nevus flammeus (port wine stain). Nevus vasculosus (strawberry hemangioma). Café au lait spots (neurofibromatosis if more than 6 marks or > 1.5 cm).

(Normal Variations) Point out and explain normal skin variations to parents.

(Color) Differentiate facial bruising from cyanosis. Central cyanosis requires suction, oxygen and further treatment. Report jaundice in the first 24 hours. Watch for respiratory problems in infants with meconium staining. Look for other signs and complications of preterm or postterm birth.

(Delivery marks) Record location, size, shape, color, type of rashes and marks. Check for facial movement with forceps marks. Watch for jaundice with bruising.

Other: Excessive lanugo (preterm). Excessive peeling, cracking (postterm). Skin tags. Pustules or other rashes (infection). "Tenting" of skin (dehydration). Excessive peeling (postterm).

Head

Suture lines palpable with small separation between the bones. Anterior fontanelle diamond shaped, 4–5 cm across, soft and flat. May bulge slightly with crying. Posterior fontanelle triangular shaped, 0.5–1 cm in size. Hair silky and soft with individual hair strands. Normal variations: Bones overriding at suture lines (molding). Caput succedaneum or cephalhematoma (pressure during birth).

Head large (hydrocephalus, increased intracranial pressure) or small (microcephaly). Widely separated bones (hydrocephalus) or suture lines not palpable (craniosynostosis). Anterior fontanelle depressed (dehydration, molding) full or bulging at rest (increased intracranial pressure). Woolly, bunchy hair (preterm). Unusual hair growth (chromosomal abnormalities).

Seek cause of variations. Differentiate caput succedaneum from cephalhematoma, and teach/reassure parents of normal outcome. Watch for jaundice with cephalhematoma. Observe for signs of dehydration with depressed anterior fontanelle, increased intracranial pressure with bulging of fontanelle and wide separation of bones at suture lines. Refer for treatment.

Ears

Ears well formed and complete. Area where the upper ear meets the head even with line drawn from inner to the outer canthus of eye. Startle response to loud noises. Alerting to high-pitched voices.

Low-set ears (chromosomal disorders). Skin tags, preauricular sinuses, dimples (kidney anomalies). No response to sound (deafness).

Check voiding if ears are abnormal. Look for signs of chromosomal abnormality if position is abnormal. Refer for evaluation if infant does not respond to sound.

Face

Symmetrical in appearance and movement. Parts proportional and appropriately placed.

Asymmetry of the jaw (pressure and position in utero). Drooping of the mouth or one side of the face, "one sided cry" (facial nerve damage). Abnormal appearance (chromosomal abnormalities).

Seek cause of variations. Check delivery history for possible cause of damage to facial nerve.

Eyes

Symmetrical. Eyes clear. Transient strabismus. Scant or absent tears. Pupils equal, react to light. Alerts to interesting sights. Follows objects 180 degrees. Doll's eye sign and red reflex present. May have subconjunctival hemorrhage or edema of eyelids from pressure during delivery.

Inflammation or drainage (chemical or infectious conjunctivitis). Constant tearing (plugged lacrimal duct). Unequal pupils. Failure to follow objects (blindness). White areas over pupils (cataracts). Setting-sun sign (hydrocephalus).

Clean and monitor any drainage; seek cause. Reassure parents that subconjunctival hemorrhage and edema will clear. Refer other abnormalities for treatment.

Nose

Both nostrils open to air flow. May have slight flattening from pressure during birth.	Blockage of one or both nostrils—check by closing the mouth and one nostril at a time (choanal atresia). Malformations (congenital conditions). Flaring, mucus (respiratory distress).	Observe for respiratory distress, report malformations.

Mouth

Mouth, gums, tongue pink. Tongue normal in size and movement. Lips and palate intact. Sucking pads. Sucking, rooting, swallowing, gag reflexes present. Normal variations: Precocious teeth. Epstein's pearls.	Cyanosis (hypoxia). White patches on cheeks or tongue (candidiasis). Protruding tongue (Down syndrome). Diminished movement of tongue, drooping mouth (facial nerve paralysis). Unilateral or bilateral cleft lip and/or palate. Absent or weak reflexes (preterm, neurological problem). Excessive drooling (tracheoesophageal fistula, esophageal atresia).	Administer oxygen for cyanosis. Expect loose teeth to be removed. Expect nystatin medication for *Candida*. Check the mother for *Candida* vaginal or breast infection. Refer anomalies for treatment.

Feeding

Good suck/swallow coordination. Retains feedings.	Poorly coordinated suck and swallow. Duskiness or cyanosis during feeding (cardiac defects). Choking, gagging, excessive drooling (tracheoesophageal fistula, esophageal atresia).	Feed slowly. Stop frequently if infant has difficulty. Suction and stimulate if necessary. Remove stomach contents if infant has distended upper abdomen and may have swallowed blood, amniotic fluid, or meconium. Refer infants with continued difficulty for further investigation.

Neck/Clavicles

Short neck turns head easily side to side. Infant raises the head when prone. Clavicles intact.	Weakness, contractures, or rigidity (muscle abnormalities). Webbing of the neck or large fat pad at back of the neck (chromosomal disorders). Crepitus, lump, or crying when clavicle is palpated, with diminished or absent movement of the arm on that side (fractured clavicle).	Fracture of the clavicle occurs especially in large infants with shoulder dystocia at birth. Immobilize the arm. Look for other injuries. Refer abnormalities.

Chest

Cylinder shape. Xiphoid process may be prominent. Symmetrical. Nipples present and located properly. May have engorgement, white nipple discharge (maternal hormone withdrawal).	Asymmetry (diaphragmatic hernia, pneumothorax). Supernumerary nipples. Redness (infection).	Report abnormalities.

Abdomen

Rounded, soft. Bowel sounds present soon after birth. Liver palpable 1–3 cm below the costal margin. Skin intact. Three vessels in the cord. Clamp tight and the cord drying. Meconium passed within 24–48 hours. Urine passed within 24 hours. Normal variation: Brick dust staining of the diaper (urate crystals).

Sunken abdomen (diaphragmatic hernia). Distended abdomen or loops of bowel visible (obstruction, infection, enlarged organs). Absent bowel sounds after the first hour (paralytic ileus). Masses palpated (kidney tumors, distended bladder). Enlarged liver (infection, heart failure, hemolytic disease). Abdominal wall defects (umbilical or inguinal hernia, omphalocele, gastroschisis, exstrophy of the bladder). Two vessels in the cord (other anomalies). Bleeding (loose clamp). Redness, drainage from the cord (infection). No passage of meconium (imperforate anus, obstruction). Lack of urinary output (kidney problems) or inadequate amounts (dehydration).

Refer abnormalities. Look for other anomalies if only two vessels are present in the cord. Tighten or replace loose cord clamp. If stool and urine output are abnormal, check to see that none were unrecorded, increase feedings, report.

Genitals—Female

Labia majora dark, covers the clitoris and the labia minora. Small amount of white mucus vaginal discharge. Urinary meatus and vagina present. Normal variations: Vaginal bleeding (pseudo-menstruation). Hymenal tags.

Clitoris and labia minora larger than labia majora (preterm) Large clitoris (ambiguous genitalia). Edematous labia (breech birth).

Check gestational age for immature genitalia. Report anomalies.

Genitals—Male

Testes within the scrotal sac, rugae on the scrotum, prepuce nonretractable. Meatus at the tip of the penis.

Testes in the inguinal canal or abdomen (preterm, cryptorchidism). Lack of rugae on the scrotum (preterm). Edema of the scrotum (pressure in breech birth). Enlarged scrotal sac (hydrocele). Small penis, scrotum (preterm, ambiguous genitalia). Urinary meatus located on the upper side of the penis (epispadius), underside of penis (hypospadius), or perineum.

Check the gestational age for immature genitalia. Report anomalies. Explain to the parents why no circumcision can be performed with abnormal placement of the meatus.

Extremities

Upper and Lower Extremities

Equal and bilateral movement of the extremities. Correct number and formation of the fingers and toes. Nails to the end of the digits or slightly beyond. Flexion, good muscle tone.	Crepitus, redness, lumps, swelling (fracture). Diminished or absent movement, especially during the Moro reflex (fracture, nerve damage, paralysis). Polydactyly (note the presence or absence of a bone in extra digits). Syndactyly (webbing), or fused or absent digits. Poor muscle tone (preterm, neurological damage, hypoglycemia, hypoxia).	Report all anomalies, look for others.

Upper Extremities

Two transverse palm creases.	Simian crease (single transverse palm crease)(Down syndrome). Diminished movement of arm with extension and forearm prone (Erb-Duchenne paralysis).	Report all anomalies, look for others.

Lower Extremities

Legs equal in length, abduct equally, gluteal and thigh creases and knee height equal, no hip click. Normal position of the feet.

Resistance when one leg is abducted, unequal thigh or gluteal creases, hip click, movement of head of the femur (Ortalani and Barlow tests) unequal leg length (developmental dysplasia of the hip). Malposition of the feet which may or may not be manually manipulated into a normal position (position in utero, talipes equinovarus).

Report all anomalies, look for others.

Back

No openings observed or felt in the vertebral column. Anus patent.

Failure of the vertebra to close (spina bifida), with or without a sac with spinal fluid and meninges (meningocele) and/or cord (myelomeningocele) enclosed. Tuft of hair over a spina bifida occulta. Pilonidal dimple or sinus. Imperforate anus.

Report abnormalities. Observe for movement below the level of the defect. If sac is present, cover with sterile dressings wet with sterile saline. Protect from injury.

Reflexes

Moro, palmar and plantar grasp, rooting, sucking, swallowing, tonic neck, Babinski, Gallant, and stepping reflexes present. See Table III-2, "Summary of Newborn Reflexes."	Absent, asymmetric or weak reflexes (neurological damage).	Observe for signs of fractures, nerve damage, or injury to the central nervous system.

Figure III-1

New Ballard Score

NEWBORN MATURITY RATING & CLASSIFICATION

ESTIMATION OF GESTATIONAL AGE BY MATURITY RATING
Symbols: X - 1st Exam   O - 2nd Exam

NEUROMUSCULAR MATURITY

	−1	0	1	2	3	4	5
Posture							
Square window (wrist)	>90°	90°	60°	45°	30°	0°	
Arm Recoil		180°	140°–180°	110°–140°	90°–110°	<90°	
Popliteal Angle	180°	160°	140°	120°	100°	90°	<90°
Scarf Sign							
Heel to Ear							

PHYSICAL MATURITY

Skin	sticky friable transparent	gelatinous red, translucent	smooth pink, visible veins	superficial peeling &/or rash, few veins	cracking pale areas rare veins	parchment deep cracking no vessels	leathery cracked wrinkled
Lanugo	none	sparse	abundant	thinning	bald areas	mostly bald	
Plantar Surface	heel-toe 40-50 mm: −1 <40 mm: −2	>50 mm no crease	faint red marks	anterior transverse crease only	creases ant. 2/3	creases over entire sole	
Breast	imperceptible	barely perceptible	flat areola no bud	stippled areola 1-2 mm bud	raised areola 3-4 mm bud	full areola 5-10 mm bud	
Eye/Ear	lids fused loosely: −1 tightly: −2	lids open pinna flat stays folded	sl. curved pinna; soft; slow recoil	well-curved pinna; soft but ready recoil	formed & firm; instant recoil	thick cartilage ear stiff	
Genitalia male	scrotum flat, smooth	scrotum empty faint rugae	testes in upper canal rare rugae	testes descending few rugae	testes down good rugae	testes pendulous deep rugae	
Genitalia female	clitoris prominent labia flat	prominent clitoris small labia minora	prominent clitoris enlarging minora	majora & minora equally prominent	majora large minora small	majora cover clitoris & minora	

SECTION THREE: Normal Newborn 211

Gestation by Dates_____wks

Birth Date_____Hour_____am/pm

APGAR_____1 min_____5 min

MATURITY RATING

score	weeks
-10	20
-5	22
0	24
5	26
10	28
15	30
20	32
25	34
30	36
35	38
40	40
45	42
50	44

SCORING SECTION

	1st Exam=X	2nd Exam=O
Estimating Gest Age by Maturity Rating	_____Weeks	_____Weeks
Time of Exam	Date_____ Hour_____ am/pm	Date_____ Hour_____ am/pm
Age at Exam	_____Hours	_____Hours
Signature of Examiner	_____ M.D.	_____ M.D.

New Ballard score. (Courtesy of Bristol-Myers Company, Evansville, Indiana. From Ballard, J.L., Khoury, J.C., Wedig, K., Wang, L., Eilers-Walsman, B.L., & Lipp, R. [1991]. New Ballard score, expanded to include extremely premature infants. *Journal of Pediatrics*, 19(3), 417–423.)

- — Scarf sign: Note the position of the elbow when the infant's hand is brought to across the body as far as possible without lifting the shoulder.
- — Heel-to-ear: Note how far the leg will extend without resistance when the foot is grasped and pulled toward the ears. Keep the hips flat.

- Physical characteristics

Assess each of the following characteristics.

- — Skin: Color, visibility of veins, peeling and cracking
- — Lanugo: Amount and placement of lanugo
- — Plantar surface: Depth of plantar creases and amount of the foot covered by creases
- — Breasts: Size and development of the nipples, areolae, and subcutaneous fat pads (or breast buds)
- — Eye/ear: Eyelids—fused or open; ear incurving and stiffness; fold ear over and assess how quickly it returns to its original state
- — Genitals: Female—Size of the clitoris, labia minora, and labia majora. Male—Location of the testes, amount and depth of rugae on the scrotum.

- Determine gestational age and size
- — Compare the total score with the corresponding gestational age.
- — Plot the gestational age, weight, length, and head circumference on intrauterine development graph (Fig. III-2).

III. COMMON NURSING DIAGNOSES FOR NEWBORNS

- Ineffective airway clearance related to excessive secretions in the respiratory passages
- Ineffective thermoregulation related to immature compensation for changes in environmental temperature

- Altered nutrition, less than body requirements related to poor infant feeding behaviors
- Risk for infection related to break in skin integrity at cord or circumcision and immature immune system
- Risk for altered parenting related to stressors involved with new parenting role
- Health-seeking behaviors related to the desire for information about infant care

IV. NURSING INTERVENTIONS

A. USING CRITICAL PATHWAYS

Critical pathways are guides developed by birth facilities to see that all the tasks necessary to help infants and mothers prepare for discharge are accomplished in the time available. Pathways are individualized by each institution based on protocols to meet the needs of their clients.

B. GIVING EARLY CARE

Early care includes assessment, assignment of an Apgar score (see p. 131), and stabilization (see p. 130).

- Provide resuscitation if necessary (see p. 436)
- Check and record vital signs.
- Provide for identification: Take footprints, apply identification bands on the infant, mother, and support person.
- Perform overall assessment (see Table III-1, "Summary of Newborn Assessments").

C. POSITIONING AND SUCTIONING SECRETIONS

- Position the infant with the head slightly lower than the extremities to drain fluid from the respiratory passages immediately after birth.

Figure III-2

Intrauterine Growth Grids

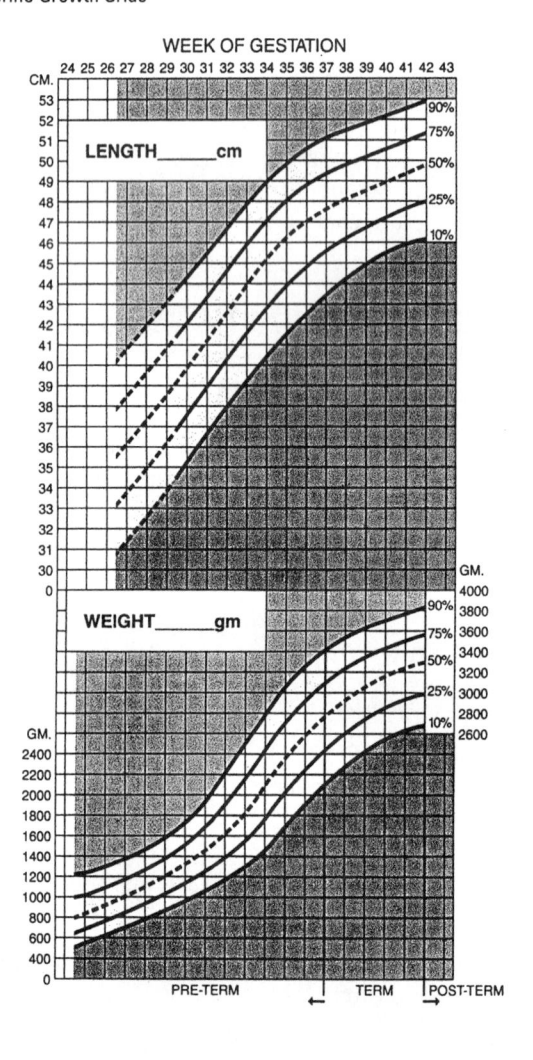

	1st Exam (X)	2nd Exam (O)
LARGE FOR GESTATIONAL AGE (LGA)		
APPROPRIATE FOR GESTATIONAL AGE (AGA)		
SMALL FOR GESTATIONAL AGE (SGA)		
Age at Exam	hrs	hrs
Signature of Examiner	M.D.	M.D.

SECTION THREE: Normal Newborn 215

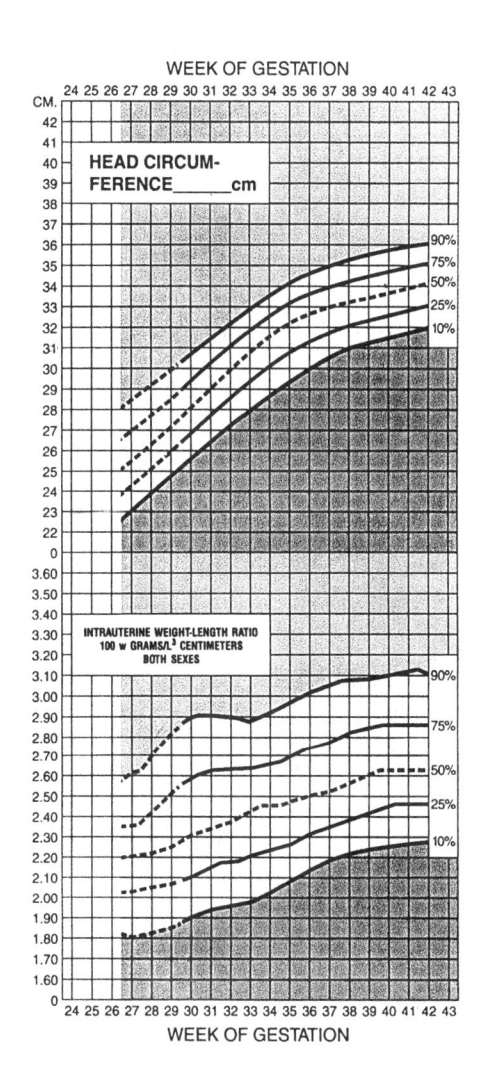

Symbols: X – 1st exam, O – 2nd exam.

(Courtesy of Bristol-Myers Company, Evansville, Indiana. Adapted from Lubchenko, L.C., Hansman, C., & Boyd, E. [1966]. *Pediatrics*, 37, 403. Adapted by permission of *Pediatrics*, Vol. 37, p. 403, 1966; and from Battaglia, F.C., & Lubchenko, L.C. [1967]. *Journal of Pediatrics*, 71, 159.)

- Return the infant to a flat position and position on the side to promote drainage of secretions.
- Use the bulb syringe frequently to suction secretions from the mouth or nose. (See "Procedure: Bulb Syringe Use," p. 445.)
- If mechanical suctioning is necessary, choose a small catheter to avoid damaging the tissues. Suction for no more than 5 seconds at a time using minimal negative pressure to avoid trauma, laryngospasm, and bradycardia.

D. MAINTAINING THERMOREGULATION

- Prevent heat loss
  — Perform initial assessments with the infant under a radiant warmer. Set the servocontrol between 36.0–36.5°C (96.8–97.7°F).
  — Dry the infant immediately after birth. Cover the infant's head with a cap when the infant is not under a radiant warmer.
  — Warm anything that comes in contact with the infant. Pad cool surfaces such as scales before placing infants on them. Warm stethoscopes and clothing before using them on the infant.
  — Bathe the infant to remove blood and excessive vernix as soon after birth as the temperature is stable. Dry quickly. Keep the infant under a warmer until the temperature is stable.
  — Wrap the infant in double warm blankets and add a hat when moving the infant to a crib.
  — Position the newborn's crib or incubator away from outside walls or windows.
  — Avoid exposing infants to drafts. Reduce traffic near radiant warmers as movement increases air currents.
  — Expose only parts of the infant's body necessary for assessment or care.
- Restore thermoregulation as necessary with warm blankets or place the infant back under a radiant warmer for a short time.

- Perform expanded assessments if temperature remains low.
  - Assess for signs of respiratory distress from the additional oxygen requirement.
  - Test the blood glucose level and feed the infant warm milk to provide glucose.
  - Observe for signs of infection, because low temperature is a common sign of infection.

E. ADMINISTERING PROPHYLACTIC MEDICATIONS

- Vitamin K
  - Given to prevent hemorrhagic disease of the newborn
  - Give only after the infant is bathed if the mother is hepatitis B- or HIV-positive
  - See Procedure: Intramuscular Injection Administration for Newborns," p. 419, and "Drug Guide: Vitamin K1 (Phytonadione)," p. 467.
- Eye treatment
  - Prophylactic antibiotic such as erythromycin is applied to the eyes to prevent ophthalmia neonatorum in case the mother is infected with gonorrhea. It also prevents Chlamydial infection.
  - See "Drug Guide: Erythromycin Ophthalmic Ointment," p. 450.
  - Mild inflammation occurs in some infants.
  - Purulent discharge from the eyes may indicate infection.

F. MAINTAINING BLOOD GLUCOSE

- Check blood glucose of infants with signs of hypoglycemia or according to agency policy. See "Hypoglycemia," p. 240.
- Feed Infants who have low glucose levels according to agency policy (e.g., if glucose screening test is 45 mg/dL or less).

- Retest according to agency policy (e.g., 1 hour after the first test and every 2 hours for the next 6 hours if level is low). See "Procedure: Blood Glucose Screening for Newborns," p. 424.
- Notify the primary caregiver if the glucose level remains low.

G. CONTINUING ASSESSMENTS

- Assess infant at the beginning of each shift.
- Focus on changes from the original assessment.
- Assess vital signs once a shift or more often if there are abnormalities.
- Weigh infants every 24 hours at the same time of day.
- Observe chest expansion and note signs of respiratory distress.
- Examine all areas of skin for new marks or changes in existing ones.
- Palpate fontanelles with infants in a slightly upright position. Note changes in molding, caput succedaneum, cephalhematoma.
- Observe eyes for inflammation or drainage.
- Note level of alertness, reflexes (Table III-2), and changes in behavior.
- Observe movement of extremities to see that it is equal.
- Check the cord for bleeding, purulent drainage, or redness at the base.
- Observe type and number of stools and frequency of voidings.
- Assess feeding behavior. Note regurgitation or feeding difficulties.

H. IDENTIFYING INFANTS AND MOTHERS

- Ensure that the infant's identification bands are in place.
- Use the imprinted number to identify the mother and the infant every time the mother and infant are separated. See "Procedure: Infant Identification," p. 431.

I. GIVING FEEDINGS

- Give (or help mothers give) the first feeding. Watch for cyanosis or choking. If either occurs, stop feeding, suction, and stimulate the infant. Continue feeding when the infant has recovered.
- Determine if the infant is feeding adequately (every 2–3 hours if breastfed, every 4 hours if formula-fed).
- Record each feeding with type, amount (or length of nursing period), regurgitation, and parents' understanding of feeding method.
- Position infants on the side after feedings to promote emptying of the stomach.

J. CARING FOR THE SKIN

- Remove the cord clamp 24 hours after birth if the end of the cord is dry.
- Teach parents to clean the cord with alcohol at least three times a day until the cord falls off at approximately 10–14 days. Demonstrate how to fold the diaper below the cord to keep it dry.
- Explain diaper area care to parents.
- Teach parents of uncircumcised boys that the foreskin may not retract for 3 years or more. It should not be forcibly retracted.

TABLE III-2

Summary of Neonatal Reflexes

METHOD OF TESTING	EXPECTED RESPONSE	ABNORMAL RESPONSE/ POSSIBLE CAUSE
Babinski		
Stroke the lateral sole of the foot from the heel to across the base of the toes	Toes flare with dorsiflexion of the big toe. Disappears by 12 months.	No response. Bilateral: CNS deficit. Unilateral: Local nerve damage.
Gallant (Trunk Incurvation)		
Lightly stroke the back, lateral to the vertebral column	Entire trunk flexes toward the side stimulated. Disappears by 1 month.	No response. CNS deficit.
Grasp (Palmer and Plantar)		
Press finger against the base of the fingers or toes	Fingers curl tightly, toes curl forward. Palmar: lessens by 3–4 months, disappears by 5–6 months. Plantar: disappears by 8–9 months.	Weak or absent. Neurologic deficit or muscle damage.
Moro		
Let the infant's head drop back approximately 30 degrees	Sharp extension and abduction of the arms with the thumbs and forefingers in "C" position. Followed by flexion and adduction to "embrace" position. Legs follow a similar pattern. Disappears by 6 months.	Absent: CNS dysfunction. Asymmetry: brachial plexus injury, paralysis, or fractured clavicle or bone of the extremity. Exaggerated: maternal drug use.

Rooting

Touch or stroke the side of the cheek near the mouth	Infant turns to the side touched. Difficult to elicit if infant is sleeping or just fed. Disappears by 3–4 months.	Weak or absent: prematurity, neurologic deficit, depression from maternal drug use.

Startle

Make a loud noise	Similar to the Moro but the hands remain clenched. Disappears by 4 months.	Weak or absent: Neurologic damage, deafness.

Stepping

Hold the infant so the feet touch a solid surface	Infant lifts alternate feet as if walking. Disappears by 4–7 months.	Asymmetry: Fracture of extremity, neurologic deficit.

Sucking

Place a nipple or finger in the mouth, rub against the palate	Infant begins to suck. Weak if recently fed. Disappears by 1 year	Weak or absent: prematurity, neurologic deficit, maternal drug use

Swallowing

Place fluid on the back of the tongue	Infant swallows fluid. Should be coordinated with sucking. Present throughout life.	Coughing, gagging, choking, cyanosis. Tracheoesophageal fistula, esophageal atresia, neurologic deficit.

Tonic Neck Reflex

Gently turn the head to one side while infant is supine	Extension of the extremities on the side to which head is turned with flexion on the opposite side. Disappears by 4 months.	Prolonged period of time in position: neurologic deficit.

K. PREVENTING HYPERBILIRUBINEMIA

- Intervene when infants feed poorly to promote stool passage, which aids bilirubin excretion.
- Notify primary caregiver of increasing jaundice so treatment may begin early.
- See "Hyperbilirubinemia," p. 234.

L. CARING FOR THE CIRCUMCISED INFANT

- Circumcision is the removal of the prepuce (foreskin) that covers the glans penis. The infant should be at least 12 hours old so that he has recovered from the stress of birth.
- Preparation
  - Obtain informed consent from the parents.
  - Inform the physician of any contraindications to circumcision.
  - Withhold feedings for 2–4 hours before the procedure to prevent regurgitation and possible aspiration.
  - Gather equipment and supplies. Place a bulb syringe nearby.
  - When the physician and equipment are ready, place the infant on a circumcision board.
  - Provide for warmth during the procedure.
  - Comfort the infant during and after the procedure.
- Aftercare
  - Gomco clamp: Place petroleum jelly or antibiotic ointment over the circumcision site. Plastibell: Do not use petroleum jelly.
  - If excessive bleeding occurs, apply steady pressure to the penis with sterile gauze and notify the physician.
- Parent teaching
  - Call the physician for signs of complications.
    - Bleeding more than a few drops with first diaper changes

- Failure to urinate
- Signs of infection: fever or low temperature, foul-smelling drainage
- Displacement of the Plastibell
— Apply petroleum jelly to the penis with each diaper change for the first 24–48 hours. If a Plastibell was used, do not apply petroleum jelly.
— Fasten the diaper loosely to prevent rubbing or pressure on the incision site.
— Do not remove the normal yellow crust that forms over the site.
— The circumcision site should be fully healed in approximately 10 days.
— If a Plastibell was used, the plastic rim will fall off in 5–8 days.

M. PROVIDING TEACHING

- Assess the parents' interaction with the infant and knowledge of infant care.
- Make a teaching plan.
- Use demonstrations and return demonstrations, videos, and pamphlets in the parents' language.
- Document all teaching performed and the parents' ability to care for the infant.
- Usual topics include handling the infant, use of bulb syringe, feeding techniques, taking an axillary temperature, elimination norms, and skin care (cord, diaper area, circumcision, bathing).

N. PREVENTING INFECTION

- Scrub hands and arms at the beginning of the shift. Wash hands before and after touching infants. Teach parents and visitors hand washing.

224 Clinical Manual for Foundations of Maternal Newborn Nursing

- Keep each infant's supplies separate from those used for other infants to avoid cross-contamination.

- Keep staff or visitors with infections away from infants. If the mother has an infection, consult with the physician as to whether the infant can be with her and can breastfeed. The presence and degree of maternal fever, organisms responsible, and medications will be considered.

- Observe for signs of neonatal infection (temperature instability, poor feeding, lethargy, or periods of apnea). See "Sepsis," p. 270.

O. PREVENTING INFANT ABDUCTION

- All personnel must wear appropriate identification at all times.

- Teach parents to allow only staff with proper identification to take their infants from them.

- Never give an infant to anyone without an identification bracelet or other proper identification.

- Never leave infants unattended in a room or hallway at any time.

- Teach parents to return infants to the nursery if they cannot be observed at all times.

- Position infants' cribs away from doorways when in the mothers' rooms.

- Transport infants only in cribs. Question anyone walking in the hallway carrying an infant.

- Question anyone with a newborn near an exit or in an unusual part of the facility.

- Be suspicious of visitors who move from room to room, ask detailed questions about nursery or discharge routines, or carry large bags or packages that could contain an infant.

- Follow unit policy for security. Keep remote exits locked, codes secret, and respond quickly if an alarm sounds.

- Alert hospital security when any suspicious activity occurs.

P. PROVIDING IMMUNIZATION FOR HEPATITIS

- Give hepatitis vaccine according to agency policy and exposure to mothers with acute or chronic hepatitis. See "Drug Guide: Hepatitis Vaccine," p. 452.

- Give hepatitis B immune globulin (HBIG) within 12 hours of birth to infants exposed to hepatitis during birth.

Q. ARRANGING NEWBORN SCREENING TESTS

- Screening tests detect inborn errors of metabolism or other genetic conditions that may cause mental retardation or other serious problems unless treated early.

- Screening for phenylketonuria, hypothyroidism, galactosemia, and hemoglobinopathies are most common.

- Tests performed on blood samples obtained during the first 24 hours of life should be repeated within 1–2 weeks of age.

R. PROVIDING FOLLOW-UP CARE

- Follow-up care should be provided within 2–3 days of discharge to all newborns discharged within 48 hours after birth.

- Care may occur in the home, clinic, or office. Home visits by a nurse and telephone contact are common.

- Explain options available to parents and help them make plans.

V. COMPLICATIONS OF NEWBORN

A. ASPHYXIA

Asphyxia is a lack of oxygen and increase of carbon dioxide in the blood.

Etiology and Predisposing Factors

- Complications during pregnancy, labor, or birth increase the risk for asphyxia.
- Maternal narcotic use shortly before birth may lead to newborn depression and failure to breathe spontaneously.

Clinical Signs

- Primary apnea consists of a few gasping breaths at birth followed by apnea and bradycardia.
- Secondary apnea consists of loss of consciousness and metabolic acidosis. Immediate resuscitation is necessary to prevent permanent damage or death.

Therapeutic Management

See "Procedure: Performing Resuscitation in Newborns," p. 436.

Nursing Considerations

- Have equipment readily available and functioning properly at all times to prevent delays.
- Begin resuscitation measures quickly, as necessary. Primary asphyxia will progress to secondary asphyxia without immediate intervention.
- Assist the physician with intubation, insertion of umbilical vein catheters, and administration of medications.
- Once the infant is stabilized, assess for further complications.
- Support parents and explain infant's condition.

B. BRONCHOPULMONARY DYSPLASIA (BPD)

Bronchopulmonary dysplasia is a serious, chronic lung condition that occurs most often in preterm infants.

Etiology and Predisposing Factors

Treatment with oxygen and mechanical ventilation may cause damage to the lungs, resulting in prolonged oxygen need. It is more common as birth weight and gestational age decrease.

Clinical Signs

- Need for prolonged treatment with mechanical ventilation
- Need for oxygen for more than 28 days of life
- X-ray: characteristic lung changes

Therapeutic Management

Treatment is supportive with gradual decrease in the amount of oxygen, bronchodilators, corticosteroids, diuretics, and antibiotics as necessary. The infant may go home on long-term oxygen therapy.

Nursing Considerations

- Assess respiratory status frequently.
- Monitor infant's blood oxygen levels and adjust oxygen as indicated.
- Determine infant response to medications.
- Teach parents for home care.

C. CLEFT LIP AND PALATE

These conditions are due to failure of the structures to close in the embryo. They may occur alone or together and affect one or both sides of the mouth.

Etiology and Predisposing Factors

Genetic and environmental factors may be involved. These conditions make up one part of a number of anomalies in some syndromes.

Clinical Signs

- Cleft lip: Minor notching of the lip or extensive cleft through the lip and into the floor of the nose
- Cleft palate: Defect in the soft palate only or extending throughout the hard and soft palates
- Cleft lip and cleft palate: One or both sides involved

Therapeutic Management

- Lip surgery within days or weeks of birth
- Palate surgery in stages, depending on degree
- Long term follow-up for orthodontia, speech therapy, hearing problems

Nursing Considerations

- Palpate the hard and the soft palate during the initial assessment to find less obvious clefts.
- Experiment with feeding techniques.
    - Breastfeeding, for interested mothers
    - Soft preemie nipples directed away from a cleft palate
    - Nipples with enlarged holes
    - Compressible bottles
    - Special long nipples that extend beyond a cleft palate
    - Nipples with extensions to cover a cleft palate
    - Medicine droppers
    - Asepto syringe with soft tubing attached
- Feed in an upright position to prevent aspiration.
- Feed slowly with frequent stops for burping.

- Wash away milk curds after feedings.
- Prevent infections.
- Support parents.
  — Show "before and after" pictures of plastic surgery.
  — Reinforce explanations of surgery.
  — Teach feeding techniques.
  — Explain need for long-term follow-up.

D. CONGENITAL CARDIAC DEFECTS

Common congenital heart defects include

- Ventricular septal defect: Small or large opening in the septum between the ventricles: this is the most common defect. It may cause pulmonary hypertension and heart failure or may close spontaneously.
- Patent ductus arteriosus: Failure of the vessel to close after birth; more common in preterm infants. Causes recirculation of blood to the lungs and pulmonary hypertension.
- Coarctation of the aorta: Narrowing of the aorta near the ductus arteriosus; causes increased pressure behind the defect and may cause heart failure.
- Transposition of the great vessels: Reversed positions of the aorta and pulmonary artery; fatal without presence of another defect that allows mixing of oxygenated and unoxygenated blood.

Etiology and Predisposing Factors

- Often unknown
- Genetic factors
- Environmental factors such as teratogens or maternal rubella or diabetes
- May occur with other anomalies

Clinical Signs

Signs depend on the type and severity of the defect.

- Cyanosis—may increase with crying or feeding
- Pallor
- Murmurs
- Tachycardia
- Tachypnea
- Dyspnea
- Choking spells
- Falling asleep during feedings
- Diaphoresis

Therapeutic Management

- Testing, such as echocardiogram, cardiac catheterization, etc., to determine the type of defect
- Oxygen
- Surgery—corrective or palliative, as indicated
- Medications, such as digitalis, diuretics, potassium, sedatives

Nursing Considerations

- Assess for changes in condition.
- Reduce infant's need for oxygen by providing frequent rest periods.
- Feed by gavage for rapid respirations. Provide oxygen during feedings if necessary.
- Maintain oxygen at lowest level possible to maintain adequate oxygenation.
- Provide parental support and education about the infant's condition and expected treatment.

- Teach parents home care, including administration of medications, and signs of complications.

E. DIAPHRAGMATIC HERNIA

Diaphragmatic hernia is a failure of the diaphragm to close during fetal life, allowing intestines to pass through the opening into the chest; may cause failure of lung development.

Etiology and Predisposing Factors

- Due to failure of the diaphragm to close before birth
- Exact cause unknown, genetic and environmental factors

Clinical Signs

Signs vary according to the size of herniation and degree of lung development.

- Mild to severe respiratory distress at birth
- Breath sounds diminished over the affected area
- Barrel chest
- Heartbeat may be displaced to the right

Therapeutic Management

- May be diagnosed prenatally by ultrasound
- Endotracheal tube for ventilation
- Gastric tube to decompress stomach
- Surgery to replace the intestines and repair the defect when stable
- Extracorporeal membrane oxygenation (ECMO) may be used

Nursing Considerations

- Position infant on the affected side to allow the unaffected lung to expand.

- Elevate the head.
- Assist with ventilation.
- Monitor the respiratory status.

F. ERYTHROBLASTOSIS FETALIS

See "Hyperbilirubinemia, Complications," p. 234.

G. ESOPHAGEAL ATRESIA AND TRACHEOESOPHAGEAL FISTULA (TEF)

In these conditions, there is most commonly a division of the esophagus into two unconnected segments (atresia) with a blind pouch at the proximal end. The proximal or distal end may be connected to the trachea, resulting in TEF.

Etiology and Predisposing Factors

- Failure of the structures to form normally before birth
- Exact cause unknown

Clinical Signs

Signs vary by the type of anomaly.

- Excessive, frothy mucus
- Drooling
- Regurgitation
- Failure of a catheter to pass into the stomach
- Coughing, choking, cyanosis with feedings
- Distended stomach

Therapeutic Management

- Suspect with hydramnios during pregnancy
- Diagnosis by symptoms and x-ray

- Continuous suction to the upper pouch
- Gastrostomy tube
- Surgery to close the fistula and join the esophageal segments
- Long-term follow-up for esophageal reflux and dilation of strictures

Nursing Considerations

- Observe all infants carefully during the first feeding.
- Use a semi-upright position to prevent aspiration of gastric fluids.
- Maintain suction equipment.
- Post-surgical care: Maintain ventilator, chest tubes, IV lines, gastrostomy feedings.

H. GASTROSCHISIS

See "Omphalocele," p. 251.

I. HYALINE MEMBRANE DISEASE (HMD)

See "Respiratory Distress Syndrome," p. 268.

J. HYDROCEPHALUS

Hydrocephalus is dilation of the cerebral ventricles with cerebrospinal fluid, which may cause compression of the brain. It may or may not be accompanied by problems with absorption or obstruction of flow of cerebrospinal fluid in the ventricles of the brain, causing compression of the brain and enlargement of the head.

Etiology and Predisposing Factors

- Genetic and environmental factors
- Increased production of cerebrospinal fluid

- Obstruction of flow of cerebrospinal fluid
- Stenosis of the aqueduct
- Neural tube defects
- Hemorrhage that causes obstruction

Clinical Signs of Hydrocephalus

- Full or bulging fontanelle
- Separation of sutures
- Head enlargement, especially in the frontal area
- Setting sun sign (sclera visible above the pupils of the eyes)

Therapeutic Management

Management consists of surgical correction and insertion of a shunt to drain the fluid. Most often ventriculoperitoneal shunt is used to drain fluid into the peritoneal cavity.

Nursing Considerations

- Measure the head circumference daily.
- Prevent pressure areas.
- Observe for signs of infection.
- Teach parents how to care for the shunt and how to recognize signs of increased intracranial pressure.

K. HYPERBILIRUBINEMIA (JAUNDICE)

Hyperbilirubinemia is an elevated level of unconjugated bilirubin, which causes jaundice. Jaundice becomes visible when the serum bilirubin reaches 5–7 mg/dL. High levels of bilirubin may stain the brain (kernicterus) and cause bilirubin encephalopathy and severe brain damage. There are three major types of jaundice: physiologic, breast-milk, and pathologic jaundice.

Physiologic Jaundice

Physiologic jaundice is considered normal in newborns.

Etiology

- Normal hemolysis of excessive erythrocytes
- Short red cell life
- Liver immaturity
- Lack of intestinal flora needed to process bilirubin

Predisposing Factors

- Delayed feeding
- Trauma resulting in bruising or cephalhematoma
- Cold stress or asphyxia

Clinical Signs

- Begins after the first 24 hours of life
- Peaks at 5–6 mg/dL between the 2nd and 4th day of life
- Falls below 2 mg/dL by the end of the first week

Breast-Milk Jaundice

Breast-milk jaundice is jaundice that occurs in the breastfed infant when physiologic jaundice should be resolving.

Etiology and Predisposing Factors

- Exact cause is unknown.
- Pregnanediol, free fatty acids, and β-glucuronidase in the breast milk may interfere with conjugation or increase absorption of bilirubin from the intestine.
- None of these are proven causes.

Clinical Signs

- Late rise in bilirubin (4th–7th day of life)
- Peaks at 15–20 mg/dL 2 weeks after birth
- May last as long as 16 weeks
- Rarely causes bilirubin encephalopathy

Therapeutic Management

- Close monitoring of bilirubin levels
- At least 8–10 feedings each 24 hours
- Phototherapy if necessary
- Discontinuation of breastfeeding for 24–48 hours may be necessary.
- Differentiate from jaundice due to insufficient intake of breast milk, which delays stooling and allows bilirubin in the stools to be deconjugated and absorbed back into the bloodstream.

Pathologic Jaundice

Etiology and Predisposing Factors

- Blood incompatibilities
  — Rh incompatibility (Rh-negative mother with an Rh-positive infant)
  — ABO incompatibility (Type O mother with a type A, B, or AB infant)
- Infection
- Hypothyroidism
- Glucuronyl transferase or other enzyme deficiency
- Polycythemia
- Biliary atresia

Predisposing Factors

- Prematurity
- Cephalhematoma
- Bruising
- Asphyxia
- Sibling with jaundice
- Breastfeeding

Clinical Signs

- Appearance of jaundice in the first 24 hours of life
- Laboratory indications of pathologic jaundice
  — Direct bilirubin above 1 mg/dL
  — Increase of total bilirubin concentration by more than 5 mg/dL/day
  — Total bilirubin over 12 mg/dL in a full-term infant or 10–14 mg/dL in a preterm infant
  — Positive direct Coombs' test
- Jaundice that persists after the second week of life

Therapeutic Management

- Phototherapy: Special fluorescent lamps or a fiberoptic phototherapy blanket or both
- Exchange transfusions: When quick reduction of dangerously high bilirubin levels is necessary
  — Removal of 5–10 mL portions of blood and replacement with donor blood
  — Complications: Infection, hypervolemia or hypovolemia, cardiac arrhythmias, hypercalcemia, and air embolism
  — Followed by phototherapy

Complications of Pathologic Jaundice

- Bilirubin encephalopathy
  - This occurs when bilirubin levels are high enough to cause kernicterus (bilirubin staining of the brain).
  - Degree of hyperbilirubinemia necessary to cause bilirubin encephalopathy is unknown; may be bilirubin over 20 mg/dL in full-term infants, lower levels in preterm infants or neonates with other complications.
  - Incidence increases when sepsis, hypoxia, or respiratory acidosis occur.
  - Bilirubin encephalopathy has a high mortality rate, with possible mental retardation, cerebral palsy, and neurologic problems in survivors.
- Erythroblastosis fetalis
  - Condition is caused by destruction of fetal red blood cells by maternal antibodies in Rh-negative sensitized women.
  - Severely affected infants may experience hydrops fetalis, a severe anemia that results in heart failure and generalized edema.
  - Less common now due to use of Rh immune globulin (Rh IgG) to prevent maternal antibody formation after exposure to Rh-positive blood.

Nursing Considerations for All Types of Jaundice

- Check for jaundice at each assessment in the birth agency and during follow-up visits. Note areas of the body involved. Jaundice of the face and neck occurs at levels up to 8 mg/dL and of the upper trunk up to 12 mg/dL.
- Teach parents the importance of adequate feedings to stimulate passage of stools and excretion of bilirubin. Intervene when infants are feeding poorly. Instruct breastfeeding mothers to nurse every 2–3 hours.
- Prevent factors that increase the risk of hyperbilirubinemia: cold stress, hypoglycemia, inadequate intake.

- Note changes in laboratory results and correlate them with the infant's age.
- Teach parents how to check for jaundice at home and to contact their care provider if it occurs.
- Avoid giving water to jaundiced infants; milk stimulates stool excretion better.
- Phototherapy
  — Position lights according to the manufacturer's guidelines to prevent overheating or burning the skin. Check the level of irradiance with a light meter once a shift.
  — Protect the eyes from retinal damage with eye patches. Check the position of patches at least every hour. Remove patches from the eyes during feedings out of the lights. Assess eyes for infection and provide visual stimulation.
  — Dress infant in only a diaper to prevent exposure of the gonads to the lights and to expose more skin area to the light. Turn frequently.
- Observe for side effects
  — Frequent loose, green stools and resulting skin breakdown and fluid loss
  — Skin rash similar to erythema toxicum
  — Temporary lactose intolerance during therapy
  — Teach parents care if home phototherapy will be used. Arrange for home visits by nurses and other follow-up care.

L. HYPOCALCEMIA

Hypocalcemia is a condition of low serum calcium.

Etiology and Predisposing Factors

- Preterm birth
- Asphyxia at birth
- Birth to an insulin-dependent diabetic mother

- Lack of or poor enteral intake
- Exchange transfusions

Clinical Signs

- Jitteriness
- Apnea, cyanosis
- Lethargy
- Poor feeding, vomiting, abdominal distention
- Seizures

Therapeutic Management

- Laboratory analysis of calcium level
- Intravenous calcium

Nursing Considerations

Consider in infants with tremors who have normal blood glucose levels.

M. HYPOGLYCEMIA

Hypoglycemia is a blood glucose level below 40 mg/dL in the full-term infant.

Etiology and Predisposing Factors

- Prematurity
- Postmaturity
- Intrauterine growth restriction
- Asphyxia
- Cold stress
- Large for gestational age
- Small for gestational age

- Maternal diabetes
- Maternal intake of ritodrine or terbutaline

Clinical Signs

- Jitteriness
- Poor muscle tone
- Sweating
- Tachypnea
- Dyspnea
- Apnea
- Cyanosis
- Low temperature
- Poor suck
- High-pitched cry
- Lethargy
- Seizures, coma
- Some infants may be asymptomatic

Therapeutic Management

Feeding usually alleviates the problem in the normal newborn. Intravenous glucose may be necessary for repeated episodes of hypoglycemia.

Nursing Considerations

- Screen infants in risk categories and those who show signs of hypoglycemia. See "Procedure: Assessing Blood Glucose in the Newborn," p. 424.
- Obtain a laboratory analysis to verify low readings on glucometers or glucose strips because they are less accurate.
- Assess for sepsis if episodes reoccur.

- Check the mother's history for diabetes.
- Assess for other complications, such as hypocalcemia, if signs continue after feeding.

N. INFANT OF A DIABETIC MOTHER

The infant of a diabetic mother (IDM) may be normal or have a number of complications.

- Macrosomia from the large supply of glucose from mother
- Trauma due to large size
- Congenital anomalies such as caudal regression syndrome or neural tube, heart, and kidney anomalies
- Respiratory distress syndrome (RDS) because high levels of insulin interfere with production of surfactant
- Hypoglycemia after birth from sudden loss of maternal glucose at birth and infant's continued insulin production
- Hypocalcemia from decreased production of parathyroid hormone
- Polycythemia
- Intrauterine growth restriction due to poor placental blood flow

Etiology and Predisposing Factors

Gestational or preexisting maternal diabetes; the level and frequency of maternal hyperglycemia and the functioning of the placenta determine severity of neonatal effects.

Clinical Signs

- Large-for-gestational-age infant with a normal length and head circumference but obese body due to enlargement of organs and fat
- Round, red face
- Poor muscle tone

- See "Signs of Hypoglycemia," p. 241.

Therapeutic Management

- Control the mother's diabetes during pregnancy to decrease complications of the fetus
- Cesarean birth if necessary due to the infant's size
- Intravenous glucose if feeding does not correct problem to prevent damage to the brain

Nursing Considerations

- Check the mother's records to determine the severity of her diabetes and how well it was controlled.
- Assess blood glucose level according to hospital policy or immediately after birth, hourly for 4–6 hours after birth, and every 4 hours until the results are normal.
- Assess for signs of hypoglycemia.
- Observe for signs of complications, trauma, and anomalies.
- Feed early and more often if hypoglycemia is a problem. Gavage-feed if sucking is poor or respirations are high.
- Keep hydrated, especially if polycythemia is present.
- Prevent cold stress, which increases the need for glucose and oxygen.
- Explain to parents the need for frequent blood tests.
- Assess for congenital anomalies such as heart and neural tube defects.

O. INTRAUTERINE GROWTH RESTRICTION (IUGR)

See "Small-for-Gestational-Age Infants," p. 277.

P. INTRAVENTRICULAR HEMORRHAGE

See "Periventricular-Intraventricular Hemorrhage," p. 252.

Q. JAUNDICE

See "Hyperbilirubinemia," p. 234.

R. KERNICTERUS

See "Bilirubin Encephalopathy," p. 238.

S. MECONIUM ASPIRATION SYNDROME (MAS)

Meconium aspiration syndrome develops when meconium enters the lungs during fetal life or at birth. It may cause obstruction of the airways, pneumonitis, air trapping, pneumothorax, or persistent pulmonary hypertension of the newborn.

Etiology and Predisposing Factors

- Meconium may be passed by a normal or hypoxic fetus.
- It enters the lungs in utero if gasping movements occur with asphyxia and acidosis.
- It is aspirated when the infant takes the first breaths at birth.
- Postmaturity increases risk.

Clinical Signs

- Mild to severe respiratory distress (tachypnea, cyanosis, retractions, nasal flaring, grunting)
- Coarse breath sounds
- X-rays: atelectasis, consolidation, and hyperexpansion from air trapping.

Therapeutic Management

- The infant's mouth and pharynx are suctioned as soon as the head is delivered and before delivery of the rest of the body.
- A laryngoscope is inserted and the trachea is suctioned before the first breath to prevent meconium from being drawn into the lower airways.

- An endotracheal tube is inserted for deep suction and ventilation. Thin meconium in a vigorous infant may not require intubation.
- Warmed, humidified oxygen or a ventilator may be used as necessary.
- Extracorporeal membrane oxygenation (ECMO), a method to oxygenate the blood while bypassing the lungs, may be necessary in some infants.

Nursing Considerations

- Notify the primary caregiver when meconium is noted in the amniotic fluid during labor.
- Ensure that equipment is available and functioning.
- Assist with care at delivery.
- Adapt nursing care to the problems presented and watch for complications.

T.   MENINGOCELE

See "Neural Tube Defects," p. 250.

U.   MYELOMENINGOCELE

See "Neural Tube Defects," p. 250.

V.   NECROTIZING ENTEROCOLITIS (NEC)

N*ecrotizing enterocolitis* is a serious condition of the intestinal tract that may lead to necrosis, perforation, and peritonitis.

Etiology and Predisposing Factors

- Exact cause unknown
- Injury to bowel and infection
- Preterm birth

Clinical Signs

- Increased abdominal girth
- Increased gastric residuals
- Decreased or absent bowel sounds
- Loops of bowel seen through the abdominal wall
- Vomiting
- Signs of infection
- Blood in the stools
- X-ray: Loops of bowel dilated with air and layers of gas in the intestinal wall

Therapeutic Management

- Preventive measures
    - Breast-milk feedings
    - Corticosteroids given to the mother during pregnancy
    - Slow advancement of feedings
    - Oral IgA
- Treatment
    - Antibiotics
    - Parenteral nutrition
    - Surgery to remove necrotic areas and perform an ostomy

Nursing Considerations

- Early recognition of signs is essential to decrease mortality.
- Withhold the next feeding and notify the physician if one or more signs are present.

W. NEONATAL ABSTINENCE SYNDROME

Neonatal abstinence syndrome is a cluster of physical withdrawal signs in a newborn exposed in utero to maternal use of drugs.

Etiology and Predisposing Factors

Maternal use of substances such as cocaine or heroin.

Clinical Signs

Signs usually begin within 48–72 hours after birth but may not occur until after 1 week. Signs vary according to the drug or combination of drugs used and the time of the last dose. Some infants show no abnormal signs.

- Behavioral signs
  - Irritability
  - Jitteriness, tremors
  - Muscular rigidity, increased muscle tone
  - Restlessness, excessive activity
  - Exaggerated startle reflex
  - Prolonged, high-pitched cry
  - Difficult to console
- Signs related to feeding
  - Uncoordinated sucking and swallowing
  - Frequent regurgitation or vomiting
  - Diarrhea
- Other signs
  - Poor sleeping patterns
  - Yawning, sneezing
  - Nasal stuffiness, sneezing
  - Tachypnea
  - Apnea
  - Seizures
  - Diaphoresis

Therapeutic Management

- Suspect maternal substance abuse with
  - A history of no prenatal care.

- — Unusual behaviors during labor and delivery.
- — Abruptio placentae (may occur after cocaine use).
- Obtain a urine specimen, preferably the first urine output (See "Procedure: Applying a Pediatric Urine Collection Bag," p. 420.)
- Meconium or hair may also be tested for drugs.
- Use scoring sheets to follow number, frequency, and severity of behaviors indicating neonatal abstinence syndrome.
- Administer sedatives as ordered for severe irritability. Tincture of opium, tincture of paregoric, Phenobarbital, oral morphine, and diazepam (Valium) are common.
- Initiate gavage or intravenous feeding as necessary for uncoordinated suck and swallow. See "Procedure: Administering Gavage Feeding," p. 417.
- Provide increased calories for excessive activity.
- Refer to social services for placement of the infant after hospitalization, as well as follow-up of the mother or other caretaker.

Nursing Considerations

Feeding

- Determine infant's ability to coordinate sucking and swallowing.
- Prevent distractions by feeding in a quiet area of the nursery.
- Swaddle during feedings to prevent excessive activity.
- Gavage-feed infants with excessive agitation, poor suck and swallow, or rapid respirations.
- Give chin and cheek support to help infant suck more efficiently.
- Position infant on the right side with the head of the bed elevated 30–45° after feedings.

- Discourage breastfeeding by mothers likely to continue drug use.

Rest

- Assess effect of agitation and irritability on rest and sleep patterns.
- Prevent overstimulation by reducing noise, bright lights, and excessive handling. Organize care to prevent disturbances.
- Swaddle the infant in a flexed position to prevent startling and agitation. Use slow, smooth movements during care.
- Provide non-nutritive suckling to help quiet infant.

Bonding

The mother may be required to enter a drug rehabilitation program before she can obtain custody of the infant. She will probably obtain custody eventually if she desires, and attachment should be facilitated.

- Assess the frequency of maternal visits and evidence of bonding behavior.
- Help the mother feel welcome when she visits. Avoid being judgmental of the mother's past behavior.
- Help the mother participate actively in infant care during visits.
- Assess the mother's infant care skills and teach where needed.
- Model parenting skills and methods of interacting with the infant.
- Provide positive feedback.
- Teach the parent or caregiver the techniques needed for care of drug-exposed infants.
    - Swaddling the infant in a flexed position to prevent excessive tremors

— Signs of overstimulation

— Usual methods of interaction by drug-exposed infants (avoiding eye contact, being unable to tolerate more than brief periods of interaction)

- Refer to programs for parenting drug-exposed infants.

X. NEURAL TUBE DEFECTS

Neural tube defects result from a failure of the vertebral arch to close.

Etiology and Predisposing Factors

- Genetic predisposition
- Associated with folic acid deficiency in mother near time of conception

Clinical Signs

- Spina bifida occulta: A dimple on the back, often with a tuft of hair over it; usually no other abnormalities. Opening may be palpated.
- Meningocele: Protrusion of meninges through the spina bifida, covered by skin or thin membrane; no paralysis because spinal cord is not involved.
- Myelomeningocele: Protrusion of meninges and spinal cord covered with membrane through the spina bifida. Degree of paralysis depends on location of the defect. Infant may also have hydrocephalus before or after surgery.

Therapeutic Management

- Folic acid before conception and during pregnancy
- Surgery for meningocele and myelomeningocele
- Shunt to divert cerebrospinal fluid if hydrocephalus develops
- Antibiotics
- Long-term follow-up with physical therapy

Nursing Considerations

- Assessments
  - Position and covering of the defect at birth
  - Movement below the level of the defect
  - Relaxation of the anal sphincter or dribbling of stool and urine
  - Integrity of the sac
  - Signs of infection
  - Signs of increasing intracranial pressure. See "Hydrocephalus," p. 233.
- Apply sterile saline dressing and plastic over the defect covered by membrane to prevent drying.
- Handle the infant carefully to prevent trauma to the sac.
- Position on the side or prone.
- Keep the site free of fecal contamination.

Y. OMPHALOCELE AND GASTROSCHISIS

Omphalocele and gastroschisis are abdominal wall defects resulting in protrusion of abdominal contents outside the abdominal cavity.

Etiology and Predisposing Factors

Weakness of the abdominal wall. In omphalocele, the intestines protrude into the base of the umbilical cord. In gastroschisis, there is a defect in the lateral abdominal wall that does not involve the cord. Other anomalies may be present, especially in omphalocele.

Clinical Signs

- Omphalocele: Enlarged cord with intestines visible through it
- Gastroschisis: Intestines outside the abdominal wall without a sac or other covering

Therapeutic Management

- Diagnosis may be made by prenatal ultrasound
- Surgery as soon as possible
- A silastic silo (pouch) may be used to replace the intestines gradually over days
- Intubation at delivery
- Gastric suction
- Parenteral nutrition
- Antibiotics

Nursing Considerations

- Cover the intestines with sterile saline dressings and plastic to prevent drying.
- Prevent infection and trauma.
- Explain to parents.
- Provide postsurgical care.

Z. PERIVENTRICULAR-INTRAVENTRICULAR HEMORRHAGE (PIVH)

Periventricular-intraventricular hemorrhage is rupture of the blood vessels around the ventricles of the brain. Severity of effects depends on the degree of hemorrhage.

Etiology and Predisposing Factors

- Gestation less than 32 weeks
- Weight under 1500 g
- Increased blood pressure
- Increased cerebral blood flow

Clinical Signs

Signs vary according to the severity of the hemorrhage.

- Lethargy
- Poor muscle tone
- Deterioration of respiratory status (cyanosis, apnea)
- Decreased hematocrit level
- Decreased reflexes
- Full or bulging fontanelle
- Seizures

Therapeutic Management

- Early and repeated ultrasonography to diagnose in infants under 32 weeks
- Maintenance of respiratory function
- Treatment of complications such as hydrocephalus
- Lumbar taps or a ventriculoperitoneal shunt to drain fluid

Nursing Considerations

- Measure the head circumference daily.
- Assess for changes in neurological status, which may be subtle.
- Avoid increases in blood pressure from excessive handling or suctioning.

AA. PERSISTENT FETAL CIRCULATION

See "Persistent Pulmonary Hypertension of the Newborn," below.

BB. PERSISTENT PULMONARY HYPERTENSION OF THE NEWBORN (PPHN)

In *persistent pulmonary hypertension of the newborn* (also called *persistent fetal circulation*) the vascular resistance of the lungs remains high after birth due to effects of inadequate oxygenation. There is vasoconstriction of the pulmonary artery and the ductus arteriosus remains dilated. A right-to-left shunt of blood through the foramen ovale and patent ductus arteriosus occurs.

Etiology and Predisposing Factors

- Hypoxia, asphyxia
- Abnormal lung development
- Maternal use of nonsteroidal anti-inflammatory agents or aspirin
- Acidosis
- Meconium aspiration
- Sepsis
- Respiratory distress syndrome
- Unknown causes

Clinical Signs

- Signs develop within 24 hours after birth
- Tachypnea, respiratory distress, and progressive cyanosis
- Decreased oxygen saturation and PaO_2
- Hypoxia that increases with handling and stimuli

Therapeutic Management

Management involves treating the underlying cause of poor oxygenation.

- High frequency ventilation, surfactant therapy, or ECMO therapy
- Liquid ventilation with nitric oxide (being investigated)

Nursing Considerations

Nursing care is similar to that for other severe respiratory disease.

CC. POLYCYTHEMIA

In polycythemia, the central hematocrit level is above 65% due to an elevated number of erythrocytes. This may cause organ damage from decreased blood flow, renal vein thrombosis, necrotizing enterocolitis, and hyperbilirubinemia.

Etiology and Predisposing Factors

- Conditions in which infants produce more erythrocytes than normal due to poor oxygenation during fetal life.
- High altitude
- Postterm infant
- Delayed clamping of the umbilical cord
- Maternal diabetes
- Intrauterine growth retardation

Clinical Signs

Signs vary depending on areas affected by the viscous blood flow.

- Ruddy skin tone
- Respiratory distress
- Hypoglycemia
- Lethargy or irritability
- Poor feeding
- Seizures

Therapeutic Management

- Adequate hydration to prevent sluggish blood flow and ischemia to vital organs
- Monitoring of bilirubin levels
- Exchange transfusion

Nursing Considerations

- Check hematocrit in infants with ruddy color.
- Ensure adequate hydration.
- Observe for jaundice or other complications.

DD. POSTMATURITY SYNDROME

Postterm infants are born after the 42nd week of gestation. They may have postmaturity syndrome and have an increased rate of complications during birth because of deterioration of the placenta.

Etiology and Predisposing Factors

- Unknown

Clinical Signs

- During pregnancy and birth
  - Diminished fetal growth
  - Oligohydramnios
  - Meconium passage
- After birth
  - Hyperalert, wide-eyed, worried look
  - Polycythemia
  - Thin, loose skin with little subcutaneous fat
  - Little or no lanugo
  - Little or no vernix caseosa
  - Dry, cracked, peeling skin

Therapeutic Management

Treatment varies according to the problems presented (asphyxia, meconium aspiration, respiratory support).

Nursing Considerations

- Check blood glucose soon after birth. Repeat at one hour of age and as indicated.
- Feed early and frequently.
- Assess temperature regulation ability and adapt nursing care as needed.
- Observe for other complications.

EE. PRETERM INFANTS

Preterm infants (also called *premature infants*) are born before the beginning of the 38th week of gestation. They may have complications such as respiratory distress syndrome, bronchopulmonary dysplasia, periventricular-intraventricular hemorrhage, retinopathy of prematurity, and necrotizing enterocolitis, which are discussed separately. Care is focused on the problem areas discussed below.

Predisposing/Etiologic Factors

See preterm labor. p. 175.

Respiratory Problems

The lungs are underdeveloped. Surfactant production may be inadequate and may lead to respiratory distress syndrome.

Clinical Signs
- Tachypnea
- Nasal flaring
- Grunting
- Gasping
- Apnea for more than 20 seconds or with change in heart rate or color
- Asymmetry or decreased chest expansion

- Intercostal, xiphoid, subcostal, or supraclavicular retractions
- Seesaw respirations
- Rales, crackles, rhonchi

Therapeutic Management

Respiratory assistance needed may vary from oxygen in a hood to mechanical ventilation.

Nursing Considerations

- Assess respiratory status. Use the Silverman-Andersen Index to evaluate the degree of respiratory distress.
- Monitor the infant's blood oxygen levels and adjust oxygen as indicated.
- Place infant in a side-lying or prone position or use a diaper roll under the shoulders when supine.
- Perform chest physiotherapy (postural drainage, percussion, and vibration) and suctioning as ordered. Observe for adverse responses such as decreased blood oxygen levels, bradycardia, or cyanosis.
- Ensure adequate hydration to keep secretions thin.

Thermoregulatory Problems

Clinical Signs

- Axillary temperature <36.5°C (97.7°F) or >37.5°C (99.5°F)
- Abdominal skin temperature <36°C (96.8°F) or >36.5°C (97.7°F)
- Poor feeding or intolerance to feedings
- Lethargy
- Irritability
- Decreased muscle tone
- Cool skin temperature
- Mottled skin

- Signs of hypoglycemia
- Signs of respiratory difficulty

Therapeutic Management

- Maintain a neutral thermal environment using radiant warmers, incubators, or open cribs as appropriate.
- Place a transparent plastic blanket over the infant to allow heat from the radiant warmer to reach the infant, decrease insensible water loss, and maintain visibility of the infant's body parts.
- Consider weaning to an open crib when infants reach about 1500 g and gain approximately 15–30 g daily.

Nursing Considerations

- Ensure that all heating devices are properly set to prevent over- or underheating.
- Use an open radiant warmer for procedures.
- Warm oxygen before administering.
- Keep portholes and doors of incubators closed as much as possible to prevent heat loss.
- Use heated blankets and a head covering when removing infants from heat sources.
- Consider infection in infants whose temperature remains unstable.
- Wean gradually.
— Decrease incubator temperature 1–1.5°C each day. Raise incubator temperature if the infant's temperature falls below 36°C.
— Transfer to an open crib when infants tolerate the incubator setting at 28°C.
— Double-wrap with warm blankets when transferring and assess temperature frequently.

— Watch for hypoglycemia or respiratory distress if the temperature falls.

Fluid and Electrolyte Balance Problems

Infants under 35 weeks gestation have immature kidneys and are prone to fluid and electrolyte balance problems. Radiant warmers and phototherapy cause increased fluid losses.

Clinical Signs

- Dehydration
    - Urine output < 1 mL/kg/hour
    - Urine specific gravity > 1.015
    - Weight loss greater than expected
    - Dry skin and mucous membranes
    - Sunken anterior fontanelle
    - Poor tissue turgor
    - Blood: elevated sodium, protein, and hematocrit levels
- Overhydration
    - Urine output > 3 mL/kg/hour
    - Urine specific gravity < 1.005
    - Edema
    - Weight gain greater than expected
    - Bulging fontanelles
    - Blood: decreased sodium, protein, and hematocrit levels
    - Moist breath sounds
    - Difficulty breathing
- Electrolyte imbalances: Signs vary according to specific electrolytes involved.

Therapeutic Management

- Fluid and electrolytes are carefully calculated and prescribed according to gestational age.

- Average fluid need is 110–140 mL/kg/day after the first 2 days of life.

Nursing Considerations

- Measure and record all intake and output: parenteral, feeding tube, oral fluids; output from urine, drainage tubes, and blood specimens taken for laboratory tests.
- Weigh diapers to measure urine output (1 gram equals 1 mL of urine).
- Check specific gravity as indicated. Normal range is 1.005–1.015.
- Assess weight daily.
- Use infusion control devices to help prevent fluid volume overload.
- Dilute intravenous medications with as little fluid as is consistent with safe administration of the drug.
- Observe for signs of dehydration, overhydration, or specific electrolyte imbalances.

Problems with Infection

Many preterm infants have one or more episodes of sepsis during their hospital stay.

Clinical Signs

See "Signs of Sepsis," p. 271.

Therapeutic Management

See "Sepsis," p. 270.

Nursing Considerations

- Have parents and staff scrub hands and arms before handling infants. Teach family members to avoid exposing infants to contagious diseases.

- Restrict use of adhesives to prevent damage to the skin. Use nontraumatizing tape and adhesives.
- Position infants and equipment to avoid undue pressure on the skin.
- Assess for signs of infection to treat early. See "Sepsis," p. 270.

Problems with Pain

Infants in the NICU setting undergo many painful procedures that cause physiologic and behavioral changes.

Clinical Signs

- High-pitched, intense, harsh cry
- "Cry face": Eyes squeezed shut, mouth open
- Grimacing
- Rigidity or flailing of extremities
- Color changes: red, dusky, pale
- Increased or decreased heart rate
- Increased respirations and BP
- Decreased oxygen saturation
- Signs of increased intracranial pressure

Therapeutic Management

Medication should be provided for the infant during painful procedures and for long-term pain. Dosage should be changed according to the infant's response.

Nursing Considerations

- Prepare infants for potentially painful procedures.
  — Wake infants slowly and gently.
  — Give ordered pain medications before the procedure.

- Use containment—swaddling, blanket rolls, or the nurse's hands—to keep the extremities in a flexed position near the mouth for sucking.
- Use comfort measures.
  - Non-nutritive sucking
  - Soft talking
  - Holding, rocking

Environmentally-Caused Stress

The bright, loud environment of the intensive care nursery can cause stress in preterm infants. It is associated with hearing loss, retinopathy of prematurity, increased energy expenditure, and changes in heart rate, oxygen saturation levels, and behavior states.

Clinical Signs

- Increase or decrease in pulse and respiratory rate
- Cyanosis, pallor, or mottling
- Flaring nares
- Decreased oxygen saturation levels
- Coughing
- Yawning
- Stiff, extended arms and legs
- Fisting of the hands or splaying of the fingers
- Alert, worried expression
- Turning away from eye contact
- Hiccoughing, regurgitation
- Fatigue

Nursing Considerations

The nurse must provide developmentally supportive nursing care.

- Assess the level of environmental stimuli and the infant's response.
- Schedule activities when the infant is awake, when possible.
- Group activities to allow rest between, but watch for signs of stress.
- Avoid routine care, such as frequent vital signs or bathing, that is not essential.
- Coordinate activities of different health care workers to prevent overstimulation.
- Keep environmental noise as low as possible.
  — Avoid talking near the incubator.
  — Set alarm volumes on low; respond quickly when they sound.
  — Open and close doors on incubators and cupboards gently.
  — Do not place objects on top of the incubator.
- Decrease light stimulation to help develop sleep cycles.
  — Position incubators away from bright lights.
  — Place infants so they are not facing lights.
  — Drape a blanket over one end to decrease light.
  — Use a dimmer switch to vary the intensity of lights.
- Schedule "quiet periods," when lights and noise in the unit are kept to a minimum.
- Schedule daytime, evening, and night naps.
- Avoid musculoskeletal problems by keeping infants in flexed positions using blankets and rolls to maintain flexion.

Problems with Nutrition

Preterm infants need 120–150 kcal/kg/day. Their small stomach capacity limits the volume that they can tolerate at each feeding.

Clinical Signs

- Poor suck, swallow, and gag reflexes
- Low blood glucose levels
- Lack of expected growth
- Excessive gastric residuals

Therapeutic Management

- Administer intravenous or gavage feedings until the infant is ready for oral feedings.
- Calories, amino acids, fatty acids, vitamins, and minerals are calculated according to the infant's gestational age, weight, and tolerance to feedings.

Nursing Considerations

- Administer intravenous and gavage feedings as ordered. See "Procedure: Administering Gavage Feeding," p. 417.
- Note signs that the infant is not yet ready for nipple feedings.
  — Respiratory rate > 60 breaths/minute
  — No rooting, sucking, or gag reflex
  — Excessive gastric residuals
- Note signs of readiness for nipple feedings, especially when infants reach 32–34 weeks and 1500–1600 g in weight.
  — Rooting
  — Sucking on gavage tube, finger, or pacifier
  — Able to tolerate holding
  — Respiratory rate < 60 breaths/minute
  — Presence of gag reflex
- Assist interested mothers with breastfeeding.
  — Teach use of breast pump and milk storage.
  — Provide privacy as the mother breastfeeds the infant.
  — Demonstrate kangaroo care for very small infants.

— Demonstrate breastfeeding techniques for small infants.

- Position the infant at a 45–60° angle with the head slightly forward and the chin slightly down.
- Place a finger on each cheek and one under the jaw at the base of the tongue to provide support during feeding.
- Feed slowly with frequent stops to burp and rest.
- Experiment with different types of nipples to find one that works best.
- Teach mothers signs of fatigue during breast or bottle feeding.
- Finish feedings by gavage if the infant becomes too fatigued.
- Position on the right side or prone with a 30° head elevation after feedings.
- Note and report adverse responses to nipple feedings.
  — Tachycardia or bradycardia
  — Increased respiratory rate or apnea
  — Markedly decreased oxygen saturation level
  — Coughing or gagging
  — Falling asleep early in the feeding
  — Feeding time beyond 25–30 minutes
  — Vomiting or diarrhea
- Observe for signs of intestinal complications.
  — Measure abdominal girth with tape at the level of the umbilicus to check for abdominal distention.
  — Test stools for reducing substance and occult blood.
- Provide rest periods before and after nipple feedings.

Parenting

The extended hospitalization of the preterm infant results in separation from parents and may interfere with parenting.

Clinical Signs

Parental behaviors that may indicate delayed bonding include.

- Using negative terms to describe the infant.
- Discussing the infant in impersonal or technical terms.
- Failing to give the infant a name or to use the name.
- Visiting or calling infrequently or not at all.
- Decreasing the number and length of visits.
- Showing interest in other infants equal to that in their own infant.
- Refusing offers to hold and learn to care for the infant.
- Decrease in or lack of eye contact and in time spent talking to or smiling at the infant.
- Decrease in previously shown attachment behaviors.

Nursing Considerations

- Allow the mother to see the infant immediately after delivery if possible.
- Allow the father/support person to be present for initial care of the infant, if possible.
- Explain all nursing care, its purpose, and the expected response.
- Use therapeutic communication techniques to support parents.
- Prepare parents for what they will see in the NICU before the first visit (equipment, sounds, how the infant will look).
- Suggest that parents touch the infant to promote development of attachment. Show them how.
- Offer realistic reassurance about the infant's condition.
- Begin kangaroo care as soon as possible. Place the infant, wearing only a diaper and hat, under the mother's clothes between her breasts.

- Explain the infant's socialization abilities based on gestational age.
- Teach parents signs of overstimulation and signs the infant is ready for more interaction.
- Involve the parents in care as soon as possible.
- Allow parents to participate in decisions about the infant.
- Assess for gradual increase in comfort and participation in care of the infant.
- Help parents prepare for discharge.
  - Give them a copy of the critical pathway, if used.
  - Teach medication administration, special procedures, and other care the infant will need after discharge.
  - Observe the parents perform care until they feel comfortable and are safe.
  - Discuss adaptations necessary in the home for care of the infant.
  - Arrange for home nursing services.

FF. RESPIRATORY DISTRESS SYNDROME (RDS)

Respiratory distress syndrome, also called *hyaline membrane disease* (HMD), is most often seen in preterm infants. Immature lungs and lack of adequate surfactant production cause atelectasis and severe respiratory difficulty.

Etiology and Predisposing Factors

- Insufficient surfactant production in the lungs
- Birth asphyxia
- Cesarean birth
- Maternal diabetes

Clinical Signs

Signs begin within hours of birth, worsen the next day, and often improve in 72 hours.

- Tachypnea
- Nasal flaring
- Retractions
- Cyanosis
- Grunting on expiration
- Decreased or wet breath sounds
- Acidosis
- Chest x-ray: "ground glass" appearance of the lungs with areas of atelectasis

Therapeutic Management

- Surfactant replacement therapy at birth or when signs occur. Repeat doses if necessary.
- Mechanical ventilation
- Correction of acidosis
- Intravenous feedings
- Other treatment as appropriate

Nursing Considerations

- Observe for signs of developing RDS at birth and during the early hours after the delivery.
- Observe for changes in the infant's condition.
- Other nursing care is supportive and depends on the infant's condition.

GG. RETINOPATHY OF PREMATURITY/ RETROLENTAL FIBROPLASIA

Retinopathy of prematurity (ROP), or *retrolental fibroplasia* (RLF), may result in visual impairment or blindness in preterm infants.

Etiology and Predisposing Factors

- Damage to retinal blood vessels and scarring
- Preterm birth, especially low birth weight
- Birth weight less than 1500 g
- Exposure to oxygen

Clinical Signs

Signs can be seen only on ophthalmic examination.

- Constriction of blood vessels of the eye
- Proliferation of new blood vessels in the retina and into the vitreous
- Hemorrhage and scarring
- Retinal detachment

Therapeutic Management

- Screening of LBW infants between 4 and 8 weeks after birth
- Cryotherapy or laser surgery if necessary

Nursing Considerations

- Adjust oxygen to smallest amounts possible to maintain infant.
- Arrange for ophthalmic examinations.

HH. SEPSIS NEONATORUM

Sepsis neonatorum is a systemic infection with bacteria in the bloodstream. Early-onset sepsis usually begins in the first 24 hours after birth and has a more rapid progression than late-onset sepsis. It often involves the respiratory system or causes meningitis. Late-onset sepsis generally develops after the first week of life and usually involves the central nervous system.

Etiology

- Group B-hemolytic Streptococcus (GBS) and Escherichia coli are the most common causes.
- Staphylococcus epidermidis, Staphylococcus aureus, Haemophilus influenzae, and Listeria monocytogenes
- Vertical infection
  - Transplacental
  - Transmitted from the mother during birth
  - Common vertical infections and their effects on the neonate are listed in Table III-3.
- Horizontal infection: Contact with infected people or objects

Predisposing Factors

- Prolonged rupture of membranes
- Prolonged labor
- Chorioamnionitis
- Preterm birth

Clinical Signs

Signs tend to be subtle and may indicate other conditions.

- General signs
  - Temperature instability (usually low)
  - Nurse's feeling that infant is not doing well
  - Rash
- Respiratory signs
  - Tachypnea
  - Apnea
  - Respiratory distress—nasal flaring, retractions, grunting

TABLE III-3

Common Vertical Infections in the Newborn

TRANSMISSION	EFFECT ON NEWBORN	NURSING CONSIDERATIONS
Viral Infections		
Cytomegalovirus		
Transplacental	Most infants asymptomatic at birth. LBW, IUGR, enlarged liver and spleen, jaundice, petechiae, mental retardation, hearing loss, blindness, epilepsy. May have no signs for months or years.	Most common perinatal infection. A major cause of mental retardation. Diagnosed by urine culture. May shed virus in saliva and urine for months. Antiviral drugs being tested.
Hepatitis B		
Usually during birth through contact with maternal blood. Also transplacental, breast milk.	Asymptomatic at birth. LBW, prematurity. Most become chronic carriers. Risk of later liver cancer.	Wash well to remove all blood before skin is pierced for any reason. After cleaning, administer hepatitis B immune globulin and hepatitis B vaccine to prevent infection.

Herpes

Usually during birth through infected vagina or ascending infection after rupture of membranes. Transplacental rarely.	Clusters of vesicles, temperature instability, lethargy, poor suck, seizures, encephalitis, jaundice, purpura. One-half to two-thirds have disseminated infection with death or severe neurological impairment very high.	Contact precautions. Obtain lesion specimens for culture. Mortality and morbidity rate high even with antiviral drugs.

Human Immunodeficiency Virus/Acquired Immunodeficiency Syndrome

Transplacental, during birth from infected blood and secretions, or from breast milk. Transmission rate in U.S. is 25–30%. Transmission less if mother takes antiviral drugs during pregnancy.	Asymptomatic at birth, signs usually apparent at 4–12 months. Enlarged liver and spleen, lymphadenopathy, failure to thrive, pneumonia, persistent Candida and bacterial infections.	Diagnosed from symptoms or at 6–18 months when antibodies from mother are gone. Wash early and before skin is punctured to remove blood. Treated with antiviral drugs and prophylaxis against other infections.

Rubella

Transplacental	Asymptomatic or IUGR, cataracts, cardiac defects, deafness, mental retardation. Damage greatest in the first trimester.	Contact precautions. Infant may shed virus for months after birth. Diagnosed by presence of antibody. No treatment.

Varicella Zoster Virus (Chickenpox)

Transplacental	Skin scarring, limb hypoplasia, eye and brain damage, IUGR, death. Damage greatest before the 20th week of gestation.	Immune globulin for infants of mothers infected just before delivery. Acyclovir. Airborne isolation of infants with lesions.

Other Infections

Group β Streptococcal Infection

During birth or ascending after rupture of membranes	Sudden onset of respiratory distress in infant usually well at birth, pneumonia, shock, meningitis. May have early or late onset.	Early identification essential to prevent death. Treated with IV antibiotics to mother in labor or to infant after birth.

Gonorrhea

Usually during birth	Conjunctivitis (ophthalmia neonatorum), with red, edematous lids and prurulent eye drainage. May result in blindness if untreated.	All infants treated with erythromycin eye ointment or other antibiotic for prevention. Previously treated with silver nitrate.

Chlamydial Infection

During birth	Conjunctivitis, pneumonia, otitis media.	Erythromycin eye ointment for prevention of conjunctivitis. Infection treated with erythromycin.

Candidiasis

Transplacental	White patches in mouth (thrush) that bleed if removed. Rash on the perineum. May be systemic.	Administer nystatin drops of cream and teach parents how to administer. Assess mother for vaginal or breast infection.

Toxoplasmosis

Transplacental	Asymptomatic, or LBW, thrombocytopenia, enlarged liver and spleen, jaundice, anemia, seizures, microcephaly, hydrocephalus, chorioretinitis. Signs may not develop for years.	Consider in infants with IUGR. Confirmed by serum tests. Treatment: pyrimethamine, sulfadiazine, and folinic acid.

Syphilis

Transplacental	Asymptomatic or enlarged liver and spleen, jaundice, lymphadenopathy, anemia, rhinitis, pink- or copper-colored peeling rash, pneumonitis, osteochondritis, CNS involvement.	Diagnosed by blood and cerebrospinal fluid testing. Administer penicillin as ordered.

Standard precautions for infection control apply to all patients and are not listed above. They include precautions for contact with blood; all body fluids, secretions, and excretions except sweat; nonintact skin; and mucous membranes. Contact precautions are used when transmission of the disease may occur from direct contact with patient's dry skin or articles in the patient's environment.

Abbreviations: LBW, low birth weight; IUGR, intrauterine growth restriction; IV, intravenous; CNS, central nervous system.

- Cardiovascular signs
  - Color changes—cyanosis, pallor, mottling
  - Tachycardia
  - Hypotension
  - Decreased peripheral perfusion
- Gastrointestinal signs
  - Decreased oral intake
  - Vomiting
  - Gastric residuals measuring over half the previous feeding
  - Diarrhea
  - Abdominal distention
  - Hypoglycemia or hyperglycemia
- Central nervous system signs
  - Decreased muscle tone
  - Lethargy
  - Irritability
  - Bulging fontanelle
- Signs that may indicate advanced infection
  - Jaundice
  - Evidence of hemorrhage (petechiae, purpura, pulmonary bleeding)
  - Anemia
  - Enlarged liver and spleen
  - Respiratory failure
  - Shock
  - Seizures

Therapeutic Management

- Cultures of blood, urine, gastric aspirate, cerebrospinal fluid
- Blood analysis: decreased neutrophils, increased bands (immature neutrophils), and decreased platelets. Elevated IgM levels in cord blood or shortly after birth indicates in utero infection.

- Chest x-ray
- Intravenous antibiotics, usually for 10 or more days
- Intravenous gamma globulin may be used in prevention and treatment of sepsis in some preterm infants.

Nursing Considerations

- Ensure that medications are administered on time.
- Plan with the laboratory for analysis of antibiotic peak and trough levels.
- Observe for complications such as shock, hypoglycemia, hyperglycemia, electrolyte imbalances, and problems in temperature regulation.
- Gavage feed if necessary.
- Prevent spread of infection to other infants by scrupulous use of medical asepsis.
- Support parents, who may be shocked at the sudden illness of their infant.

II. SMALL-FOR-GESTATIONAL-AGE INFANTS (SGA)

Small-for-gestational-age infants are below the 10th percentile in size because of intrauterine growth restriction (IUGR). Infants may be preterm, full-term, or postterm.

Etiology and Predisposing Factors

- Congenital malformations
- Chromosomal anomalies
- Fetal infections
- Poor placental function
- Maternal pregnancy-induced hypertension, severe diabetes
- Maternal substance abuse

Clinical Signs

- Symmetric growth restriction: Entire body is proportionately small.
- Asymmetric growth restriction
    - Normal size head that appears large
    - Normal length
    - Weight below that expected for gestational age
    - Long, thin appearance
    - Loose skin with longitudinal thigh creases
    - Sparse hair
    - Thin cord
    - Dry skin

Therapeutic Management

- Prevention by good prenatal care
- Treatment as problems occur

Nursing Considerations

- Assess for hypoglycemia.
- Feed frequently to provide extra calories.
- Assess temperature regulation.
- Other care is similar to that for preterm or postterm infant.

JJ. SPINA BIFIDA OCCULTA

See "Neural Tube Defects," p. 250.

KK. TRACHEOESOPHAGEAL FISTULA (TEF)

See "Esophageal Atresia," p. 232.

LL. TRANSIENT TACHYPNEA OF THE NEWBORN (TTN)

Transient tachypnea of the newborn, also called *respiratory distress syndrome, type* II, is a condition of rapid respirations with decreased lung compliance and air trapping in full or preterm infants. The condition usually resolves in a few days.

Etiology

- Exact cause unknown
- May be due to a delay in absorption of fetal lung fluid
- May be mild immaturity of surfactant production

Predisposing Factors

- Maternal analgesia
- Bleeding
- Diabetes
- Cesarean birth
- Asphyxia

Clinical Signs

- Respirations as high as 150/minute
- Retractions
- Nasal flaring
- Grunting
- Mild cyanosis
- Chest x-ray: Hyperinflation and presence of fluid in the fissures between the lobes and in the pleural space

Therapeutic Management

- Treatment is supportive.
- Administer sufficient oxygen to prevent cyanosis.

- Feed intravenously or by gavage, while the respiratory rate is high to prevent aspiration and conserve energy.
- Observation for RDS and sepsis because signs are similar.
- Administer ordered antibiotics until sepsis is ruled out.

SECTION FOUR

Postpartum

I. POSTPARTUM ADAPTATIONS

A. REPRODUCTIVE SYSTEM

Uterus

Involution begins when muscle fibers contract around maternal blood vessels at the site left denuded when the placenta separated.

- Fundus of the uterus is palpable about the level of the umbilicus soon after childbirth.
- Uterus becomes smaller, and fundus descends about 1 centimeter (one fingerbreadth) a day; so by 10–14 days the uterus should be in the pelvic cavity and no longer palpable above the symphysis pubis. See Figure IV-1.

Afterpains

- Afterpains are particularly uncomfortable for multiparas because of intermittent contraction of uterine muscles that have been stretched repeatedly.
- Afterpains are also severe during breastfeeding when oxytocin, which is necessary for the milk-ejection reflex, causes strong contraction of uterine muscles.

Lochia

Lochia decreases in amount and changes color over time.

- Lochia rubra is dark red and lasts 2–3 days.

Figure IV-1

Involution of the Uterus (Height of the uterine fundus decreases by approximately 1 cm/day.)

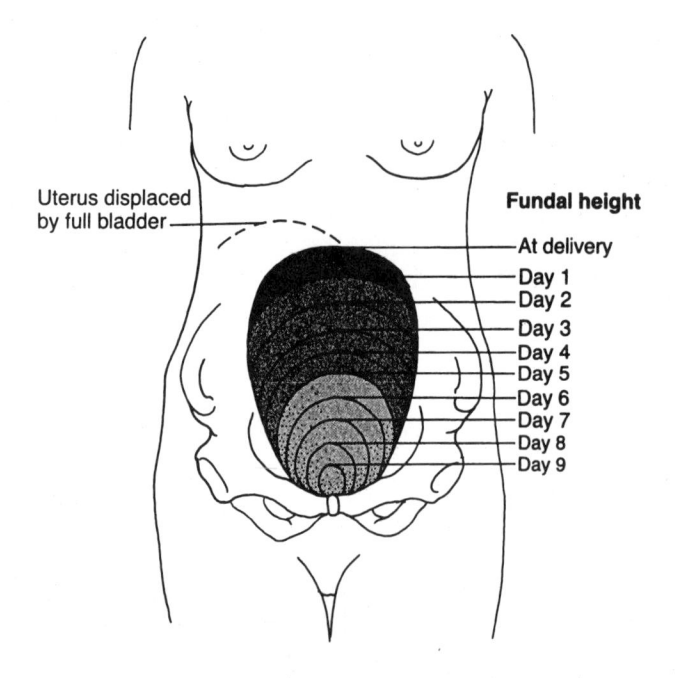

Uterus displaced by full bladder

Fundal height
- At delivery
- Day 1
- Day 2
- Day 3
- Day 4
- Day 5
- Day 6
- Day 7
- Day 8
- Day 9

- Lochia serosa, a serosanguineous discharge that is pink or brown in color, lasts from about days 4–10.

- Lochia alba, the final discharge, is creamy or whitish in color and may persist until the 3rd or 4th week.

- The odor of lochia is "musty," "earthy," or "fleshy." A foul odor suggests infection.

- Bright red color in the presence of firm fundus suggests bleeding laceration.

Perineum

Some edema and bruising of the perineum can be expected following childbirth. An episiotomy is often made to facilitate childbirth. Sutures used to close the incision are absorbed; there is no need to remove them. Lacerations may also occur and require suturing. Lacerations are classified according to the amount of tissue involved.

- *First degree* involves superficial vaginal mucosa or perineal skin.

- *Second degree* involves deeper tissue and may include perineal muscles.

- *Third degree* extends into the rectal sphincter.

- *Fourth degree* extends through the sphincter and into the rectal mucosa.

B. CARDIOVASCULAR SYSTEM

Blood Volume

On the average, 500 mL of blood is lost during vaginal births and 1000 mL in cesarean births. The woman can tolerate this loss without ill effects because

- Vascular volume increases that occur during pregnancy.

- Blood from the uteroplacental unit returns to central circulation when the placenta is expelled.

Blood Values

- Red blood cells, hemoglobin, and hematocrit remain near prebirth levels despite normal blood loss during childbirth due to hemoconcentration that follows postpartal diuresis.

- The increase in factors that promote clotting, coupled with a decline in factors that promote lysis of clots, puts the new mother at risk for thrombus formation.

- White blood cell count increases from the normal range of 5,000–10,000/mm^3 to 20,000–30,000/mm^3. Neutrophils, which rise in response to inflammation, pain, and stress, account for most of the increase.

C. VITAL SIGNS

Temperature

- Temperature of 38° C (100.4° F) is common the first 24 hours following childbirth and may be caused by dehydration or the normal stress response.
- Infection should be suspected if the elevation persists for longer than 24 hours or if it exceeds 38° C.

Blood Pressure

Blood pressure should remain near prepregnancy levels due to the effect of progesterone and other hormonal factors that increase resistance to angiotensin (a vasoconstrictor) during pregnancy and the early postpartum period.

Orthostatic hypotension occurs due to a rapid reduction in intra-abdominal pressure after childbirth that results in dilation of blood vessels supplying the viscera.

- Resulting engorgement of abdominal blood vessels contributes to a rapid fall in blood pressure when the woman moves from a recumbent to an upright position.
- Mothers often say they feel dizzy or lightheaded when they stand.
- Without assistance, they are at risk to faint and suffer injury.
- Hypotension may also indicate excessive blood loss; therefore, making careful assessments for hemorrhage (location and firmness of the fundus, amount and color of lochia, pulse rate, and blood pressure) is essential.

Pulse and Respirations

- Pulse and respirations should remain within normal limits.
- Bradycardia may occur as a result of increased vascular volume; this reflects an increase in cardiac return and a consequent rise in stroke volume that allows a reduced pulse rate.
- Tachycardia may be the first indication of hypovolemia.

D. BREASTS

Following childbirth, levels of estrogen and progesterone decline. This decrease allows prolactin, which stimulates milk production, to rise. Although colostrum is present from the second trimester of pregnancy, milk is generally not produced until 2–3 days following childbirth. A second hormone, oxytocin, stimulates the milk-ejection (let-down) reflex.

E. CHANGES IN ELIMINATION

Bladder and Kidneys

- Decreased sensitivity to fluid pressure in the bladder due to loss of muscle tone, plus trauma to the urethra, bladder, and urinary meatus that often occurs during childbirth, interfere with emptying the bladder.

- The bladder fills quickly as the body rids itself of excess fluid by diuresis.

- The woman may be completely unaware of a severely distended bladder.

- A distended bladder lifts and displaces the uterus and is one of the major causes of postpartum hemorrhage.

- Signs of a distended bladder:
  - Fundus is located above baseline level (i.e., when bladder is empty)
  - Fundus displaced from midline
  - Excessive lochia
  - Bladder discomfort
  - Bulge of bladder above symphysis pubis
  - Frequent voidings of less than 150 mL of urine (indicating urinary retention with overflow)

- Acetone in urine in the early postpartum period suggests dehydration that may occur as a result of exertion during labor.

- Mild proteinuria is usually the result of catabolic processes of involution.

Bowel

Constipation and painful defecation may occur in the postpartal period.

- Bowel tone, which was diminished during pregnancy as a result of progesterone, remains sluggish for several days.
- Restricted food and fluid intake during labor may result in small, hard stools.
- Pain from perineal trauma, episiotomies, and hemorrhoids interferes with effective bowel elimination.

F. MUSCLES, JOINTS, AND SKIN

- Exertion in labor may result in muscle fatigue and aches, particularly of the shoulders, neck, and arms.
- Levels of the hormone relaxin gradually subside and ligaments and cartilage of the pelvis begin to return to their prepregnancy position, causing hip or joint pain that interferes with ambulation and exercise.
- Skin changes, such as the "mask of pregnancy," spider nevi, and palmar erythema, disappear when the hormones of pregnancy decline following childbirth.
- Striae gravidarum (stretch marks) fade to silvery lines but do not disappear altogether. Stretch marks may be removed by laser therapy at a later time.

II. PSYCHOSOCIAL ADAPTATIONS

A. PUERPERAL PHASES

Following childbirth, the mother passes through three phases as she replenishes her energy and gains confidence in her role as mother.

- *Taking-in* occurs during the first hours after childbirth, is characterized by passive, dependent behavior. The mother is often focused on her own care rather than the infant. She "takes in" attention and physical care. Her primary needs are for fluid, food, and deep restorative sleep.

- *Taking-hold* occurs gradually as the mother becomes more independent and assumes care of herself. She gradually shifts her attention from her needs to those of the infant.

- *Letting-go* is a time of relinquishment as the mother gives up idealized expectations of the birth experience and the infant of her fantasies. She is then able to accept this infant, who may be very different from the infant she dreamed of during pregnancy.

B. BONDING AND ATTACHMENT

- Bonding is the initial attraction felt by the parents when they are able to hold the infant soon after birth.

- Attachment is a process that follows a progressive course and occurs over time. It is facilitated by
  — Positive feedback, such as mutual gazing of parents and infant, the ability to console the infant, and the infant's response to parental touch and voice.
  — Close and prolonged contact between parents and infant.

C. MATERNAL TOUCH AND VERBAL INTERACTION

Maternal touch indicates the progress of maternal attachment as it progresses from "fingertipping" as the mother becomes acquainted with her child to enfolding as the she becomes more comfortable with her role as mother.

Verbal behaviors also indicate maternal attachment. Most mothers

- Speak to the infant in a high-pitched voice.

- Progress from calling the baby "it" to "he" or "she" and then to using the given name.

- Paternal behaviors parallel those of the mother during the initial contact with the infant.

D. INFANT COMMUNICATION CUES

Infants actively participate in communication through signals or cues that are sometimes called reciprocal attachment behaviors. Infant cues can be verbal or nonverbal. Verbal cues include crying and cooing. Nonverbal cues include

- Making eye contact and engaging in prolonged mutual gazing.
- Moving the eyes and attempting to "track" the parent's face.
- Grasping the parent's fingers.
- Moving in rhythm to parent's pattern of speech (entrainment).
- Rooting, latching onto the nipple, and finally suckling.
- Being comforted by parent's voice or touch.

Parents' interpretation of and response to infant cues is known as "reciprocity" and may take several weeks to develop.

E. FACTORS THAT AFFECT ADAPTATION

Factors that can interfere with family adaptation to the birth of an infant include

- Lingering fatigue or discomfort (perineal, incisional, etc.).
- Lack of knowledge of infant needs.
- Previous experience with infants.
- Maternal age (<18 years usually require more assistance).
- Maternal personality (calm, patient mother has easier time).
- Temperament of infant (easily consoled, enjoys cuddling versus irritable, difficult to console).
- Availability of strong support system.

III. NURSING ASSESSMENTS

Because of the risk of postpartal hemorrhage, frequent and thorough physical assessments are a priority during the first hours following childbirth. When physical safety of the mother is assured, psychosocial assessments become equally important. See Table IV-1, "Postpartum Nursing Assessment."

TABLE IV-1

Postpartum Nursing Assessment

ASSESSMENT	EXPECTED FINDINGS	NURSING ACTIONS
Physiologic Adaptation		
Uterus		
Assess the uterine fundus. See "Procedure I.," p. 428.	Fundus should be firm, midline, and located midway between the symphysis pubis and the umbilicus immediately after the placenta is expelled. It then rises to the level of the umbilicus. It should remain firm and begin to decrease in size by the second postpartal day.	Help woman empty bladder so the uterus can contract firmly. Begin at umbilicus and palpate gently until fundus is located. Reassess to be sure uterus remains contracted when massage is stopped.
Lochia		
Evaluate lochia for amount, character, and odor. Note how often pads are saturated, and observe perineum for constant trickle that indicates excessive flow.	Amount should be moderate (approximately 8 pads per day). A few small clots are normal during the first day or two.	If excessive flow is suspected, save all pads and bedliners so an accurate estimation of blood loss can be made by weight (1 gm = 1 mL).

Note: Blood can pool under the woman's hips. Ask her turn so linen and bed liners can be seen. Excessive flow in the presence of a contracted fundus suggests a laceration of the cervix or vagina.

Perineum

Observe the perineum and episiotomy; see "Procedure H.," p. 427.

Slight edema or bruising is normal. There should be no redness, or drainage. Edges of the episiotomy should be approximated.

Notify primary caregiver if there are signs of infection ing, such as pain or bulging of tissue that indicate formation of a hematoma.

Vital Signs

Blood Pressure (BP)

Measure BP in the same arm with the mother in the same position each time to avoid inaccurate data. Be consistent in use of Korotkoff's 4th or 5th sound to determine diastolic pressure.

BP should remain near prepregnancy level. Elevation suggests pregnancy-induced hypertension. Decline may indicate excessive bleeding.

Review chart to to determine prepregnancy BP. Help mother ambulate for the first few times to prevent injury as a result of orthostatic hypotension.

Pulse

Count radial or apical pulse with mother at rest.

Pulse rate of 50–90 is considered normal. Bradycardia is not unusual.

Tachycardia, which may result from a difficult labor, excitement, or hemorrhage, requires additional assessments of fundus and lochia.

Respirations

Count with mother at rest.

Normally 16–24 per minute.

If decreased, assess for effects of medication; if increased, check for other signs of respiratory infection or for source of anxiety.

Temperature

From 36.2–38°C (98–100.4°F) is considered normal for the first 24 hours if there are no other signs of infection.

Report elevation that is higher or that persists for longer than 24 hours.

Breasts

Palpate the breasts and inspect the skin and areola. Observe nipples closely for cracks, tenderness, or soreness. Observe breastfeeding techniques.

Breasts should be smooth and soft (initially), somewhat firm (filling), or firm (full of milk). Protruding nipples facilitate breastfeeding.

Women with flat or inverted nipples may require special assistance with breastfeeding. Cracks may allow microorganisms to enter and cause infection.

Elimination

Bladder

Observe and measure first voidings. Palpate the uterine fundus and note amount of lochia. Observe for palpable bulge above symphysis pubis.

First voiding should be more than 150 mL. Fundus should be firm, near the level of the umbilicus, and midline. Lochia should be no more than moderate.

Review signs of distended bladder (p. 285) Help mother void; catheterize if necessary.

Bowel

Ask about usual pattern of bowel elimination and determine when she had the last bowel movement. Observe number and size of hemorrhoids.

Softly formed stool by the third day after childbirth is expected.

Infrequent, hard stools or painful defecation may require administration of stool softeners. Teach measures to reduce pain of hemorrhoids and to prevent constipation.

Lower Extremities

Inspect the legs for areas of redness, heat, or tenderness. Palpate pedal pulses.

The legs should be free of areas redness, heat, or tenderness. Pedal pulses should be equal bilaterally.

Help mother ambulate ASAP. Apply support hose as indicated. Report any abnormal signs.

Laboratory Values

Check hemoglobin, hematocrit, RBC, WBC, Rh factor, and rubella titer.	A drop of 1 g in hemoglobin or 3% in hematocrit is considered normal. Larger declines suggest excessive intrapartal bleeding. WBC may be elevated; RBC near pregnancy levels.	Administer Rho-GAM to unsensitized Rh-negative mother with Rh-positive infant. Administer rubella vaccine to mother who is not immune (titer <1:8).

Psychologic Adaptation

Puerperal Phases

Taking-in	Passive, dependent on nurses for assistance; recounts birth experience over and over; does not initiate care of the infant.	This is a time to "mother the mother." Provide nourishment and time for rest.
Taking-hold	More autonomous, assumes self-care; seeks information about infant care.	Foster independence; promote attachment by involving mother in infant care.
Letting-go	Relinquishes role as childless person; adapts to body changes; begins to see self as mother.	Provide anticipatory guidance for this phase, which may occur after discharge from birth facility.

Interaction with Infant

Maternal touch	Fingertipping, palming, enfolding, consoling behaviors, holding "en face."	Provide ample opportunity for contact with infant.
Verbal interaction	Speaks in high voice; uses given name; coos to attract and hold attention of infant.	Model how to make eye contact and interact with infant.
Response to infant cues	Prompt, gentle, consistent.	Point out infant signals and model appropriate responses.

RISK ASSESSMENT

Two of the most common complications of the puerperium are hemorrhage and infection. Nurses must be aware of factors that increase the risk of these complications so they can expand their vigilance to protect the mother.

Risk Factors for Hemorrhage

- Multiparity (>3)
- Overdistention of the uterus
- Precipitous labor (<3 hours)
- Retained placenta
- Placenta previa or abruptio placentae
- Induction or augmentation of labor
- Administration of tocolytics to stop uterine contractions
- Operative procedures (vacuum extraction, forceps, cesarean birth)

Risk Factors for Infection

- Operative procedures
- Multiple cervical examinations
- Prolonged labor (>24 hours)
- Manual extraction of the placenta
- Diabetes mellitus
- Indwelling catheter
- Anemia

IV. COMMON NURSING DIAGNOSES

- Pain related to uterine contractions (afterpains), perineal trauma, breast engorgement, or hemorrhoids

- Effective breastfeeding related to basic knowledge and maternal confidence
- Risk for ineffective breastfeeding related to lack of understanding of breastfeeding techniques
- Alteration in skin integrity (nipple) related to incorrect positioning during breastfeeding
- Altered patterns of urinary elimination related to temporary loss of sensation and decreased muscle tone of the bladder
- Constipation related to knowledge deficit of measures to promote bowel elimination
- Risk for altered health maintenance related to knowledge deficit of self-care or signs of complication
- Risk for infection related to impaired tissue integrity and tissue trauma from childbirth
- Health seeking behaviors regarding self-care, newborn care, health maintenance, prevention of complications
- Risk for alteration in parenting related to fatigue, discomfort, lack of knowledge of infant care
- Risk for alteration in family processes related to lack of knowledge of infant needs and behaviors

V. NURSING INTERVENTIONS

Nursing interventions focus on preventing hemorrhage or injury, promoting comfort, and providing health education.

A. PREVENTING HEMORRHAGE

Initial Assessments

- Every 15 minutes for the first hour following childbirth
  — Palpate fundus for uterine tone and position.
  — Assess lochia for amount and color.
  — Determine vital signs.

- Repeat assessments every 30 minutes for next two hours (more frequently if condition warrants).
- Continue assessments every 4 hours for 12–24 hours (or according to facility protocol).

Massaging the Uterus

If the uterus is soft or boggy, massage the uterus to stimulate uterine contraction and restore firm tone.

- Place the non-dominant hand above the symphysis pubis to anchor and support the lower segment of the uterus.
- Compress and massage the fundus with the dominant hand.
- Attempt to express clots only when the uterus is firm (pushing against a boggy uterus could cause uterine inversion).
- Stop massage when uterus becomes firm.
- Reevaluate fundus frequently to be sure it remains firm.

Administering Oxytocin

If massage fails to restore uterine tone, expect to administer intravenous oxytocin preparation, methylergonovine maleate, or prostaglandin to control bleeding. See pages 312-315 for further information about management of postpartum hemorrhage.

Ensuring Bladder Elimination

Several measures help the perineal muscles relax and stimulate the sensation of needing to void.

- Assist to bathroom as soon as able to ambulate; allow plenty of time, and provide privacy.
- Place the mother's hands in running water.
- Pour warm water over the mother's vulva.
- Provide hot tea or fluids of choice.
- Ask the mother to blow bubbles through a straw.
- Encourage her to urinate in the shower or sitz bath.

- Catheterize if there are signs of bladder distention and she is unable to void.

B. PREVENTING INJURY

Women may be lightheaded because of medication, blood loss, fatigue, or orthostatic hypotension. To prevent falls that can result in injury, nurses should

- Advise the mother to call for assistance before getting out of bed for the first time.
- Keep bed in locked position with side rails up until she is fully recovered from anesthesia or analgesia.
- Elevate the head of the bed for a few minutes before the mother attempts to stand.
- Help her sit on the side of the bed, and then to stand slowly to allow blood pressure to stabilize before she is fully upright.
- Instruct her to move her feet constantly when she first stands to increase venous return from the lower extremities.
- Help the mother ambulate as soon as possible.
- Remain accessible and provide emergency bells for use during showers or sitz baths, when heat may add to the problem.
- Lower her to sitting or lying position if she becomes lightheaded. This increases blood flow to the brain and prevents fainting.

C. PROMOTING COMFORT

Perineal Trauma and Hemorrhoids

- Use glove filled with ice or chemical cold pack for the first 12 hours following childbirth.
  — Wrap ice pack in disposable glove or paper before applying to the perineum.

- Leave in place until ice melts; then remove it for 10 minutes before applying another pack.
- Begin sitz baths according to facility protocol (usually 12–24 hours after delivery). Cool water reduces pain caused by edema; warm water increases circulation and promotes healing.
- Teach mother to use topical medications to decrease perineal discomfort. Instruct her to hold the nozzle of anesthetic spray 10–12 inches from her body and direct it toward the perineum.
- Advise the mother to squeeze her buttocks together before sitting and to lower her weight slowly to lessen pain in the perineal area. Many mothers also benefit from an air cushion or "doughnut" to relieve pressure when sitting.
- Teach the mother to reinsert hemorrhoids if necessary.
  - Put on finger cot or unsterile glove and apply lubrication to the finger.
  - Lie on her side, place lubricated finger against the hemorrhoids and apply steady, gentle pressure against hemorrhoids.
  - Hold them in place for 1–2 minutes; after this, the anal sphincter should hold them in place.
- Apply soothing witch-hazel compresses or an anesthetic cream to hemorrhoids or insert antihemorrhoidal suppositories for relief of discomfort.
- Administer analgesics as directed.

Afterpains

- Suggest that the woman lie in a prone position with a small pillow under the abdomen. This constant pressure causes the uterus to remain contracted and relieves pain of intermittent contractions.
- Instruct her to take analgesics at least one-half hour before breastfeeding, and reassure the woman that the medication will do no harm to the infant.

D. PROVIDING HEALTH EDUCATION

Process of Involution

- Teach the mother how to locate and palpate the fundus and how to estimate the amount of lochia.
- Demonstrate the expected rate of uterine descent.
- Recommend that the woman note the firmness and location of the fundus at least once a day.
- Instruct in expected color, quantity, and duration of lochia

Hand Washing

Emphasize the importance of thorough handwashing before touching the breasts, after diaper changes, after bladder or bowel elimination, and always before handling the infant.

Breast Care for Nonlactating Mothers

- Explain that she must avoid breast stimulation to suppress lactation. For instance, when showering, she should protect her breasts from the cascade of warm water.
- Remind her to wear a tight support bra or breast binder to reduce circulation and filling of the breasts.
- Recommend that she apply ice to prevent engorgement or to reduce discomfort if her breasts become engorged.

Formula Feeding

- Available formulas include cow's milk- or soy-based formula, or protein hydrolysate.
- Available forms include ready-to-use, concentrated (must be diluted), and powdered (must be mixed according to directions).
- Equipment (bottles and nipples) depends on mother's preference.
- Preparation may be single bottle or 24-hour supply; cap and refrigerate formula until needed.

- Sterilization is unnecessary if water supply is safe. If water supply is unsafe, sterilize equipment by boiling for 5 minutes.

- Boil water for diluting formula separately.

- Wash bottles and nipples with hot sudsy water, rinse well, and air dry. Bottles may be washed in dishwasher, but nipples tend to deteriorate quickly unless washed by hand.

- Position the infant in a semi-upright position (such as cradle hold).

- Keep nipple filled with formula to prevent swallowing of air. Infants typically take 0.5–1 ounce per feeding the first day and 2–3 ounces per feeding by third day.

- Burp infant after every half ounce at first.

- Place infant in a side-lying position after feedings.

- Feed every 3–4 hours, but avoid rigid schedule.

- Do not prop the bottle; doing so increases the risk of aspiration and promotes the growth of bacteria that can lead to ear infections and dental caries when the teeth are in.

- Discard formula not used within an hour because of bacterial growth.

- Avoid heating formula in microwave because the heating is uneven and may result in burning the infant. Test formula temperature by placing a few drops from the bottle on the inner arm.

Breastfeeding

- Help the mother assume a comfortable position; use pillows to support her arm and the infant and to protect an abdominal incision.

- Teach side-lying, cradle, and football holds. See Figure IV-2 A, B, and C.

- Position infant facing the breast with as much of the areola as possible in the infant's mouth.

300 Clinical Manual for Foundations of Maternal Newborn Nursing

Figure IV-2

Positions for Breastfeeding

A.

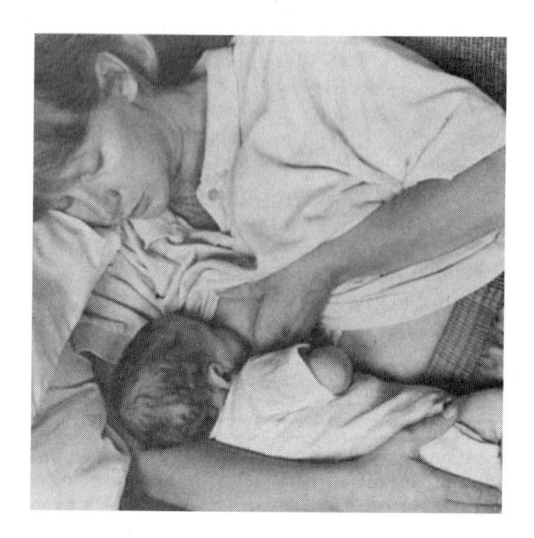

Side-lying position

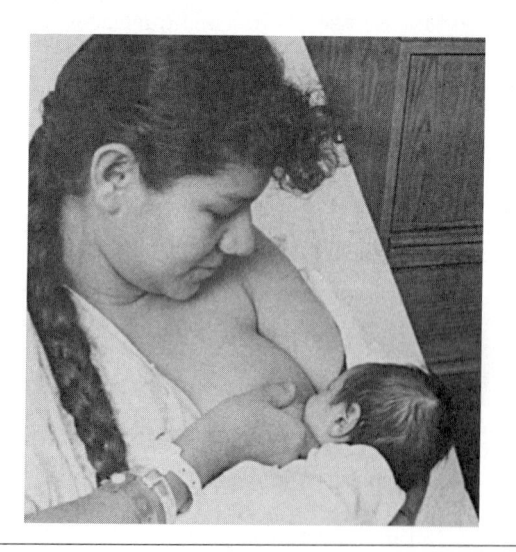

B.

Cradle hold position

SECTION FOUR: Postpartum 301

C.

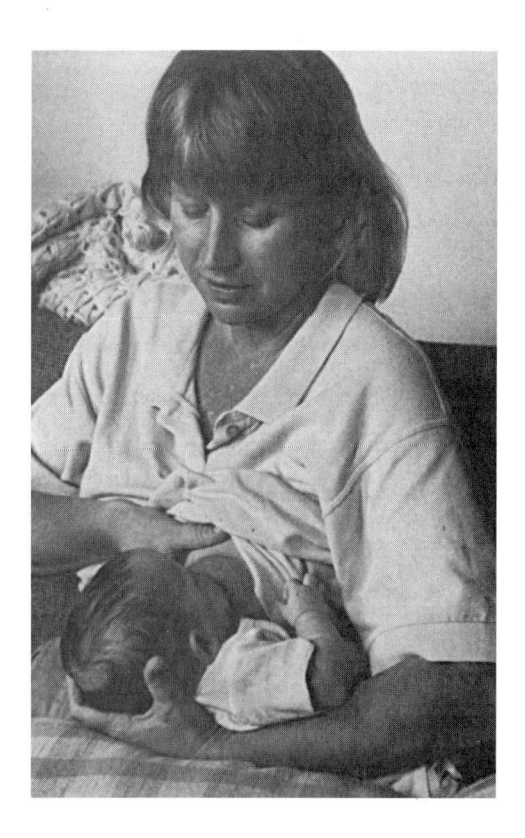

Football hold position

- Evaluate infant suckling, which should be smooth and continuous with only occasional pauses.
- Take the infant off the breast and start again if suckling is short, choppy, and without audible swallowing sounds.
- Advise the mother to feed the infant when the breasts feel full or when the infant indicates hunger rather than following a schedule.
- Explain that she should not restrict the duration of breastfeeding, but she should allow adequate time for both breasts to be emptied at each feeding.
- Remind her that keeping breasts dry between feedings helps prevent tissue damage, and wearing a good bra provides necessary support.

Common Problems of Breastfeeding

Sleepy Infant

- Teach mother measures to awaken infant gently (changing diaper, removing blankets until infant is awake, rubbing cheeks or hair, talking, playing, washing infant's face with lukewarm washcloth).
- Recommend burping infant frequently to reduce feeling of fullness.
- Suggest expressing colostrum onto nipple to interest infant in feeding.

Nipple Confusion or Preference

These problems may occur in infants who have received bottles and confuse the tongue movements needed for the two types of feedings. Teaching includes:

- Avoid all bottles unless absolutely necessary.
- Avoid pacifiers.
- Nurse more frequently to stimulate milk production and help infant learn proper suckling.

Suckling Problems

Infants may suck on the end of the nipple, fail to open the mouth widely enough, have dimpling of the cheeks, or make smacking noises. Teaching includes:

- Rub nipple against lower lip to stimulate infant to open mouth widely.
- Wait until infant opens mouth widely before inserting nipple.
- Check position: Much of areola should be in mouth, and lips should be 1–1.5 inches from nipple base.
- Remove infant and start again if latch is incorrect.

Sore Nipples

Nursing interventions to prevent sore nipples include

- Ensure that infant is positioned correctly at the breast.
- Check infant's mouth for the white patches of *Candida* infection (thrush). If present, notify the health care provider to obtain medication for mother and infant.
- Check for allergies and irritations caused by breast creams.

Teaching includes:

- Avoid using soap or other drying agents on the nipples.
- Avoid creams that must be removed before feedings.
- Change wet nursing pads promptly.
- Avoid nipple shields that decrease milk flow to the infant.
- Begin feeding with the least sore side.
- Vary the position of the infant during feeding (the area of the nipple directly in line with the infant's nose and chin is most stressed during a feeding).
- Apply warm-water compresses, colostrum, or breast milk after feeding.
- Expose the nipples to air between feedings.

Engorgement

To prevent engorgement, which may occur when the milk comes in or if feedings are not of sufficient frequency or length, teach the mother to

- Breastfeed every 2–3 hours day and night for an average of 15 minutes per feeding.
- Use a breast pump to empty breasts if breastfeeding must be interrupted.
- Apply ice packs to reduce edema and pain (using a clean glove or plastic bag filled with crushed iced and covered with washcloths).
- Apply heat with compresses, or shower prior to feedings.
- Massage breasts before feedings to stimulate let-down reflex.
- Express milk by hand or use breast pump before feedings if areola is too hard for infant to grasp.

Flat or Inverted Nipples

Infants may have difficulty grasping flat or inverted nipples. Teaching includes

- Use breast shells to help make nipples protrude.
- Roll the nipples between thumb and forefinger to make them protrude just before feedings.
- Use a breast pump just before feedings to draw out inverted nipples.
- Put the baby to breast immediately after pumping when the nipple is erect.

Interruption of Breastfeeding

To maintain milk supply when breastfeeding must be interrupted temporarily

- Teach mother how to use breast pump.

- Instruct her to pump for 15–20 minutes for at least 8 sessions each day.

- Demonstrate breast massage before pumping to increase flow of milk.

- Provide sterile containers for the milk so that the infant can be fed the milk. Instruct in special nursery requirements.

Assessing Infant Milk Requirements

Signs the infant is getting enough milk

- Swallowing is audible (a soft "ka" or "ah" sound).

- Mother's breast gets softer during the feeding.

- Milk is seen in the baby's mouth or dripping from the mother's breast.

- Infant has at least 2–6 wet diapers a day for the first 2 days and 6–8 wet diapers by the fifth day. Urine is light yellow in color, not concentrated.

- Infant passes at least 3 stools daily during the first month; stools are yellow in color by the end of the first week.

- Infant seems satisfied after feedings.

- Infant has gained weight at the first well baby check-up.

Perineal Care

Teach some method for perineal cleansing as soon as possible. Although methods may vary, these are the most common.

- Fill a squeeze bottle with warm water and spray over the perineum from front to back.

- Avoid separating the labia so water does not enter the vagina.

- Pat dry with toilet paper or a moist antiseptic towlette.

- Dry from front to back to prevent contamination from the anal area toward the vaginal introitus.

- Cleanse the perineum after each voiding or defecation, and change the perineal pads at the same time.
- Wash the hands thoroughly.

Kegel Exercise

Teach the mother to contract muscles around the vagina (as though stopping the flow of urine) for a few seconds, then relax. Suggest that she breathe through an open mouth to avoid pushing down as she does the exercise. She should do this contraction-relaxation cycle 10 times in each series. Emphasize that the series may be repeated 5 times each day during the postpartum period.

Bowel Elimination

- Emphasize the importance of adequate fluid, dietary fiber, and progressive exercise.
- Encourage the mother to establish a regular pattern of bowel elimination.
- Teach measures to reduce perineal or hemorrhoidal pain (sitz baths, witch-hazel compresses, or appropriate ointments).
- Advise her to act on any urge to defecate and to take adequate time.
- Reassure her that she will not damage the repaired episiotomy wound by bearing down gently.
- The physician may order a stool softener, such as Docusate, or a stimulant, such as bisacodyl suppository.

Body Mechanics

- Encourage the mother and father to find a location for infant care that does not require bending.
- Suggest mild exercises, such as abdominal breathing, head lifts, and knee and leg rolls to improve muscle tone. She may begin these exercises within a few days of childbirth.

- Advise her to reduce or stop exercising if lochial flow increases or if she becomes uncomfortable or fatigued.

Sexual Activity

- Suggest that she avoid sexual intercourse until the physician or nurse-midwife has conducted a postpartal examination.
- Advise her that intercourse should be gentle because the vaginal and perineal areas may remain tender.
- Recommend that she use a lubricant if vaginal dryness is a problem.
- Caution her that she can become pregnant during the puerperium, whether or not she is breastfeeding.
- Identify need for family planning (see p. 349).

Return of Ovulation and Menstruation

	OVULATION	MENSTRUATION
Nonlactating women (average time)	10 weeks	7–9 weeks
Lactating women (depends on duration of lactation)	17–28 weeks	30–36 weeks

Signs and Symptoms that Should Be Reported

New mothers and at least one member of the family should know the signs and symptoms that should be reported to the health care provider as soon as possible.

- Fever
- Localized area of redness, swelling, or pain in either breast that is not relieved by support or analgesics
- Persistent abdominal tenderness or feelings of pelvic fullness or pelvic pressure
- Persistent perineal pain
- Frequency, urgency, or burning on urination

- Changes in character of lochia (increased amount, resumption of bright-red color, passage of clots, foul odor)
- Localized tenderness, redness, or warmth of the legs

Promoting Bonding and Attachment

- Provide early, unlimited contact between parents and newborn.
- Position infant so that eye contact with parent is possible.
- Point out reciprocal attachment behaviors of the infant.
- Help breastfeeding mothers put the infant to breast.
- Model appropriate behaviors (holding close, using high-pitched voice and soothing tone).
- Provide comfort and ample time for rest so mother can replenish her energy and be free of discomfort as she assumes care of the newborn.

VI. NURSING CARE FOLLOWING CESAREAN BIRTH

A. NURSING ASSESSMENT

Assessments must be modified and expanded when the mother has a cesarean birth. See Table IV-2, "Nursing Assessments Following Cesarean Birth."

TABLE IV-2

Nursing Assessments Following Cesarean Birth

PHYSIOLOGIC CHANGES: EXPECTED FINDINGS	HOW TO ASSESS EXPECTED FINDINGS	ABNORMAL FINDINGS: NURSING ACTIONS
Respiratory Effort		
Epidural narcotics, which can cause respiratory depression, are often used for pain relief. Immobility and decreased respirations may result in pooling of bronchial secretions.	If apnea monitor is not used, evaluate respiratory rate and depth at least every half hour for first 24 hours. Auscultate breath sounds.	Respiratory rate <12 per minute. Diminished depth or adventitious breath sounds. Notify anesthesiologist; elevate head of bed, administer oxygen and be prepared to administer narcotic antagonist.
Abdomen		
Decreased peristalsis occurs as a result of operative procedure.	Auscultate for bowel sounds. Palpate fundus gently to prevent discomfort. Abdomen should be soft, bowel sounds present, passing flatus within 1–2 days.	Abdominal distention, no bowel sounds (listen in all four quadrants), unable to pass flatus.
Surgical Incision		
A transverse incision in the lower uterine segment is most common.	Use acronym REEDA to assess surgical wound.	Report any signs of infection.
Intake and Output		
Intravenous fluids are usually given, and an indwelling urinary catheter is left in place for the first 24 hours.	Monitor rate of IV flow and condition of IV site. Evaluate amount, color, and clarity of urine.	Adjust intravenous infusion rate as directed. Edema, redness, or pain at IV site may make it necessary to stop infusion and restart at another site.

B. MOST COMMON NURSING DIAGNOSES

- Pain related to surgical incision or abdominal distention
- Activity intolerance related to incisional pain, effects of anesthesia
- Ineffective airway clearance related to immobility, depressed respirations
- Risk for altered parenting related to discomfort, difficulty in moving or positioning infant

C. NURSING INTERVENTIONS

Providing Comfort

Patient-controlled analgesia (PCA) and epidural analgesia are two methods used for pain relief. Respiratory depression may occur if opioids are used for analgesia. Some women experience itching if morphine sulfate is used for analgesia. Antihistamines, such as diphenhydramine, or narcotic antagonists, such as naloxone, are often used to control itching.

Overcoming Effects of Immobility

- Splint the abdomen with a small pillow to reduce discomfort.
- Help the mother turn, cough, and breathe deeply every two hours to prevent pooling of bronchial secretions.
- Encourage her to move her feet and legs to improve peripheral circulation.
- Help her sit and dangle the legs after about 8 hours and walk as soon as possible to prevent thromboembolic complications and to prevent abdominal distention.

Relieving Abdominal Distention

- Encourage slow resumption of oral intake, beginning with ice chips, progressing to liquid, and then to regular diet once the mother expels flatus.

- Advise mother to avoid carbonated beverages, use of straws, and gas-forming foods.
- Teach pelvic lifts (a flat, supine position with knees bent, lifting the pelvis from the bed) to reduce distention.
- Insert rectal tube or suppositories to help expel flatus from the distal colon.
- Obtain order for simethicone to reduce flatus formation.

Reinstating Normal Activities

After 24 hours, several normal functions usually return, and mothers are able to participate more actively in their own care.

- Discontinue intravenous infusion and provide liquid diet.
- Remove indwelling urinary catheter and monitor first two voidings to be sure bladder is empty.
- Remove dressing and staples according to facility protocol.
- Encourage ambulation and as much self-care as is comfortable for the mother.
- Provide ample opportunity for parent-infant contact and assist mother with infant feeding.

Assisting with Infant Feeding

- Find comfortable position for holding infant.
  - Suggest football hold or side-lying position for breastfeeding.
  - Place pillow on lap to protect incisional area from weight of infant.
  - Help the mother change position to breastfeed on both sides.

VII. POSTPARTUM COMPLICATIONS

A. POSTPARTUM HEMORRHAGE

Postpartum hemorrhage is loss of more than 500 mL of blood following vaginal childbirth or loss of more than 1000 mL following cesarean birth.

Etiology

- Uterine atony
- Trauma to the birth canal
- Retained placental fragments
- Subinvolution or infection

Predisposing Factors

- Overdistention of the uterus from any cause (multiple gestation, large infant, hydramnios)
- Multiparity
- Prolonged labor
- Precipitate labor
- Induced or augmented labor
- Use of assistive devices (forceps, vacuum extractor)
- Cesarean birth
- Manual removal of the placenta
- Previous postpartum hemorrhage
- Administration of oxytocin, magnesium sulfate, beta-adrenergic tocolytic agents, antihypertensive medications, and halothane (an anesthetic agent)

Clinical Signs

- Fundus that is soft, "boggy," or difficult to locate

- Uterus that does not remain firm when massage is stopped
- Fundus is located above umbilicus or displaced from the midline
- Excessive lochia (saturation of more than 1 perineal pad per hour, constant steady trickle)
- Tachycardia, tachypnea
- Falling blood pressure
- Skin cool and pale

Priority Nursing Assessments

- Review chart for history of predisposing factors.
- Evaluate firmness and location of fundus.
- Assess blood loss; weigh pads, bedliners, and linen (1 gram = 1 mL). Excessive bleeding when the fundus is firm suggests cervical or vaginal laceration.
- Examine perineum for bluish discoloration, bulging, or tender areas that might indicate hematoma. Deep, unrelieved pelvic pain implies vaginal or retroperitoneal hematoma that cannot be seen.
- Measure vital signs (including mean arterial pressure and pulse pressure) at least every 15 minutes. Tachycardia and falling pulse pressure are early signs of hypovolemia; however, blood pressure may remain normal as hypovolemia develops because of vasoconstriction that shunts blood to vital organs during the initial phase of hypovolemic shock.
- Evaluate bladder (distended bladder hinders effective uterine contraction) and urinary output (less than 30 mL per hour suggests inadequate vascular volume).
- Analyze laboratory reports (decreasing hematocrit and hemoglobin indicate blood loss).

Therapeutic Management

- Maintain intravenous access and start second IV with large-bore catheter that is capable of carrying whole blood.

- Draw blood for hemoglobin and hematocrit, blood type and crossmatch, coagulation studies (fibrinogen, prothrombin time, and fibrinogen degradation products), and blood chemistries.

- Place in supine position. Avoid Trendelenburg position, which may interfere with respiratory and cardiac function.

- Massage uterus while supporting lower uterine segment. See Figure IV-3.

Figure IV-3

Technique for Fundal Massage

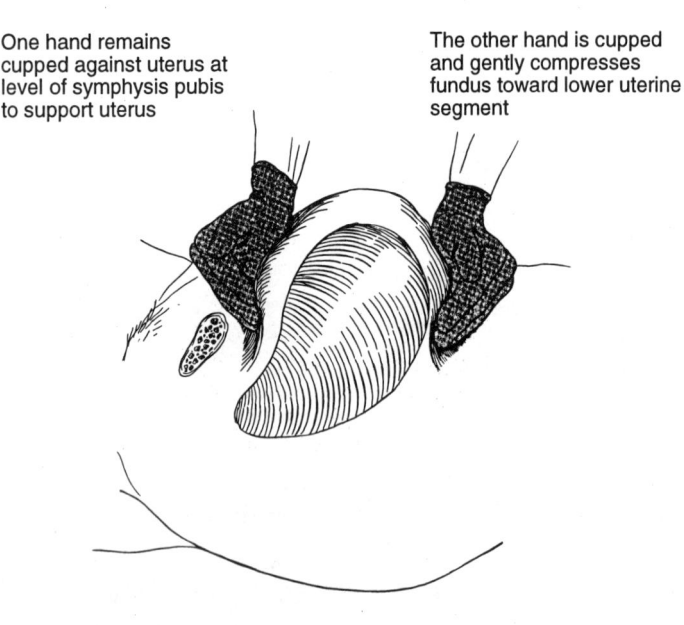

One hand remains cupped against uterus at level of symphysis pubis to support uterus

The other hand is cupped and gently compresses fundus toward lower uterine segment

- Insert indwelling catheter to empty bladder and allow accurate measurement of output.

- Administer intravenous fluids, volume expanders, and blood as directed.

- Administer prescribed drugs, such as oxytocin, prostaglandins, or methylergonovine maleate.

- Administer intramuscular drugs, such as methylergonovine and prostaglandin.

- Apply pulse oximeter to determine oxygen saturation; administer oxygen by snug face mask at 6 L/min or as directed by physician or facility protocol.

- Anticipate further medical interventions (uterine packing, ligation of uterine, ovarian, or hypogastric arteries, or hysterectomy if other measures fail to control bleeding.

Nursing Considerations

Carry out prescribed medical orders.

- Monitor the condition of the woman, and communicate with the health care provider.

- Provide explanations and emotional support for the woman and her family.

- Obtain signed consents for specific surgical procedures or blood transfusions.

B. SUBINVOLUTION

Subinvolution refers to a slower than expected return of the uterus to its prepregnancy size following childbirth.

Etiology

The most common causes of subinvolution are

- Retained placental fragments.
- Pelvic infection.

Clinical Signs and Symptoms

The clinical signs and symptoms of subinvolution are usually not obvious for several days or weeks after the mother has been discharged from the birth facility. The most common are

- Prolonged lochial discharge.
- Irregular or excessive uterine bleeding.

- Pelvic pain or feelings of pelvic heaviness.
- Backache, fatigue, persistent malaise.
- Uterus that feels larger and softer than expected for a particular time.

Therapeutic Management

Medical treatment is tailored to correct the cause of subinvolution. Oral methylergonovine maleate 0.2 mg every 3–4 hours for 24–48 hours provides sustained contraction of the uterus. Infection responds to antimicrobial therapy. Uterine curettage may be necessary if treatment is not effective.

Nursing Considerations

Because subinvolution develops well after the mother has gone home, nursing responsibilities focus on providing education.

- Teach the mother (and significant other) how to locate and palpate the fundus in relation to the umbilicus.
- Remind the mother that the uterus should get smaller and should descend by about one fingerbreadth every day.
- Request return demonstrations until the mother is confident of her ability to locate the fundus.
- Explain normal duration and progressive changes in lochia (from rubra to serosa to alba).
- Instruct woman to report if the uterus does not become smaller, if there is a deviation from expected pattern or duration of lochia, or if a foul odor (suggesting infection) is noted.

C. THROMBOEMBOLIC DISORDERS

The three most common thromboembolic disorders are (1) superficial venous thrombosis, (2) deep vein thrombosis, and (3) pulmonary embolism. A *thrombus* is a collection of blood factors, primarily platelets and fibrin on a vessel wall. Once started, the thrombus can enlarge with successive layering of platelets, fibrin, and blood cells as blood flows past the clot. When an inflammatory process also occurs in the vessel wall, it is termed *thrombophlebitis*.

Etiology

Three major causes of thrombosis

- Venous stasis
- Hypercoagulable blood
- Injury to the innermost layer (intima) of the blood vessel.

Predisposing Factors

- Varicose veins
- Obesity
- Smoking
- Age >35 years
- More than 3 pregnancies
- Cesarean birth
- Immobility associated with antepartum bedrest
- Diabetes mellitus
- Prolonged time in stirrups in second stage of labor

Superficial Venous Thrombosis

Clinical Signs and Symptoms

Symptoms are usually confined to the calf area and include swelling, tenderness, redness, and warmth. It may be possible to palpate the enlarged, hardened vein.

Therapeutic Management

Treatment includes analgesics, rest, and elastic support hose. Elevate the lower extremity to improve venous return, and apply warm packs to promote healing. After symptoms disappear, allow the woman to ambulate gradually. Recommend that she avoid standing for long periods of time and continue to wear support hose to prevent venous stasis. Anticoagulant therapy is usually not required and there is little chance of pulmonary embolism if the thrombosis occurs and remains in the superficial veins of the lower leg.

Deep Vein Thrombosis (DVT)

Clinical Signs and Symptoms

- Severe leg pain, edema, and paleness of affected leg
- Elevated temperature, chills
- Tachycardia
- Positive Homan's sign may or may not be present and is not a reliable indicator of DVT.

Diagnosis is usually based on Doppler flow studies and impedance plethysmography.

Therapeutic Management

In addition to treatment for superficial thrombophlebitis, anticoagulant therapy is needed for DVT.

- Administer intravenous heparin as directed.
- Monitor activated partial thromboplastin time (APTT) so that the heparin dose can be adjusted to maintain a therapeutic level of 1.5–2.5 times control.
- Have protamine sulfate on hand for heparin overdose.

After several days, anticoagulation therapy for the postpartum woman may be changed to warfarin (Coumadin). Prothrombin time and international normalized ratio (INR) are used to monitor coagulation time when warfarin is used. An appropriate INR for DVT is 2.0–3.0.

Nursing Considerations

Nurses can do a great deal to prevent thrombus formation.

- Help mother ambulate frequently and as early as possible.

- Perform range of motion and assist with passive exercises if mother is unable to ambulate.

- Instruct mother to avoid using pillows or knee gatch to prevent pressure on popliteal space and consequent pooling of blood in lower leg.

- Obtain an order for anti-emboli stockings for women with varicose veins, a history of thrombophlebitis, or cesarean birth.

- Pad stirrups during childbirth to prevent prolonged pressure against the popliteal angle during second stage of labor.

- Provide information to prevent hemorrhage when anticoagulant therapy is used for a prolonged time.
  — Instruct the mother to report bleeding, including epistaxis, blood in the urine, bleeding gums, or increased vaginal bleeding.
  — Teach measures to prevent excessive anticoagulation, such as schedule of medication, side effects, importance of taking medication as directed.
  — Caution that over-the-counter medications, such as aspirin and nonsteroidal anti-inflammatory drugs, increase the risk of hemorrhage.
  — Recommend that she take only medications prescribed by physician who is aware that she is taking anticoagulants.
  — Suggest that she use a soft toothbrush, floss her teeth gently, and postpone dental appointments until therapy is completed.
  — Recommend a depilatory, which is safer than a razor, to remove unwanted hair while she is on anticoagulant therapy.

Pulmonary Embolism

Pulmonary embolism is a rare but potentially life-threatening complication of DVT. It occurs when fragments of a blood clot dislodge and are carried to the pulmonary artery or one of its branches. This occludes the vessel and obstructs the flow of blood into the lungs.

Clinical Signs and Symptoms

Signs and symptoms depend on how much pulmonary tissue is affected. The most common signs and symptoms are sudden, sharp chest pain; tachycardia; tachypnea; pulmonary rales; cough; and hemoptysis.

Therapeutic Management

Treatment is aimed at dissolving the clot and maintaining pulmonary circulation.

- Administer intravenous heparin or thrombolytic drugs, such as streptokinase or urokinase.
- Give oxygen (8–10L/min) to decrease hypoxia.
- Elevate the head of the bed slightly to reduce dyspnea.
- Administer analgesics to relieve pain.
- Initiate pulse oximetry to evaluate oxygen saturation.
- Obtain critical care nursing for support of ventilation and cardiovascular status.

Nursing Considerations

- Be aware of the signs and symptoms of pulmonary embolism and be vigilant in assessments of women with thrombosis.
- Report any sign of embolism to the health care provider.
- When signs of embolism are present, obtain assistance, position the woman to reduce dyspnea, and begin oxygen administration.
- The nurse should remain with the woman and provide information and support to a family that usually becomes increasingly fearful and anxious.

D. PUERPERAL INFECTIONS

The most common puerperal infections are metritis, wound infections, and mastitis.

Predisposing Factors

Factors that increase the risk of puerperal infection are

- Cesarean birth
- Trauma (precipitate birth, large infant, forceps, vacuum extractor)
- Prolonged rupture of membranes
- Prolonged labor
- Catheterizations
- Excessive number of vaginal examinations
- Retained placental fragments
- Hemorrhage
- Poor general health (anemia, excessive fatigue, frequent illnesses)
- Poor nutrition (inadequate intake of protein, vitamin C)
- Poor hygiene
- Other medical conditions such as diabetes mellitus

Metritis

Etiology

Metritis, infection of the uterus following childbirth, is usually due to organisms that ascend to the uterus from the lower genital tract.

- Group B *Streptococcus*
- *E. Coli*
- Bacteroides
- *Staphylococcus*

Clinical Signs and Symptoms

- Fever (temperature equal to or >38°C, or 100.4°F) after the first 24 hours following childbirth, occurring on at least 2 days during the first 10 days postpartum

- Chills often accompany fever, which may reach 39.4°C (103°F)

- Lethargy, general malaise, anorexia

- Abdominal pain, cramping, and uterine tenderness

- Purulent, foul-smelling lochia

- Tachycardia

- Subinvolution

Therapeutic Management

Initial medical management includes intravenous administration of broad-spectrum antibiotics. Specimens from blood, endocervix, and uterine cavity are cultured to determine specific second-line antibiotic therapy. Oral antibiotics may be used to complete the course of treatment. Antipyretics are often administered for fever, and oxytocins are administered to promote involution.

Nursing Considerations

- Place mother in Fowler's position to promote drainage of lochia.

- Give medications as directed, and observe for signs of improvement or the development of new symptoms, such as nausea and vomiting, abdominal distention, absent bowel sounds, or severe abdominal pain, that indicate the development of complications.

- Provide comfort measures such as warm blankets, cool compresses, sponge baths, cold or warm drinks.

- Help mother pump breasts to maintain milk supply if it is necessary to isolate her from the infant.

- Instruct mother (and family) in measures to prevent the spread of infection.

Wound Infections

Any break in the skin or mucous membranes provides a portal of entry for bacteria. The most common sites for wound infections include

- Episiotomies
- Perineal lacerations
- Cesarean incisions

Clinical Signs and Symptoms

Signs of infection include localized areas of redness, warmth, swelling, tenderness, and pain. In addition, the edges of the wound may pull apart, and there may be seropurulent drainage from the wound. If untreated, systemic signs such as fever and malaise may develop.

Therapeutic Management

Initial medical management includes administration of broad-spectrum antibiotics until a report of the antibiotic-sensitive organism is determined. The physician or nurse-midwife may remove some sutures and pack the wound with iodoform gauze to allow drainage from the wound.

Nursing Considerations

Wound infections may require readmittance to the hospital or home health care visits. Mothers require reassurance, supportive care, and comfort measures.

- Administer analgesics as necessary
- Apply warm compresses to wound or teach how to take sitz baths to provide comfort and to improve circulation and thus promote healing.
- Teach the importance of frequent perineal care and thorough handwashing.

- Instruct to take adequate fluid and food necessary for healing.
- Teach side effects of medication, and signs of worsening condition.

Mastitis

Mastitis is an infection of the lactating breast. It occurs most often in the second and third weeks following birth. It is more common in mothers nursing for the first time and usually affects only one breast.

Etiology

- *Staphylococcus aureus* from the infant's nose and throat or may be carried on the hands of the mother or the medical or nursing staff.
- Engorgement and stasis of milk frequently precede mastitis.

Clinical Signs and Symptoms

- Localized area of redness and inflammation
- Fatigue and aching muscles
- Fever

Therapeutic Management

- Antibiotics
- Antipyretics
- Analgesics
- Supportive measures, such as breast support and ice packs
- Continuing to empty breast by breast-feeding or gentle pumping if affected breast is too sore for breastfeeding.

Nursing Considerations

A major responsibility for nurses is to teach measures that prevent mastitis.

- Demonstrate how to position the infant correctly for breastfeeding.
- Encourage breastfeeding at least every 2–3 hours for the first 2 weeks.
- Recommend that the woman avoid formula supplements, which may make the infant less interested in breastfeeding.
- Suggest that she change nursing pads as soon as they are wet.
- Instruct her to avoid continuous pressure on the breasts from tight bras or infant carriers.

Once mastitis occurs, nursing measures are aimed at increasing comfort and helping the mother maintain lactation.

- Recommend that the woman apply moist heat to increase comfort and circulation.
- Emphasize that breasts should be emptied completely at each feeding to prevent stasis of milk.
- Teach her how to express milk or to use a breast pump if breastfeeding must be temporarily curtailed on the affected side.
- Recommend that she take at least 3000 mL of fluid each day.

Septic Pelvic Thrombophlebitis

Septic pelvic thrombophlebitis occurs when infection spreads along the venous system and thrombophlebitis develops. It occurs more often in women with wound infections, and it usually involves the ovarian, uterine, or hypogastric veins.

Clinical Signs and Symptoms

- Pain in the groin, abdomen, or flank
- Fever, tachycardia
- Gastrointestinal distress or decreased bowel sounds

Laboratory studies—including CBC with differential, blood chemistries, coagulation studies, and cultures—exclude other diagnoses.

Therapeutic Management

Readmittance to the hospital is usually necessary. Primary treatment includes anticoagulation therapy with intravenous heparin and intravenous antibiotics. Supportive care is similar to that for deep venous thrombosis and includes monitoring for safe levels of anticoagulation therapy and for signs of pulmonary embolism.

E. AFFECTIVE DISORDERS

Postpartum Blues

Postpartum blues, the so-called "baby blues," is a common transient, self-limiting mood that usually occurs within 1–10 days following childbirth and lasts no longer than 2 weeks.

Etiology

The cause is unknown; however, wide fluctuations in hormones are believed to contribute.

Clinical Signs and Symptoms

- Mood instability
- Weeping
- Fatigue
- Anxiety

Nursing Considerations

- Acknowledge feelings and offer support.
- Explain that what the woman is experiencing is normal.
- Reassure her that the feeling will abate within a few days.
- Encourage continued contact with other adults.
- Explain the importance of adequate rest and nutrition.

Postpartum Depression

Etiology and Predisposing Factors

- Cause is unknown; predisposing factors are believed to be
  - Hormonal fluctuations.
  - Medical problems, such as pregnancy-induced hypertension, preexisting diabetes mellitus, or thyroid dysfunction, during pregnancy.
  - A history of depression, mental illness, or alcoholism either in the woman or in her family.
  - Difficult relationship with significant other resulting in lack of support.
  - Feelings of isolation or anger.
  - Fatigue, sleep deprivation, financial worries.

Clinical Signs and Symptoms

Postpartum depression is distinguished from the normal labile emotions of pregnancy and the puerperium by the number, intensity, and persistence of the symptoms. A majority of the symptoms mentioned are intensely and consistently experienced for at least 2 weeks. Common signs and symptoms include

- Loss of interest in surroundings.
- Loss of usual emotional response toward her family.
- Intense feelings of unworthiness, guilt, and shame.
- Generalized fatigue, difficulty concentrating.
- Anorexia and sleep disturbances.
- Tense, irritable appearance.
- Not picking up on infant cues or signals.

Therapeutic Management

Primary care is a combination of psychotherapy, social support, and medications such as antidepressants.

Nursing Considerations

- Allow ample time to convey a caring attitude.
- Recommend that the woman acknowledge her feelings and insist that others acknowledge them also.
- Help mother increase sensitivity to infant cues.
- Emphasize need for continued communication with partner.
- Encourage continued contact with other adults.
- Explain the importance of adequate rest and nutrition.
- Help her identify and contact appropriate support groups.

Postpartum Psychosis

Clinical Signs and Symptoms

The woman with postpartum psychosis loses contact with reality and experiences delusions, hallucinations, and disorientation. Common themes for delusions are associated with childbirth, the newborn's health, or sexuality. Paranoia and strong aggressive feelings may be present.

Therapeutic Management

This mother requires hospitalization, supportive psychotherapy, and antipsychotic or antidepressant drugs. Careful monitoring of the mother's reaction to the drugs is necessary because hormonal imbalances may affect the maternal response.

VIII. THE CHILDBEARING FAMILY WITH SPECIAL NEEDS

A. ADOLESCENT PREGNANCY

Implications for Maternal Health

Pregnancy presents significant health risks for adolescents.

- Pregnancy-induced hypertension

- Anemia
- Nutritional deficiencies, particularly vitamins A, D, B_6, folic acid, riboflavin, calcium, and iron
- Cephalopelvic disproportion (if under 15 years of age)

Psychological Implications

Pregnancy among adolescents is often unplanned and unwanted. Young teenagers have not completed the developmental tasks of adolescence and often do not have well-developed problem solving skills. They may not have developed a strong sense of identity and are usually dependent on their parents for financial and emotional support. Adolescents often have difficulty adapting to the physiological changes of pregnancy. They may be particularly upset by physical changes such as weight gain, hyperpigmentation, and striae gravidarum. Moreover, many young adolescents experience conflicts that involve their own plans and wishes versus the needs of the infant.

Fathers are often unprepared for the pregnancy, which may interfere with their future plans. Many fathers provide assistance with the offspring; however, many cannot, leaving the tasks of caring for the child to the mother and her family.

Implications for Fetal-Neonatal Health

An infant born to a teenage mother is at higher risk for two major complications.

- Prematurity and the resulting consequences, such as respiratory distress syndrome, hypothermia, and hypoglycemia
- Low birth weight (<2500 g)

Impact on Parenting

Adolescent mothers are at risk to become non-nurturing parents. They may exhibit:

- Less sensitivity to infant cues and signals
- Fewer instances of mutual gazing

- Less verbal interaction
- Less touch
- Inappropriate parental behaviors, such as pinching, poking, or picking at the infant
- Unrealistic expectations of the infant (will smile, sleep through the night, always be consolable)

Assessment

Assessment of pregnant teenagers is similar to that of older clients in many respects and should include a thorough health and family history. In addition, the assessment should focus on the following specific areas.

- Compliance with recommended prenatal care (keeping prenatal appointments, taking vitamin and iron supplementation, attending recommended prenatal classes)
- Hgb and Hct to detect iron deficiency anemia
- Blood pressure, urinalysis, assessment for rapid weight gain, and generalized edema that suggest development of pregnancy-induced hypertension
- Sexually transmissible diseases
- Life-style behaviors such as poor nutrition, smoking, or alcohol or other drug use
- Knowledge of growth and development of infants
- Knowledge of infant needs
- Cognitive development and ability to make long-term plans
- Family support

Nursing Diagnoses

- Self-concept disturbance related to conflict between identity development and maternal tasks of pregnancy
- Body image disturbance related to physiological changes of pregnancy

- Altered nutrition: Less than body requirements, related to lack of knowledge of nutritional needs
- Altered nutrition: More than body requirements, related to frequent consumption of fast foods and high-fat snacks
- Risk for altered parenting related to impaired mother-infant attachment, inability to form long-range plans, or unrealistic expectations of the infant
- Altered family processes related to integration of infant into existing family structure

Antepartum Nursing Interventions

- Eliminate barriers to health care
  - Determine the most convenient time and location for appointments.
  - Find ways to maintain positive attitudes of health care workers when adolescents do not comply with recommendations for prenatal care.
- Apply appropriate principles of teaching-learning.
  - Recognize the importance of peer groups.
  - Form small groups with like concerns.
  - Encourage questions and repeat material as needed.
  - Use audiovisual aids, which may be more helpful than reading material for this age group.
  - Maintain open, friendly posture and convey empathy.
- Allow time to counsel about specific problems such as stress reduction.
- Provide instructions about infant growth and development, with particular emphasis on infant cues and signals that require prompt, gentle response.
- Promote family support; important topics include
  - Who will help care for the infant.
  - Future plans for returning to school.
  - Financial assistance from infant's father and family.

- Refer to appropriate national and community resources.
  - Well-baby clinics
  - Programs for school-aged mothers offered by high schools
  - Aid to Families with Dependent Children (AFDC)
  - Women, Infants, Children (WIC)
  - Church and community organizations
  - Nutrition for the Pregnant Adolescent
- Emphasize the benefits of good nutrition for the health of both the mother and infant.
- Reinforce the value of nutritional supplements, such as iron and vitamins, particularly folic acid.
- Provide information about the best food choices, such as milk and milk products, chicken, fish, fruits, vegetables, whole grain cereals, bread, and pasta.
- Explain that foods that are broiled, roasted, or barbecued are lower in fats than foods that are fried.
- Recommend curtailing salty foods, such as olives, pickles, and chips, to prevent or decrease fluid retention.
- Suggest cutting down on fried foods (French fries, onion rings) and substituting baked potatoes with broccoli, cheese, or meat fillings.
- Consider snacks and fast foods, which provide about one fourth of a teenager's calories, when planning nutrition.
  - Recommend yogurt, fresh fruit, popcorn, or cheese and crackers for nutritional snacks.
  - Suggest adding tomatoes and lettuce to hamburgers and deleting dressings that are high in fat and calories.
  - Point out that a milkshake provides more nutrition than carbonated beverages, which are high in sodium and phosphorus.

Intrapartal Care

Supportive nursing interventions are particularly necessary for adolescents, who often have a fear of hospitals and inadequate information about the birth process.

- Nurturing attitude that includes frequent physical contact, reassurance that she will not be left alone, and involvement of the father or other family members
- Acknowledgment of feelings and concerns
- Ongoing information about the labor and delivery process
- Demonstrations of relaxation and breathing techniques
- Attention to physical comfort and pain relief
- Frequent encouragement and reassurance

Postpartum Interventions

The adolescent mother requires the same nursing care as an adult woman. However, her developmental level may make it necessary to focus more on the following interventions.

- Self-care measures (breast and perineal care, comfort measures)
- Measures to promote maternal role acquisition
  — Provide extended contact with the newborn.
  — Instruct in safe and effective parenting skills (feeding, bathing, diapering, and dressing).
  — Teach how to protect the infant from accidents; teach the signs and symptoms of illness that should be reported to health care worker (see pages 207-308).
  — Remind that crying indicates a need, and a consistent gentle response will not spoil the infant.
  — Emphasize that in addition to food, sleep, and comfort, infants also need appropriate stimulation (cuddling, hearing the parents' voices, looking at their faces).
  — Teach that infants also signal when they have had enough stimulation (gaze aversion, yawning, splaying the fingers, hiccoughing, etc.).

- Help to identify support system to assist with child care.
- Emphasize the importance of follow-up appointments and immunizations.

B. DELAYED PREGNANCY

Maternal-Fetal Implications

Women who delay childbirth until 35 years or older are sometimes referred to as "elderly primigravidas," or "older mothers." The term "mature primigravida," however, is preferred by many. The mature primigravida is at higher risk for

- A delay in becoming pregnant due to normal aging of the ovaries and the increased incidence of reproductive tract disorders.
- Chromosomal abnormalities, particularly trisomy 21.
- Complications due to preexisting diseases, such as hypertension, diabetes mellitus, and uterine myomas (fibroids).
- Obstetric complications such as multiple gestation, preterm labor, dysfunctional labor, and cesarean birth.
- Small-for-gestational age infant.

Advantages of Delayed Pregnancy

Most women over 35 years of age who become pregnant have planned the pregnancy after careful thought. They often have resources that include

- Psychosocial maturity.
- Self-confidence.
- Financial security.
- A high level of empathy and flexibility in childrearing attitudes.
- Problem-solving skills.

Disadvantages of Delayed Pregnancy

- Need more time to recover from childbirth
- Have less energy than younger counterparts
- May lack family and peer support
- Experience a feeling of social isolation during early weeks following childbirth

Nursing Considerations

Because the fetus of a mature primigravida is at increased risk for chromosomal abnormalities, she will need information about available diagnostic tests. Although only physicians, certified nurse-midwives, and nurses with special preparation in genetics should provide genetic counseling, all nurses must be prepared to reinforce and clarify information that has been provided.

- Chorionic villus sampling
- Amniocentesis
- Ultrasonography
- Alpha-fetoprotein screening (see page 36)

Several days may pass between the performance of a diagnostic test and when results of the test are known. Nurses must provide an opportunity for the woman and her family to express their concerns and provide information and support.

First-time mothers over the age of 35 years are especially receptive to

- Prenatal classes.
- Childbirth education.
- Cesarean birth classes.
- Breastfeeding classes.
- Infant care demonstrations and return demonstrations.
- Printed materials that describe infant growth and development and how to provide nurturing care for the infant.

C. SUBSTANCE ABUSE

When the pregnant woman takes a substance, by drinking, smoking, snorting, or injecting it, the fetus receives the same substance and experiences the same effects. The fetus, however, is unable to metabolize the drug as efficiently as the expectant mother and experiences more severe effects for a longer period of time. Table IV-3 summarizes the maternal, fetal, and neonatal effects of specific drugs. Although five highly abused substances are presented separately, it must be remembered that it is rare for only one drug to be used. Those who use one drug frequently use others as well.

TABLE IV-3

Effects of Commonly Abused Substances

MATERNAL EFFECTS	FETAL/NEONATAL EFFECTS
Tobacco	
Nicotine causes vasoconstriction; reduces placental blood flow; carbon monoxide inactivates hemoglobin resulting in hypoxia; decreased maternal appetite; increase in spontaneous abortions.	Prematurity; low birth weight; smaller head circumference; delayed neurological and intellectual development; hyperactivity, shorter attention span.
Alcohol	
Increased incidence of second trimester abortion; intoxication; decreased maternal appetite.	Fetal Alcohol Syndrome (prenatal and postnatal growth restriction, CNS impairment, specific craniofacial dysmorphic features); prematurity; low birth weight; withdrawal syndrome during neonatal period (apnea, abdominal distention, cyanosis, tremors, or convulsions); long-term learning problems.

Cocaine

Short-acting stimulant causes vasoconstriction so heart rate, blood pressure, and demand for oxygen increase; stimulates uterine contractions; increase in abruptio placentae, premature rupture of membranes, and stillbirth; lack of prenatal care is a hallmark.

Causes the same physical stress on fetus producing tachycardia, decreased beat-to-beat variability, fetal overactivity, and intrauterine growth restriction; neonatal effects include tremors, tachycardia, irritability, muscular rigidity, exaggerated startle reflex; infants are difficult to console and exhibit learning disabilities, delayed language and motor development; higher risk for necrotizing enterocolitis and SIDS.

Marijuana

Maternal anemia, inadequate maternal weight gain; often paired with other drugs such as cocaine and alcohol.

Neonate may exhibit hyperirritability, unusual sensitivity to light. Difficult to prove effects due solely to marijuana use because of multi-drug use by many.

Heroin

CNS depressant that produces physical addiction; poor general health and nutrition; anemia; high incidence of STDs, hepatitis, and HIV as a result of sharing unclean needles.

Intrauterine hypoxia; prematurity, growth restriction, and stillbirth; infants exhibit neonatal abstinence (withdrawal) syndrome that produces tremors, jitteriness, seizures, hypertonicity and continuous crying, uncoordinated sucking and swallowing reflexes, vomiting, and diarrhea; long-term learning problems are common.

Assessment

Health care professionals must approach the diagnosis of substance abuse with a high index of suspicion. It is estimated that 2.25 million women in the United States are problem drinkers and that 20–30 percent of women of childbearing age smoke cigarettes. Use of illicit drugs is lower; however, 10% represents a reasonable minimal estimate.

Signs and Symptoms

Although any of these signs and symptoms may occur in women who have never abused drugs, the most common signs and symptoms indicating drug use are

- Seeking prenatal care late in pregnancy.
- Failing to keep appointments.
- Inconsistent follow-through with recommendations.
- Defensive or hostile behaviors.
- Anger or apathy regarding the pregnancy, particularly in the third trimester.
- Inadequate weight gain.
- Needle punctures, thrombosed veins, or signs of cellulitis.

History

The medical and obstetrical history should focus on

- Previous episodes of medical problems such as depression, seizures, cellulitis, hypertension, or suicide attempts.
- Current problems such as insomnia, panic attacks, exhaustion, and heart palpitations.
- Previous obstetrical problems such as spontaneous abortions, premature births, abruptio placentae, and stillbirths.
- Current obstetrical problems such as STDs, vaginal bleeding, and an inactive or hyperactive fetus.
- All forms of drug use, including cigarettes, over-the-counter drugs, prescribed medications, alcohol, and illicit drug use.
- Pattern of drug use, which can range from occasional binges to daily dependence.

Toxicology Screening

Screening for metabolites of drugs may be indicated for pregnant woman, new mothers, and newborn infants. Screening for metabolites is usually performed on

- Urine.
- Hair.
- Meconium from the infant.

Nursing Diagnoses

- Risk for altered health maintenance related to lack of knowledge of the effects of substance abuse on self and fetus
- Altered health maintenance related to inability to manage stress without the use of drugs
- Risk for altered nutrition: less than body requirements, related to anorexia and lifestyle that does not emphasize nutrition
- Risk for infection related to lifestyle experiences that involve exposure to pathogens
- Ineffective individual coping related to physiological and psychological demands of pregnancy and childbirth

Antepartum Management

Effective interventions for substance abuse require the combined efforts of nurses, physicians, social workers, law enforcement agencies, and numerous community and federal agencies.

- Allow time to get acquainted with the expectant mother to get a picture of what stressors may contribute to the pattern of substance abuse.
- Maintain feelings of concern, empathy, and helpfulness.
- Examine own reactions to reduce feelings of anger or judgmental behavior.
- Provide accurate information about the effects of substances such as tobacco, alcohol, and illicit drugs.
- Focus on helping her remain drug free day by day.
- Describe how the newborn benefits when the mother abstains from drugs.

- Verify compliance with recommended treatment regimens, such as chemical-dependence referral programs.
- Coordinate care among various service providers, such as group therapy and prenatal classes.
- Help the woman identify personal and family strengths.
- Acknowledge her actions when she abstains from drugs for even a short time.

Intrapartum Management

Nurses who work in labor and delivery units must become skilled at recognizing drug-induced signs and symptoms.

Signs of Recent Use of Cocaine

- Physical signs
  - Profuse sweating
  - High blood pressure
  - Irregular respirations
  - Dilated pupils
  - Increased body temperature
  - Sudden onset of severely painful contractions
- Emotional signs
  - Angry, caustic, or abusive reactions to those attempting to provide care
  - Emotional lability
  - Paranoia
- Fetal signs
  - Tachycardia
  - Excessive fetal activity

Signs of Recent Use of Heroin

The pregnant woman addicted to heroin often comes to the delivery unit intoxicated from a recent drug administration. When the drug begins to wear off, withdrawal symptoms may be observed.

- Withdrawal symptoms
  - Yawning
  - Diaphoresis
  - Rhinorrhea
  - Restlessness
  - Excessive tearing of the eyes
  - Nausea, diarrhea

Intrapartum Management

Intrapartum management focuses on preventing injury to mother and fetus during labor and childbirth.

- Assign two nurses to admit the woman to the unit; one nurse helps the woman into bed and initiates physical care, while the other acts as communicator.
- Set limits (no smoking, must remain in bed after membranes rupture, etc.).
- Initiate seizure precautions (keep bed locked in lowest position possible, pad side rails to prevent injury, have suction and oxygen equipment readily available, etc.).
- Reduce environmental stimuli as much as possible.
- Maintain therapeutic pattern of communications; acknowledge feelings; avoid confrontations.
- Provide pain control.
  - Use drugs such as morphine, hydromorphine, and meperidine with caution.
  - Avoid drugs, such as butorphanol, that may cause acute withdrawal symptoms.
  - Use nonpharmacological nursing interventions such as sacral pressure, back rubs, and continuous support.
- Administer methadone to prevent withdrawal during labor in woman who is addicted to heroin or to woman who usually receives methadone at a chemical-dependence center.

Postpartum Management

- Observe infant for signs of drug exposure or abstinence syndrome (wakefulness, irritability, tachypnea, temperature variation, frantic crying, hyperreflexia, diarrhea, poor sucking reflex).
- Obtain urine, meconium, or hair sample for toxicology on newborn as soon after birth as possible.
- Continue to observe mother for signs of withdrawal.
- Address legal implications if metabolites of drugs are found in maternal or newborn samples. These implications may include
  — Removing infant from mother's care until she completes a program of drug rehabilitation.
  — Placing the infant with alternative caregivers until long-term care can be obtained for the mother.
- Promote effective care of the infant
  — Emphasize that infants are easily stressed and demonstrate stress in a variety of ways (yawning, sneezing, hiccoughing, averting their gaze, gagging, grunting, and crying).
  — Instruct caregivers that newborns are often hyperexcitable and over-stimulation can result in frantic crying.
  — Teach measures to prevent frantic crying such as gentle handling, soft voices, swaddling with hands brought to midline, avoiding simultaneous visual and auditory stimuli, and vertical rocking.
  4. Recommend the caregiver hold the infant in a semi-sitting position with the arms forward in slight trunk flexion for feeding.
  5. Demonstrate how to support the chin and cheeks if the infant has trouble sucking. See Figure IV-4.
  6. Acknowledge feelings of frustration and rejection that caregivers often feel when they are unable to console or feed an infant without difficulty

Figure IV-4

Method of Positioning the Nurse's Hands to Provide Cheek and Jaw Support for Feeding Preterm Infants

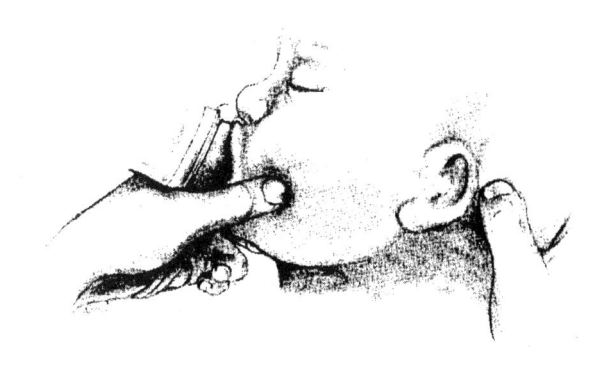

D. PHYSICAL ABUSE OF WOMEN DURING PREGNANCY

Physical abuse occurs in a cycle that consists of three phases.

- A tension-building phase, during which the man engages in increasingly hostile behaviors such as throwing objects, pushing, swearing, threatening
- A battering phase, when the man explodes in violence to hit, beat, or rape the woman
- A honeymoon phase, when the batterer is contrite and remorseful and promises never to do it again

Signs of Physical Abuse

- Nonverbal signs: Facial grimacing, slow and unsteady gait, vomiting, abdominal tenderness, absence of facial response
- Injuries: Welts, bruises, swelling, lacerations, burns, vaginal or rectal bleeding; evidence of old or new fractures of the nose, face, ribs, or arms
- Vague somatic complaints: Anxiety, depression, panic attacks, sleeplessness, anorexia

- Discrepancy between history and type of injuries; wounds do not match the woman's story; multiple bruises in various stages of healing; bruising on the arms (which she may have raised to protect herself); old, untreated wounds

Assessment

Women often seek care during the "honeymoon phase" of the violence cycle. During this time, the man typically appears overly solicitous (hovering husband syndrome) and eager to explain any injuries the woman exhibits. Nurses must be aware that introducing the subject of violence in the presence of the man places the woman in danger. It is essential to

- Separate the woman from the man for the interview.
- Reassure the woman that confidentiality will be absolute.
- Ask questions directly ("Did you get these injuries from being hit?").
- Evaluate and document all signs of injury, past and present.
- Be alert for nonverbal cues of physical abuse.
- Keep in mind that the woman may fear for her life because abusive episodes tend to escalate.

Most Common Nursing Diagnoses

- Fear related to possibility of severe injury to self and/or children
- Pain related to injuries received during violent episode
- Post-trauma response related to assault
- Rape-trauma syndrome related to violent sexual penetration against the victim's will and consent

Management

- Help the woman make concrete plans to protect her safety and the safety of all children if she returns to the shared home.
  — Suggest obtaining an extra set of keys for her car.

- — Recommend keeping keys and necessities packed and hidden until needed.
- — Emphasize the importance of locating the nearest safe house or shelter and making specific plans for going there when the cycle of violence begins.
- — Advise making arrangements with a trusted person who will respond to a call for help; suggest memorizing the person's telephone number.
- Reinforce that she is not to blame for violence against her.
- Teach basic family processes.
  - — Violence is not normal.
  - — Physical abuse is against the law.
  - — Violence usually escalates and is repeated.
  - — Battered women have alternatives.
- Refer to community agencies that are available to help the victim (police departments, community shelters, counseling agencies, and social services).
- Accept the decisions of the battered woman and acknowledge that she must act on her own timetable.
- Inform her that resources are available for her partner, but he must admit abuse and seek assistance before help can be offered; initiating referrals before he asks for help will increase the danger to the woman if her partner feels he has been betrayed.

E. BIRTH OF AN INFANT WITH CONGENITAL ANOMALIES

When an infant is born with anomalies, the parents are often overwhelmed with feelings of shock and disbelief. Before they can form attachment with the newborn, they must grieve for the perfect infant they expected.

Management

Physicians and nurses are aware that the timing and manner of being told of the anomalies influences the emotional response of parents.

- Tell (and show) the parents as soon after childbirth as possible.
- Remain with the parents during the initial phase of shock and denial.
- Promote bonding and attachment.
  — Communicate acceptance of the infant by handling gently and presenting the infant as precious.
  — Emphasize the normal aspects of the infant.
  — Allow long periods of uninterrupted time between parents and infant (as the infant's condition permits).
- Maintain an atmosphere that encourages families to express their feelings.
  — Listen carefully and reflect the content of feelings expressed.
  — Be aware that cultural and religious beliefs affect the expressions of grief.
- Provide accurate information about follow-up treatments or procedures that may be necessary.
- Answer questions as honestly as possible; find a more experienced health care worker if unsure of information.
- Encourage communication between family members; include fathers (and grandparents if desired) in discussions and demonstrations of care.
- Teach necessary home care (e.g., how to feed infant with cleft palate or how to position an infant with meningocele).
- Help parents prepare siblings for changes the newborn will make in family functioning.
- Refer to community and national resources such as National March of Dimes or Crippled Children's Services of the Public Health Department.

F. BIRTH OF A STILLBORN INFANT

Birth of a stillborn infant evokes a strong grief response in the family. Initial reactions include

- Denial and disbelief.
- Anger toward family, medical personnel, or self.
- Guilt (feelings that they might have prevented the infant's death).
- Profound sadness and mourning.

Management

- Bring the infant and parents together while the infant is still warm and soft if possible.
  - Wash the infant and apply baby lotion or powder if necessary.
  - Wrap the infant in a soft, warm blanket.
  - Keep the infant in a warmed incubator if some time elapses before the parents can have contact; if this is not possible, tell the parents the infant's skin will feel cool.
- Encourage parents to keep the infant as long as they wish, and make them feel free to unwrap the infant.
- Permit parents to progress at their own speed when inspecting the infant.
- Allow as much privacy and time as the parents and other family members need to be together.
- Prepare a "memory packet" that might include a photograph, footprints, the birth bracelet, a crib card with the infant's name, weight, and length, and a lock of hair.
- Keep memory packet on file if the parents do not want to take it home at this time.
- Acknowledge the basic rights of the baby
  - To be recognized as a person who was born and died.
  - To be named.
  - To be seen, touched, and held by the family.
  - To have life-ending acknowledged.
  - To be put to rest with dignity.

- Refer to groups who have had similar experiences (Resolve through Sharing, Aiding a Mother Experiencing Neonatal Death (AMEND), and Helping After Neonatal Death (HAND).

SECTION FIVE

Women's Health Care and Reproductive Issues

I. FAMILY PLANNING

More than half of all pregnancies are unintended and of those, half are due to incorrect contraceptive use or contraceptive failure. Nurses have major roles in educating women about family planning.

A. CONSIDERATIONS WHEN TEACHING ABOUT CONTRACEPTION

- Offer teaching about contraception during any contact with women.
- Provide privacy for discussion.
- Include the woman's partner, if she wishes.
- Assess the woman's knowledge, satisfaction, and concerns about her contraceptive method.
- Answer questions and correct misunderstandings.
- Help women/couples analyze various contraceptive methods if they wish (see Table V-1). Include:
  — Safety
  — Protection from sexually transmissible diseases
  — Effectiveness
  — Convenience
  — Education needed
  — Side effects
  — Interference with spontaneity
  — Availability

TABLE V-1
Contraceptive Effectiveness, Failure and Discontinuation Rates

METHOD	EFFECTIVENESS RATE (ACTUAL OR TYPICAL USE)	% FAILURE RATE (ACTUAL OR TYPICAL USE)	% FAILURE RATE (IDEAL OR PERFECT USE)	% DISCONTINUATION RATE AT ONE YEAR
		Sterilization		
Tubal Ligation	99.6	0.4	0.4	
Vasectomy	99.85	0.15	0.1	
		Hormones		
Hormone Implants	99.91	0.09	0.09	15
Injectable Hormones	99.7	0.3	0.3	30
Oral Contraceptives	97	3		28
Combined Estrogen/Progestin			0.1	
Progestin Only			0.5	
		Intrauterine Devices		
Progesterone	98	2	1.5	19
Copper	99.2	0.8	0.6	22
		Condoms		
Male	88	12	3	37
Female (Reality)	79	21	5	44
		Diaphragm		
	82	18	6	42

		Cervical Cap	
Parous Women	64	36	26	55
Nulliparous Women	82	18	9	42
		Spermicides	
Gel, Foam Films, Suppositories	79	21	6	57
		Natural Family Planning	
	80	20		
Calendar			9	33
Basal Body Temperature			3	
Symptothermal			2	
Postovulation			1	
Coitus Interruptus (Withdrawal)	81	19	4	
No contraceptive use	15	85	85	

Percent of women who may be expected to avoid or become pregnant with use of each method from typical and perfect use during the first year. Discontinuation rate is the rate at which women who do not wish to become pregnant stop using a method by the end of one year of use. The discontinuation rate often rises with each year of use. Reprinted and modified with the permission of the Population Council, from James Trussell et al., "Contraceptive Failure in the United States: An Update," *Studies in Family Planning*, 21(1) (Jan/Feb 1990): 52 and Hatcher, et al. (1994) Contraceptive Technology. 16th ed.

- Expense
- Religious and personal beliefs
- Culture
- Client preference

- Show examples of contraceptive devices, if possible.
- Provide demonstrations and ask for return demonstrations.

B.   CERVICAL CAP

The cervical cap is a small, flexible latex cup that fits over the cervix and remains in place by suction.

Advantages

- Avoids systemic hormones
- May fit women who are unable to use a diaphragm
- Effectiveness: 82% for nulliparous women
- Requires less spermicide than a diaphragm
- No need for added spermicide for repeated intercourse
- No pressure against the bladder
- Less noticeable than a diaphragm
- Can remain in place for 48 hours

Disadvantages

- Sizes are limited
- Women with cervical abnormalities may not be able to use it
- Effectiveness: 64% for multiparous women
- Must be fitted by a nurse practitioner, nurse-midwife, or physician
- Can be dislodged during intercourse
- Insertion or removal may be difficult for some women
- Possibility of toxic shock syndrome

Teaching

- May be inserted ahead of time to decrease interference with spontaneity.
- Should not be removed for 6 hours after last intercourse.
- Feel the cervix to check placement before and after intercourse.
- Should not be used during menses or in women with a history of toxic shock syndrome
- A Pap smear is required 3 months after the original fitting because some users develop cervical neoplasia. If normal, yearly examinations are enough.
- Must be refitted each year and after birth, abortion, or surgery.

C. CONDOM, MALE

The male condom covers the penis during intercourse, preventing sperm from entering the vagina. It may be coated with spermicide. Latex condoms provide the best protection available (other than abstinence) from STDs. Natural membrane condoms are less effective against STDs. Polyurethane condoms can be used by people allergic to latex.

Advantages

- Readily available without a prescription
- Inexpensive per use
- Can be carried inconspicuously by the man or the woman.
- Help protect against STDs
- Avoid use of systemic hormones
- Effectiveness rate: 88%

Disadvantages

- Interfere with spontaneity

- May interfere with sensation
- Latex allergies may occur
- May be affected by vaginal medications
- May break or slip off during intercourse or withdrawal
- For single use only

Teaching

- Use during any possible exposure to an STD, even if another contraceptive technique is practiced or if the woman is pregnant.
- Reservoir tips and water-based lubricants help prevent breakage.
- Check expiration dates; may deteriorate after 5 years.
- Lubrication may increase comfort for the woman.
- Use water-soluble lubricants or spermicides. Oil-based products (such as petroleum jelly or baby oil) cause deterioration of the latex.
- Apply the condom before any contact between the penis and the vagina.
- Squeeze the air out of the tip of the condom.
- Leave a half inch of space at the tip as the condom is rolled onto the erect penis.
- Withdraw the penis from the vagina before it becomes soft while holding the condom in place.
- Use a new condom each time intercourse is repeated.

D. CONDOM, FEMALE

The female condom is a polyurethane sheath inserted into the vagina with a flexible ring at each end. One ring fits over the cervix like a diaphragm and the other ring extends outside the vagina to partially cover the perineum.

Advantages

- First contraceptive device to allow women some protection from STDs without relying on the male condom
- Avoids systemic hormones
- Easy to obtain and carry
- Relatively inexpensive per use

Disadvantages

- Less effective than male condom (only 79%)
- Many women object to it on esthetic grounds
- Single use only

Teaching

- Hold the outer ring in place during insertion and removal of the penis.
- Do not use with a male condom.

E.   DEPO-PROVERA

See "Hormone Injections," p. 361.

F.   DIAPHRAGM

The diaphragm is a latex dome surrounded by a spring or coil that is inserted over the cervix by hand or with a plastic introducer. It prevents passage of sperm while holding spermicide in place.

Advantages

- Avoids systemic hormones
- Effectiveness: 82%
- May be inserted ahead of time to decrease interference with spontaneity

Disadvantages

- Pressure on the urethra may cause urinary tract infections
- Noticeable or uncomfortable when in place for some women
- Allergies to latex or history of toxic shock syndrome preclude use
- Must be fitted by a nurse practitioner, nurse-midwife, or physician
- Correct size may not be available for all women
- Some women have difficulty with insertion or removal
- Possibility of toxic shock syndrome

Teaching

- Inspect the diaphragm for small holes by holding it up to a light.
- Spermicidal cream or gel should be used inside the dome and around the rim with each use.
- Emptying the bladder before insertion decreases irritation and pressure.
- A squatting position or placing one foot on a chair makes insertion and removal easier.
- The front rim should fit behind the pubic bone, and the cervix should be felt through the center of the diaphragm.
- If more than 6 hours elapse between insertion and intercourse or if intercourse is repeated, more spermicide should be inserted into the vagina without removing the diaphragm.
- Leave in place at least 6 hours after last intercourse but no more than a total of 24 hours to reduce risk of infection.
- Douching with the diaphragm in place is unnecessary and lessens effectiveness.
- Wash with mild soap and dry well after each use.

- Some medications used for vaginal *Candida* infections may damage the diaphragm.
- Women should be checked for size changes yearly, after weight gain or loss of more than 10 pounds, and after each pregnancy or abortion.
- Replace every two years.

G. EMERGENCY CONTRACEPTION

Emergency contraception is used to prevent pregnancy after unprotected intercourse. A large dose of oral contraceptives is used to prevent normal endometrial development and may interfere with fertilization and tubal transport. The method is also called *postcoital contraception*.

Advantages

- May be used for contraceptive failure, rape, or incorrect or lack of contraceptive use
- Reduces the risk of pregnancy by 75%

Disadvantages

Side effects include nausea and vomiting.

Teaching

- Emergency contraception must be taken as soon as possible and not later than 72 hours after unprotected intercourse.
- A second dose is taken 12 hours after the first dose.
- Antiemetics may be given for nausea.

H. HORMONE IMPLANT

Hormone Implants consist of six flexible capsules about 1.5 inches long (the size of a match) that are inserted subcutaneously into the upper inner arm under local anesthetic. They release progestin continuously to inhibit ovulation and development of the endometrium and cause cervical mucus changes that impede penetration by sperm.

Advantages

- Effectiveness: 99.91%
- Reversible
- Effective for 5 years
- Long-term cost relatively low
- No estrogens
- Unrelated to coitus, always in place
- Covered by Medicaid and by some insurances
- Prompt return of fertility after removal

Disadvantages

- Initial cost high if no insurance available
- Removal may be difficult if the capsules are deeply implanted
- Practitioners must be trained in both insertion and removal
- Breastfeeding women generally advised to wait six weeks
- May not be as effective in women weighing more than 150 pounds
- Should not be used by women with conditions contraindicating oral progestins
- No protection from STDs
- Slightly visible

Teaching

- Side effects include
  — Irregular, midcycle, or prolonged bleeding (usually decreases by one year).

- Headaches.
- Weight gain.
- Acne.
- Dizziness.
- Mood changes.
- See practitioner for treatment of side effects.

I. INTRAUTERINE DEVICES

Intrauterine devices (IUDs) are inserted into the uterus to provide continuous pregnancy prevention. Two types are available in the United States.

- Copper T 380A (ParaGard)
  - Has a copper wire on the device
  - Effective for 10 years
- Progestasert
  - Releases progestin continuously
  - Effective for 1 year

Advantages

- Safe for use during lactation
- Relatively low long-term cost
- In place at all times
- Effectiveness: 98%

Disadvantages

- Cannot be inserted for six weeks after birth
- Expensive at the time of insertion
- Should be used only by women in mutually monogamous relationships and at low risk for STDs
- Complications
  - Expulsion

- Perforation of uterus
- If pregnancy occurs, may have ectopic pregnancy, spontaneous abortion, or preterm delivery.

- Contraindications
  - Nulliparous women
  - Recurrent pelvic infections
  - History of ectopic pregnancy
  - Bleeding disorders
  - Uterine abnormalities

Teaching

- Side effects
  - Cramping and bleeding with insertion
  - Menorrhagia (increased bleeding during menstruation)
  - Dysmenorrhea (painful menstruation)
- Ibuprofen may relieve cramping.
- Check for the plastic strings weekly during the first 4 weeks, then monthly after menses, and for signs of expulsion (cramping or unexpected bleeding).
- Pelvic infections may occur, especially in women with more than one partner.
- See a health care provider if signs of infection occur.
  - Unusual vaginal discharge
  - Vaginal pain or itching
  - Low pelvic pain
  - Fever
- Report signs of pregnancy to rule out ectopic pregnancy and remove IUD.
- Schedule a yearly Pap smear.
- Check for anemia if menses are heavy. May need to take iron.

J. HORMONE INJECTIONS

Depo-Provera, (medroxyprogesterone acetate or DMPA) is an injectable progestin that is given by deep intramuscular injection. The site should not be massaged after injection, as this accelerates absorption. The injection should be given within 5 days of the beginning of the menstrual period.

Advantages

- Prevents ovulation for 14 weeks
- Only four doses a year are needed
- Effectiveness: 99.7%
- Convenient
- No estrogen
- Unrelated to coitus

Disadvantages

- Must be repeated on time to keep up effectiveness
- Should not be used by women with contraindications for other hormone contraceptives
- Delay in return of fertility is 4–9 months after discontinuation
- No protection from STDs

Teaching

- Side effects
  — Menstrual irregularities: spotting, breakthrough bleeding
  — Amenorrhea in 50% of women at one year
  — Weight gain: approximately 4 pounds/year
  — Headaches
  — Hair loss

- If received after first five days of menstrual cycle, use another contraceptive for the rest of the cycle.
- Usually not started until six weeks after delivery for breastfeeding women.
- Return for injections every three months.

K. MEDROXYPROGESTERONE ACETATE

See "Hormone Injections," p. 361.

L. NATURAL FAMILY PLANNING METHODS

Natural family planning methods are also called *fertility awareness* or *periodic abstinence* methods. They are based on predicting ovulation by physiological changes and avoiding coitus when fertilization is likely to occur. They may also be used to help women become pregnant.

Advantages

- Acceptable to most religions
- Help women learn about normal body changes
- Avoid the use of drugs, chemicals, and devices
- Effectiveness: 80% if used perfectly

Disadvantages

- Couples must be highly motivated
- Couples must avoid intercourse for as much as half the menstrual cycle
- Extensive education required
- Very unforgiving method; errors likely to result in pregnancy

Teaching

- Teaching must be specific to the individual method.

- Method may be used to determine fertile period and another contraceptive method can be used at that time.
- See Table V-2 for specific methods.

M. NORPLANT

See "Hormone Implant," p. 357.

N. ORAL CONTRACEPTIVES

Oral contraceptives (OCs) contain estrogen and progestin or progestin alone. Combination contraceptives prevent ovulation, cause cervical mucus to become too thick for sperm to penetrate, and make the endometrium less hospitable to implantation. Progestin-only oral contraceptives are useful for women who must avoid estrogen, but they are less effective at inhibiting ovulation.

Advantages

- Effectiveness: 97%
- Can be used by healthy women at any age
- Unrelated to coitus
- Reduces ovarian and endometrial cancer
- Regulates menstrual cycles and reduces blood loss
- Decreases incidence of some conditions

Disadvantages

- No protection against sexually transmissible diseases (STDs)
- May increase susceptibility to some STDs
- Return of fertility may take 2–3 months after discontinuation
- Increases incidence of some conditions

TABLE V-2

Natural Family Planning Methods

INSTRUCTIONS	CAUTIONS
Calendar Method	
Keep track of menstrual cycles for 6 months. Subtract 18–20 days from the shortest cycle and 10 days from the longest cycle. Avoid intercourse on those days.	Least reliable of all natural methods; many factors, such as stress or illness, may affect time of ovulation.
Basal Body Temperature (BBT) Method	
Chart the oral temperature each morning before getting up or increasing activity. Watch for a rise of approximately 0.2°–0.45°C (0.4°–0.8°F) indicating ovulation has occurred. Avoid intercourse for 3 days before and after the rise.	Unreliable because BBT can be affected by stress, illness, interrupted sleep, etc.; difficult to know when the temperature will rise; intercourse on the day before rise may result in pregnancy.
Cervical Mucus (Billings or Ovulation) Method	
Assess the cervical mucus daily by wiping the vaginal orifice with tissue. Watch for clear, slippery, stretchy (Spinnbarkeit) mucus (like egg white). Avoid intercourse from the time the mucus appears until the evening of the fourth day after the height of mucus change.	Intercourse is not allowed during menses because some women enter the fertile period before the end of the menses; allowed only every other day from menses until fertile period because semen interferes with mucus assessment.
Symptothermal Method	
Combines calendar, BBT, and cervical mucus methods. Notes symptoms of ovulation (weight gain, abdominal bloating, mittelschmerz, increased libido).	More effective than other methods alone, if cautions for all methods are followed.
Postovulation	
Combines all methods, but avoids intercourse from menses until the end of the fertile period.	Abstinence is necessary for more than 1/2 of cycle; most effective method, but difficult to achieve.

Teaching

- Should not be used by women with a history of any of the following.
  - Thrombophlebitis or thromboembolic disorders
  - Cerebrovascular or cardiovascular diseases
  - Any estrogen-dependent cancer or breast cancer
  - Benign or malignant liver tumors
- Should not be used by women who currently have any of the following.
  - Any of the above conditions
  - Impaired liver function
  - Suspected or known pregnancy
  - Undiagnosed vaginal bleeding
  - Heavy cigarette smoking (more than 15/day in women >35; any use of cigarettes is discouraged and should be evaluated individually)
- Side effects
  - Nausea
  - Headaches
  - Breast tenderness
  - Breakthrough bleeding
  - Weight gain or loss
  - Fluid retention
  - Amenorrhea
  - Acne
  - Chloasma
- It is important to maintain hormone levels by taking pills at the same time each day.
- Use another contraceptive method during the first week of the first cycle until the blood hormone levels are established.
- Side effects often decrease after the first few months of use. Changing the dose of estrogen or progestin may help.

- Follow specific instructions from the health care provider for what to do when OCs are missed. If more than one pill is missed, another contraceptive method should be used for at least 7 days.

- Combination OCs should only be used after milk production is well established for breastfeeding women. Progestin-only contraceptives do not affect milk production.

- OC interaction with other drugs may decrease effectiveness of both (e.g., some antibiotics or anticonvulsants). Inform health care provider of all medications being used.

- A yearly pelvic examination and Pap smear, breast examination, and blood pressure measurement are important.

- The acronym ACHES can help remember signs that should be reported immediately.
    — A: Abdominal pain (severe)
    — C: Chest pain, dyspnea, hemoptysis
    — H: Headache (severe), weakness or numbness of extremities
    — E: Eye problems (visual changes such as blurred or double vision or visual loss, speech disturbance)
    — S: Severe leg pain or swelling (calf or thigh)

O. POSTCOITAL EMERGENCY CONTRACEPTION

See "Emergency Contraception," p. 357.

P. SPERMICIDES

Spermicides come in many forms. Creams and gels are used with mechanical barriers such as the diaphragm or cervical cap. Foams, suppositories, and vaginal film may be used alone. They are inserted into the vagina just before sexual intercourse and are effective for about 1 hour. Vaginal films and suppositories must melt, which takes approximately 15 minutes, before they become effective.

Advantages

- Readily available without a prescription
- Inexpensive per use
- Easy to use
- May provide some protection against some STDs
- Provide lubrication
- Avoids use of systemic hormones

Disadvantages

- Should be used with condoms
- Messy
- Some feel they interfere with sensation
- Only 79% effective if used alone

Teaching

- Sensitivity may cause genital irritation, which may increase risk of infection.
- Douching should be avoided for at least 6–8 hours after intercourse.
- More spermicide is needed if coitus is repeated.

Q. STERILIZATION

Male or female sterilization is permanent and effective. It should be used only by those who understand that reversal surgery is difficult, expensive, usually not covered by insurance, and often unsuccessful.

Tubal Ligation

Tubal ligation involves mini-laparotomy or laparoscopic surgery to block the Fallopian tubes.

Advantages

- Effectiveness: 99.6%
- Can be performed with a cesarean birth
- Convenient if performed during the immediate postpartum period, when the fundus is near the umbilicus and the fallopian tubes are directly below the abdominal wall
- Can be performed at other times as outpatient surgery

Disadvantages

- Requires surgery
- General anesthesia is most common, but regional or local anesthesia may be used
- Expensive at the time of the surgery, but ends future contraception costs

Teaching

If tubal ligation is to be performed soon after childbirth, the consent forms must be signed well before labor begins.

Vasectomy

Vasectomy involves cutting the vas deferens through a small incision in the scrotum so that semen no longer carries sperm.

Advantages

- Effectiveness: 99.85%
- Can be performed in a physician's office under local anesthesia
- Less expensive than tubal ligation

Disadvantages

- Requires surgery
- Expensive at the time of the surgery, but less expensive than tubal ligation and ends future contraception costs.

Teaching

- Apply ice to the area, and watch for excessive swelling or bleeding.
- Complete sterilization does not occur until all sperm have left the system, which may be a month or more.
- Semen specimens should be analyzed until two specimens show no sperm present.

R. TUBAL LIGATION

See "Sterilization," p. 367.

S. VASECTOMY

See "Sterilization," p. 367.

II. INFERTILITY

Infertility is the inability to conceive after 1 year of unprotected regular sexual intercourse. A more workable definition is the inability to conceive at the time desired.

A. MALE FACTORS

- Sperm abnormalities
  — Low numbers (fewer than 20 million per milliliter of semen)
  — Excessive numbers of abnormally-formed sperm
  — Abnormal sperm movement
  — Inability to penetrate the ovum
- Abnormal erections
- Abnormal ejaculation
  — Retrograde
  — Semen deposited near vaginal outlet
  — Premature ejaculation
- Abnormal seminal fluid
  — Does not liquefy
  — Abnormal amount
  — Abnormal composition

B. FEMALE FACTORS

- Ovulation abnormalities
  — Dysfunctional hormonal stimulation of the ovary to mature and release an ovum
  — Failure of the ovaries to respond to hormonal stimulation
  — Abnormal ova
- Fallopian tube abnormalities
  — Tubal obstruction
  — Abnormal tubal motility to move the ovum to the uterus

- Cervical abnormalities
    - Failure to secrete thin, slippery mucus at ovulation
    - Scarring from infections or surgery

C. REPEATED PREGNANCY LOSS

- Abnormal fetal chromosomes
- Abnormal cervix or uterus
    - Malformations
    - Scarring
    - Myomas (benign tumors)
- Endocrine abnormalities
    - Luteal phase defect
    - Hypo- or hyperthyroidism
    - Poorly controlled diabetes
- Immunological abnormalities
    - Woman's body does not tolerate the foreign tissue of the embryo
    - Autoimmune disease
- Environmental agents
    - Radiation therapy
    - Alcohol
    - Isotretinoin (Accutane)
- Infections

D. INFERTILITY EVALUATION

Evaluation of infertility generally proceeds from the simpler tests to the more complex ones. If the woman is nearing the end of her reproductive years, testing may be accelerated.

TABLE V-3

Selected Diagnostic Tests in Infertility

TEST/PURPOSE	NURSING IMPLICATIONS
Male	
Semen Analysis	
Evaluates structure and function of sperm and composition of seminal fluid. Semen volume 2.0-6.0 ml pH 7.2- 7.8 Sperm concentration: 20 million/ml or more Motility: 50% or more with normal forms Morphology: 60% or more with normal forms Viability: 50% or more live Liquefaction: within 30 min Leukocytes (white blood cells): Fewer than 1 million/ml Fructose: 150-600 mg/dl	Explain purpose of semen analysis: three or more specimens are usually collected over several weeks' time for more accurate analysis. Explain to the man that he should collect the specimen by masturbation after a 2- to 3-day abstinence; semen may be collected in a condom if masturbation is unacceptable. Teach the man to note the time the specimen was obtained so the laboratory can evaluate liquefaction of the semen; the specimen should be transported near the body to maintain warmth and should arrive in the laboratory within 1 hr.
Endocrine Tests	
Evaluate function of hypothalamus, pituitary gland, and the response of the testicles. Assays are made to determine testosterone, estradiol, luteinizing hormone (LH), and follicle-stimulating hormone (FSH) levels. Additional tests may be made on the basis of history and physical findings.	Teach the man about the relationship between hypothalamic and pituitary function and sperm formation; LH stimulates testosterone production by Leydig cells of the testes, and FSH stimulates Sertoli cells of the testes to produce sperm.

Ultrasonography

Evaluates structure of prostate gland, seminal vesicles, and ejaculatory ducts by use of a transrectal probe.

Teach the man that ultrasonography uses sound waves to evaluate these structures; no radiation is involved.

Testicular Biopsy

An invasive test for obtaining a sample of testicular tissue; identifies pathology and obstructions.

Explain the purpose of the test; a local anesthetic is used, and there should be little discomfort.

Sperm Penetration Assay

Evaluates fertilizing ability of sperm; assesses ability of sperm to undergo changes that allow penetration of a hamster ovum from which the zona pellucida has been removed.

Explain the purpose of the test; abnormal penetration does not necessarily mean that the sperm cannot fertilize a human ovum.

Female

Ovulation Prediction

Uses any of several methods to identify the surge of LH, which precedes ovulation by 24-36 hr; this enables the timing of intercourse to coincide with ovulation and identifies the absence of ovulation.

Explain the purpose of the tests (commercial ovulation predictor kits, basal body temperature, and cervical mucus assessment).

Teach the woman to follow the instructions on the commercial product.

Teach her how to do the basal body temperature and cervical mucus assessment (see procedure, "Teaching a Woman Fertility Awareness," p. 440).

Ultrasonography

Evaluates structure of pelvic organs.
Identifies ovarian follicles and release of ova at ovulation.
Evaluates for presence of ectopic or multifetal preg-

Teach the woman that ultrasonography uses sound waves to evaluate these structures; no radiation is involved.
Explain preparations needed for specific evaluations.

Post-coital Test

Evaluates characteristics of cervical mucus and sperm function within that mucus at time of ovulation. Ultrasonography ensures proper timing for test.

Explain that the test is performed 6–12 hours after intercourse; the woman may have to rearrange her personal or work commitments each time this test is done.

Endocrine Tests

Evaluates functions of hypothalamus, pituitary gland, and ovary.

Assays are made to determine LH, ESH, estrogen, and progesterone levels.

Additional hormone evaluations may be done on the basis of the history and physical findings.

Explain the purpose of each test: FSH and LH stimulate ovulation; estrogen and progesterone prepare uterine endometrium for implantation of a fertilized ovum. Explain the importance of timing within the cycle to provide best information.

Hysterosalpingogram (HSG)

X-ray that uses contrast medium to evaluate the structure and patency of the uterus and fallopian tubes.

The test is performed after the menstrual period during the first half of the cycle to avoid flushing menstrual debris through the tubes into the pelvic cavity and to avoid disrupting a pregnancy that might be in place.

Explain the purpose of the test. Contrast medium is injected through the cervix, and x-ray films are made at the same time.

Endometrial Biopsy

An invasive test for obtaining a small sample of endometrial tissue; determines whether endometrium is responding properly to estrogen and progesterone stimulation from ovary.

Explain the purpose of the test. The test is done 2–3 days before the woman expects her menstrual period; some cramping may occur, but it should be relieved with mild analgesics, such as ibuprofen.

Hysteroscopy and Laparoscopy

Examines uterine interior and pelvic organs with an endoscope; general anesthesia is used.

Identifies abnormalities (polyps, endometrial adhesions). Some surgical procedures may be done via the endoscope.

Explain the purpose of the test and any procedures that will be done at the same time. The woman takes nothing by mouth and should urinate before the procedure. Carbon dioxide gas, used to separate pelvic organs for better visualization, may cause temporary shoulder pain.

E. INFERTILITY THERAPY

- Medications

TABLE V-4

Medications Used for Infertility Therapy

DRUG	USE
Bromocriptine (Parlodel)	Corrects excess prolactin secretion by anterior pituitary, which causes inadequate progesterone production by corpus luteum, thus inhibiting normal implantation of embryo.
Clomiphene (Clomid)	Induction of ovulation
Chorionic gonadotropin, human (hCG; Pregnyl)	Used with menotropins to stimulate ovulation in the female or sperm formation in the male; stimulates progesterone production by corpus luteum
Gonadotropin-releasing hormone (GnRH; Lutrepulse)	Stimulates release of follicle-stimulating hormone (FSH) and luteinizing hormone (LH) from the pituitary gland in men and women who have deficient GnRH secretion by their hypothalamus; FSH and LH, in turn, stimulate ovulation in the female and stimulate testosterone production and spermatogenesis
Leuprolide (Lupron)	Reduces endometriosis; adjunct to drug given to stimulate ovulation
Menotropins (FSH and LH; Pergonal)	Stimulates ovulation and spermatogenesis (given with hCG)

Nafarelin (Synarel)	Reduces endometriosis
Progesterone	Promotes implantation of embryo
Urofollitropin (Metrodin)	Stimulates ovulation (given in conjunction with hCG)

- Surgery
  - Correct male varicocele
  - Relief of obstructions
- Therapeutic insemination with the partner's or donor semen
- Surrogate mother
- Advanced reproductive techniques
  - In vitro fertilization: Inducing ovulation and retrieving ova; mixing ova with sperm; returning fertilized ova to the uterus 2 days later
  - Gamete intrafallopian transfer: Retrieving ova, placing ova and sperm in fallopian tube, where fertilization occurs
  - Tubal embryo transfer: Retrieving ova and fertilizing outside the body; replacing in fallopian tubes to enter uterus naturally
- Microsurgery: allows placement of the sperm within the ovum or its surrounding zona pellucida

F. NURSING CARE OF THE INFERTILE COUPLE

- Assisting communication
  - Encourage expression of their feelings.
  - Encourage partners to accept their own feelings, both positive and negative.
  - Discuss differences in the partners' communication styles.
  - Encourage partners to be open with each other.

- Increasing the couple's sense of control
  — Encourage them to identify how their previous ways to deal with stresses can help them in this situation.
  — Reinforce positive coping skills that reduce stress.
  — Teach relaxation techniques (visualization, moderate exercise).
  — Explain procedures and purposes in understandable language. Reinforce any medical explanations already given. Encourage questions.
  — Help them explore their options at each decision point.
- Reducing isolation
  — Refer the couple to support groups.
  — Encourage re-establishment of ties with relatives and friends if these have been disrupted.
- Promoting a positive self-image
  — Explore areas of competence other than conception.
  — Encourage them to maintain activities such as hobbies.
  — Explore whether their careers are a source of stress or an avenue for positive self-perception.

III. WOMEN'S HEALTH CARE

A. HEALTH MAINTENANCE

Health maintenance refers to measures that can be taken to prevent or detect disorders. The most useful measures are individual health history, family history, physical examination, screening procedures, and immunizations.

Individual Health History

The health history should focus on particular habits and lifestyle factors that promote or interfere with long-term health.

- Diet (low-fat, with adequate nutrients and fiber)
- Exercise (weight bearing, aerobic)

SECTION FIVE: Women's Health Care and Reproductive Issues 379

- Use of tobacco or alcohol
- Long-term use of prescription and over-the-counter medications
- Safety and injury precautions (use of seat belts, non-skid area rugs, sunscreen, etc.)
- Use of illicit drugs (types, frequency, date of last use)
- Sexual practices (age of first sexual experience, family planning methods, monogamous relationship, multiple partners, or partner with multiple contacts)

Family History

A family history may reveal a risk profile for specific diseases such as heart disease, osteoporosis, or cancer (particularly breast and colon cancer).

Physical Assessment

Although a physical examination should include every body system, particular emphasis is placed on the following.

- Measurements of vital signs (for hypertension, fever, tachycardia, or bradycardia)
- Weight (should be within 10 percent of ideal weight for height according to weight charts)
- Height and loss of height (associated with osteoporosis)
- Auscultation of heart sounds for rate and rhythm, and to detect murmurs
- Auscultation of lungs for adventitious sounds such as rales or wheezes
- Inspection and palpation of the breasts for lumps, masses, dimpling, or nipple discharge
- Observation and palpation of extremities for edema, varicosities, equality of pedal pulses
- Palpation of abdomen for tenderness, masses, or distention

- Explanation and instruction for pelvic examination
  - Schedule a pelvic examination between menstrual periods.
  - Do not have sexual intercourse for 48 hours prior to the exam.
  - Do not douche or use vaginal medications, sprays, or deodorants that might interfere with interpretation of cytology specimens that are collected.
  - Void just prior to the examination.
  - A lithotomy position with the head slightly elevated is necessary. Some practitioners offer the woman a mirror so she can observe the examination.
- Examination of external genitalia
  - Observation of the vulva for character and distribution of hair and the degree of development or atrophy of the labia
  - Evaluation of cysts, tumors, or inflammation of Bartholin's gland
  - Inspection of urethra and Skene's glands for exudate
  - Collection of any exudate for laboratory analysis
- Speculum examination to inspect the vagina and cervix
  - Warming and lubricating the speculum with warm water only to avoid interfering with the examination of cervical cytology or other vaginal exudate
  - Evaluation of the size, shape, and color of the cervix
  - Collection of purulent cervical discharge for culture
  - Collection of material for cervical cytologic smear (Papanicolaou) should be taken before speculum is withdrawn
- Bimanual examination for information about the uterus, fallopian tubes, and ovaries
- Inspection of the anus for hemorrhoids, inflammation, or lesions
- Digital examination of the rectum to determine sphincter tone and to prepare a slide for detection of occult blood

Screening Procedures

- Breast self-examination (BSE) is a supplement to screening by professional examination and mammography. BSE should be performed monthly about a week following the onset of menses, when hormonal influences on the breasts are at a low level. See "Procedure: How to Perform BSE," p. 433.

- Professional breast examination is similar to BSE; however, professional examiners may detect questionable areas that the woman misses. While the woman is in an upright position, the health professional should
  - Inspect the breasts for size, symmetry, and color, or skin changes.
  - Observe the nipples and areola for differences in size, color, unilateral retraction of a nipple, or asymmetrical nipple direction.
  - Ask the woman to raise her hands above her head to inspect the sides and underneath portions of the breasts.
  - Direct the woman to place her hands on her hips and press down; this action may reveal skin dimpling or masses.
  - Palpate each axilla for enlarged or tender lymph nodes.

- Help the woman into a supine position and place a small pillow or folded towel under the shoulder to stretch and flatten the breast tissue on that side.
  - Use the flat part of the first three fingers to palpate the breast, rotate the fingers against the chest wall; palpate the tissue that extends into the axilla; repeat on opposite side.
  - Compress the nipples and collect a sample of any discharge for culture and examination of cells.

> **Clinical Tip:** Normal breast tissue may feel firm, lumpy, nodular, or tender. A discrete mass that can be felt or measured (often likened to a raisin, watermelon seed, or grape) is abnormal and requires further evaluation.

- Mammography is currently recommended every 1–2 years for women aged 40–49 and annually for women over the age of 50 (ACOG, 1996). It is the only screening procedure that can detect breast lumps long before they are palpable.

- Vulvar self-examination (VSE) should be performed monthly by all women over the age of 18 and by those under 18 years who are sexually active.
  - Instruct the woman to sit in a well-lighted area and use a hand-held mirror to see the external genitalia.
  - Suggest that she inspect and palpate the area in a systematic manner, starting at the mons pubis and progressing to the labia, clitoris, and perineum. She should inspect the anus.
  - Emphasize that new moles, warts, or growths of any kind, as well as ulcers, sores, changes in skin color or itching should be reported to the health care provider as soon as possible.

- Papanicolaou (Pap) test is a reliable screening test for cervical cancer. Cytology findings are reported by the Bethesda system, which addresses 3 elements.
  - Specimen adequacy
  - General categorization (normal or abnormal)
  - Descriptive diagnosis of abnormal cytology that uses the following terminology: (a) atypical squamous cells of undetermined significance; (b) squamous intraepithlial lesion (SIL), which is subdivided into low-grade SIL and high-grade SIL (previously categorized as carcinoma in situ); and (c) squamous cell cancer

- Fecal occult blood testing (FOBT) is a useful screening measure for colorectal cancer. To prevent false FOBT results, the woman should be advised to
  — Collect a specimen from 3 consecutive stools.
  — Return slides as directed.
- Laboratory screening tests depend on the history and risk assessment of the woman, but might include the following.
  — Testing for sexually transmissible diseases (STDs) is recommended for those with (a) a history of multiple sexual partners; (b) a sexual partner with multiple contacts; (c) sexual contact with people with culture-proven STD; (d) a history of repeated episodes of STDs.
  — HIV testing should be offered to those (a) seeking treatment for STDs; (b) who use IV drugs; (c) who have a bisexual partner or a partner who is HIV-positive; (d) who have been exposed to blood or other body fluids in their line of work.
  — Testing for rubella antibodies should be performed during the childbearing years to determine immunity.
  — Lipid profile is appropriate for women with a family history of coronary heart disease (particularly during the postmenopausal years, when estrogen deficit results in an increase in low-density lipoproteins and a decrease in high-density lipoproteins).
  — Urinalysis is routinely performed to detect infection of urinary tract.
  — Fasting glucose test should be performed if the woman is (a) obese; (b) has a history of gestational diabetes; or (c) has a family history of diabetes mellitus.
  — Tuberculosis (TB) skin test should be performed for all women (a) with HIV infection; (b) in close contact with people known or suspected to have TB; (c) born in a country with high TB prevalence; (d) with low income; (e) with alcoholism; (f) who use IV drugs; or (g) who work in high-risk areas such as hospitals and health care clinics.

- Thyroid function test is recommended if there are signs of thyroid dysfunction, such as heart palpitations or heat intolerance, or a family history of thyroid dysfunction.
- Serum CA 125 should be checked if the woman has a family history of ovarian cancer.
- Transvaginal ultrasound may be used to diagnose disorders of the ovaries or fallopian tubes.
- Colonoscopy is recommended for women with a family history of colon cancer.

Immunizations

Recommended immunizations include

- Tetanus-diphtheria booster.
- Measles mumps rubella (MMR) for women of childbearing age with no evidence of immunity.
- Hepatitis B vaccine for high-risk groups (IV drug use, current recipients of blood products, health-related job with exposure to blood products, household or sexual contact with hepatitis B carrier, sexual activity with multiple partners)
- Pneumococcal vaccine should be offered to those who are immunosuppressed or who have sickle cell disease, Hodgkin's disease, alcoholism, cirrhosis, or multiple myeloma.
- Influenza vaccine is recommended annually for those over 55 years.

B. BREAST DISORDERS

Diagnosis

Methods used to determine if a lesion or lump in the breast is benign or malignant include

- Ultrasound examination to distinguish fluid-filled cysts from solid tissue that is potentially malignant.

- Needle aspiration biopsy to remove fluid from suspected cyst for analysis of cells.
- Surgical biopsy is performed if
  - Bloody fluid is removed from cyst on aspiration.
  - Cyst fails to disappear completely after aspiration.
  - Cyst reoccurs.
  - Solid dominant mass is not diagnosed.
  - Nipple discharge is bloody .
  - Nipple is persistently ulcerated or crusted.
  - Skin is swollen and red (suggests inflammatory breast cancer).
  - Mammography findings are suspicious (ACOG, 1996).

Risk Factors for Breast Cancer

- Advanced age
- Previous history of breast cancer
- Nulliparity
- Delayed childbearing (after 30 years)
- Early menarche (before age 12)
- Late menopause (after age 53)
- Family history of breast cancer
- Genetic factors (BRCA1 and BRCA2) (ACOG, 1996)

Psychosocial Implications of Breast Cancer

Common psychosocial concerns of women who have breast cancer are

- Fear of death.
- Anxiety about treatment and quality of life.
- Changes in body image.
- The effect on sexuality.

- Side effects of therapy.
- The effect on family relationships and work responsibilities.

Staging of Breast Cancer

Although confirmation of malignancy is the first step in evaluating the woman with cancer, staging is necessary to understand the extent of the cancer. Staging is based on a TNM (tumor, node, metastasis) system. Stages progress from stage 1, indicating a small tumor without lymphatic involvement or metastases, to stage 4, which indicates spread to lymph nodes and metastasis to other organs.

Management

Treatment depends on many factors, including the location and size of the tumor, extension into surrounding tissue, and involvement of the lymphatic system. Body organs such as the bones, brain, and liver are scanned prior to treatment to detect metastasis. A combination of surgical excision and adjuvant therapy is often recommended.

Surgical Treatment

- Breast conservation treatment involves wide local excision (sometimes called lumpectomy) of the tumor to microscopically clean margins.
- Simple mastectomy is removal of the breast.
- Modified radical mastectomy is removal of breast tissue, axillary nodes, and some chest muscles; however, the pectoralis major is preserved.

Adjuvant Therapy

Adjuvant therapy is supportive therapy that includes radiation, chemotherapy, or antiestrogen hormonal therapy such as tamoxifen.

Breast Reconstruction

Breast reconstruction may be immediate or delayed. The most common methods are listed.

- Tissue expansion is a method in which a prosthesis is filled with saline in small increments to slowly expand the tissue. An implant is inserted when the desired size is reached.
- Autogenous grafts, which carry their own blood supply, are recommended when radiation leaves the wound unsuitable for implants. They may also be more suited to the woman with large breasts or the woman who objects to implants.
- Nipple-areola reconstruction may use skin from the opposite nipple, skin that covers the prosthesis mound, or skin from other body tissue. Many surgeons inject pigment into the area to create an areola.

Nursing Considerations

The woman who is diagnosed with breast cancer should be able to depend on nurses for accurate information and emotional support. Nurses must allow time for the woman to express her feelings and worries. Many women and their families experience a great deal of confusion and frustration as they try to coordinate appointments and information from a variety of specialists, such as surgeons, radiologists, and oncologists. Nurses must convey a sense of empathetic understanding as they help the woman, and her family if she desires, participate in decisions about her care. Moreover, nurses are often responsible for providing information about the preoperative and postoperative periods.

- Usual time in the hospital or surgical facility (1–2 days; however, some surgical procedures including mastectomies, are performed in outpatient clinics)
- Function of pressure dressing and drainage tubes (to prevent further bleeding and edema)

- A description of the wound (may be red and raised for first few weeks); and when stitches should be removed

- How to minimize the risk of infection (keep wound dry and clean); signs of wound infection to report at once (purulent drainage, heat, tenderness)

- How the wound heals (redness and edema gradually subside, fluid from drainage tube lessens, wound gradually becomes a thin scar)

- Side effects of adjuvant therapy (nausea, fatigue, hair loss)

- Explanation of arm exercises that may be recommended to prevent lymphedema and to maintain mobility of the arm

- Information about groups that provide support (Reach to Recovery and Encore)

C. ABNORMAL UTERINE BLEEDING

Normal menstruation occurs every 24–35 days and lasts 2–7 days. Abnormal bleeding occurs more frequently, lasts longer, or is excessive in amount.

Etiology

The most common causes of abnormal bleeding are

- Pregnancy complications, such as spontaneous abortion.

- Anatomic lesions, such as cervical polyps or uterine myomas.

- "Break-through" bleeding that may occur when oral contraceptives are used.

- Systemic disorders, such as diabetes mellitus or hypothyroidism.

- Failure to ovulate (dysfunctional uterine bleeding).

Management

Management depends on the cause, but may include

- Use of progestin-estrogen combination oral contraceptives that suppress ovulation and allow a more stable endometrial lining to form.
- Surgical therapy, such as dilation and curettage, to remove polyps or to diagnose endometrial hyperplasia.
- Myomectomy for uterine fibroids.
- Hysterectomy if fibroids are large, bleeding persists, and the woman no longer desires to become pregnant.
- Laser ablation to remove endometrial lining.
- Iron supplementation to treat iron-deficiency anemia.

Nursing Considerations

Nurses are often responsible for encouraging women to seek medical attention promptly when abnormal bleeding occurs. Nurses may help the woman keep a record of bleeding episodes and the amount of blood lost. Moreover, nurses can emphasize the importance of adequate nutrition and provide information about diagnostic procedures, such as ultrasound examination and endometrial biopsy, that may be necessary.

D. PAIN ASSOCIATED WITH MENSTRUAL CYCLE

Primary Dysmenorrhea

Primary dysmenorrhea ("cramps") refers to menstrual pain without identified pathology. It occurs during ovulatory cycles and most often affects young, nulliparous women.

Etiology

- Excessive production of prostaglandin during luteal phase of menstrual cycle
- Diffusion of prostaglandin into endometrial tissue, causing uterine ischemia, hypoxia, and muscle contraction

Signs and Symptoms

- Colicky, spasmodic pain of the lower abdomen that occurs within hours of the onset of menses
- Sharp pain may radiate from the abdomen to the lower back or down the legs
- Nausea, vomiting, or diarrhea may accompany discomfort

Management

- Oral contraceptives that decrease amount of endometrial growth and thus reduce the production of endometrial prostaglandins
- Prostaglandin inhibitors such as ibuprofen (Motrin, Advil) or naproxen (Naprosyn, Anaprox)

Nursing Considerations

- Recommend nonpharmacologic measures such as frequent rest periods, application of heat to lower abdomen, moderate exercise, and well-balanced diet.
- Instruct that prostaglandin inhibitors are more effective if taken before onset of menses.
- Suggest that they be taken with meals to decrease gastric irritation.

Endometriosis

Etiology

The cause of endometriosis is unknown, although various theories have been advanced, including the following.

- Menstrual discharge contains viable endometrial cells that can attach to sites outside the uterus.
- Endometrial cells are disseminated primarily by retrograde menstruation or reflux of menstrual flow through the fallopian tubes.
- Endometriosis represents an autoimmune process that has a genetic basis.

- Although the cause is unknown, the pathologic process is clear.
- Tissue that is identical to that in the endometrium is present outside the uterus. The tissue proliferates during the follicular and luteal phases of the menstrual cycle and then sloughs during menstruation. Unlike menstruation, however, the bleeding occurs in a closed cavity, causing pressure and pain. Cyclic bleeding initiates chronic inflammatory changes throughout the pelvis and can cause infertility.

Signs and Symptoms

- Abdominal pain that is deep and constant, unlike the spasmodic pain of primary dysmenorrhea
- Dyspareunia (especially with deep penetration)
- Rectal pain
- Diarrhea, constipation, feelings of rectal pressure
- Infertility

Management

Treatment is aimed at interrupting the menstrual cycle so that bleeding is impeded. Therapeutic measures may include

- Oral contraceptives to induce a pseudopregnancy and prolonged amenorrhea.
- Gonadotropin inhibitor such as danazol that causes atrophy of endometrial tissue, anovulation, and amenorrhea
- Drugs that interfere with the production of gonadotropin-releasing hormones (Lupron, Zoladex, Synarel) when taken daily
- Laparoscopy for lysis of adhesions and laser vaporization of lesions
- Hysterectomy with bilateral salpingo-oophorectomy if the woman no longer wishes to conceive; estrogen replacement therapy if all lesions are removed

Nursing Considerations

Nurses must provide information and support for the woman who often lives with a great deal of cyclic pain and uncertainty about future fertility. Common nursing responsibilities include

- Validation that the woman is not pregnant; therapy should begin during menstrual cycle.

- Education about expected side effects of medication, such as hot flushes, weight gain, oily skin.

- Instruction to notify health care provider of unusual side effects, such as headache, dizziness, rapid weight gain (> 5 pounds per week) swelling of fingers or feet, jaundice, dark urine, or clay-colored stools.

- Recommendation not to delay pregnancy if the woman wishes to conceive.

E. PREMENSTRUAL SYNDROME (PMS)

Signs and Symptoms

- Complaints of PMS can be divided into behavioral and physical symptoms. See Table V-5, "Symptoms of Premenstrual Syndrome."

Criteria for Diagnosis

- Signs and symptoms must be cyclical and recur in the luteal phase of the menstrual cycle.

- The woman should be symptom-free during the follicular phase of the cycle, and there must be at least 7 symptom-free days.

- Symptoms must severe enough to have an impact on work, lifestyle, and relationships.

- Diagnosis must be based on charting of symptoms as they occur rather than recall of symptoms that occurred in the past; see Figure V-1 for one type of calendar on which symptoms may be recorded.

TABLE V-5

Symptoms of Premenstrual Syndrome (PMS)

PHYSICAL SYMPTOMS	PSYCHOLOGICAL SYMPTOMS
Edema	Anxiety
Weight gain	Depression
Abdominal bloating	Irritability
Constipation	Mood swings
Hot flashes	Aggressive behavior
Breast pain	Increased appetite
Headache	Food cravings
Acne	Fatigue
Rhinitis	Difficulty concentrating
Heart palpitations	Insomnia

Etiology

Although the cause is unknown, there are several theories, including

- Imbalance between estrogen and progesterone.
- Abnormal production of prostaglandins.
- Low levels of endorphins.
- Fluid imbalance.
- Nutritional deficiency.

Management

Treatment is based on the symptom profile of each individual woman, and there is little agreement on what is effective. Examples of medical therapy include

- Mild potassium-sparing diuretics.
- Prostaglandin inhibitors.
- Nutritional supplements such as calcium, magnesium, vitamin E, and Vitamin B_6.
- Progesterone supplementation.
- Bromocriptine to reduce breast tenderness and swelling.

394 Clinical Manual for Foundations of Maternal Newborn Nursing

Figure V-1

Calendar for Premenstrual Syndrome (PMS) Symptoms

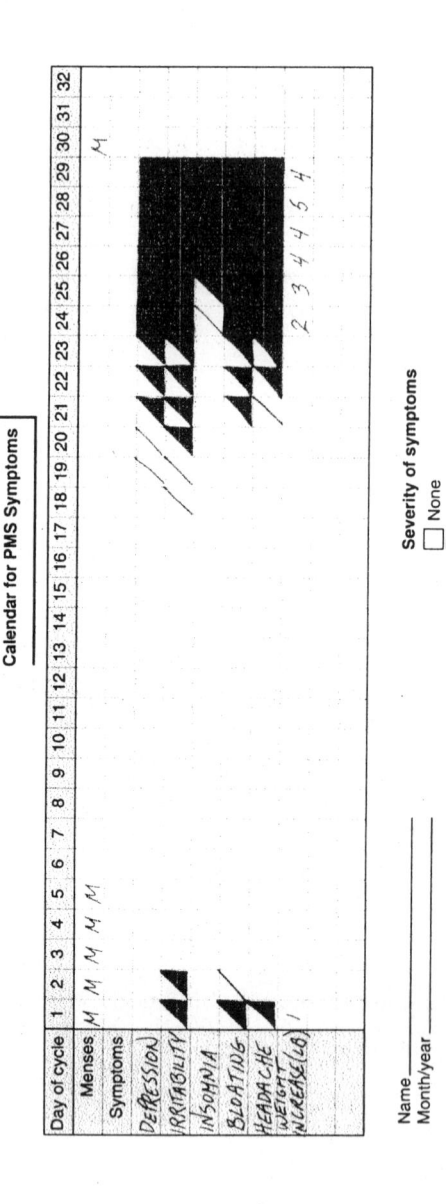

Calendar for PMS Symptoms

Day of cycle	1	2	3	4	5	6	7	8	9	10	11	12	13	14	15	16	17	18	19	20	21	22	23	24	25	26	27	28	29	30	31	32
Menses	M	M	M	M	M																									M		
Symptoms																																
Depression																																
Irritability																																
Insomnia																																
Bloating																																
Headache																																
Weight Increase (Lb)	1																						2		3	4	4	5	4			

Severity of symptoms

☐ None
◰ Mild
◨ Moderate
■ Severe

Name _____
Month/year _____

- Evening primrose oil.
- Anti-anxiety medications (usually reserved for severe anxiety that does not respond to other therapy).

Nursing Considerations

Nurses can educate the family about lifestyle changes that may alleviate symptoms of PMS. The most common measures include the following.

- Decrease consumption of caffeine or other stimulants.
- Avoid simple sugars, which can cause rebound hypoglycemia.
- Restrict intake of salty foods, which increase fluid retention.
- Drink at least 2000 mL of water each day to maintain hydration.
- Eat six small meals per day to prevent episodes of hypoglycemia.
- Avoid alcohol, which can aggravate depression.
- Increase physical exercise for sense of well-being.
- Reduce stress by guided imagery, conscious relaxation techniques, warm baths, and massage.
- Adhere to a regular schedule for sleep and engage in relaxing activities prior to bedtime.
- Make concrete plans to obtain relief when she feels she is losing control or fears she may harm herself or a child.

F. INDUCED ABORTION

Techniques used to induce abortion depend on the length of gestation. The three most common techniques are

- Vacuum aspiration (to 13 weeks)
- Dilation and evacuation (13–16 weeks)
- Labor induction (after 16 weeks)

Methods in the future may include

- Administration of RU486 within the first 7 weeks of gestation, followed by administration of prostaglandin.
- Administration of methotrexate and misoprostol.

Nursing Considerations

Nurses must be knowledgeable about the legal implications of induced abortions in areas where they practice. For example, some states have laws that affect minors seeking an abortion. Other states have waiting periods and restrict abortion to specific periods of gestation. Moreover, nurses are often responsible for providing information about self-care measures following induced abortion. Major points of information include the following.

- Normal activities may be resumed, but strenuous work or exercise should be avoided for a few days.
- Bleeding or cramping may occur for a week or two; medical advice should be sought if either becomes severe.
- Sanitary pads, rather than tampons, should be used for the first week.
- Douching should be avoided for at least a week.
- Intercourse should be restricted for about a week.
- Birth control measures are necessary if sex is resumed.
- Menstruation usually resumes in 4–6 weeks.
- Temperature should be taken twice a day; temperature above 37.8°C (100°F) should be reported to health care provider.
- Follow-up appointment in 2 weeks is necessary.

G. MENOPAUSE

Menopause is the permanent cessation of menstruation after the loss of ovarian function. When the ovaries cease to function, the ovarian hormones, estrogen and progesterone, fall. The average age of menopause in North America is 51 1/2 years.

Signs and Symptoms of Menopause

Many of the signs and symptoms of menopause are due to a deficiency in estrogen.

- Amenorrhea
- Vasomotor instability (hot flushes, palpitations)
- Atrophic changes of the external genitalia, resulting in dyspareunia, atrophic vaginitis, or cystitis
- Adverse changes in serum lipids (increase in low-density lipoproteins, decrease in high-density lipoproteins) that increase the risk of coronary heart disease
- Decrease in bone density

Psychological responses to menopause vary widely, and a clear connection to estrogen deficiency has not been established.

- Depression
- Irritability
- Insomnia
- Fatigue
- Loss of libido

Hormone Replacement Therapy (HRT)

Hormone replacement therapy is recommended for many women in the United States and Canada. The type of hormone replacement depends on whether the woman has an intact uterus.

- Estrogen alone is prescribed for women who have had a hysterectomy and thus do not have the concern of endometrial hyperplasia.
- Estrogen and progesterone are prescribed for women who retain the uterus and are at risk for endometrial hyperplasia.

Benefits of HRT

- Controls hot flushes
- Prevents genital atrophy
- Protects against coronary heart disease
- Protects against bone loss (osteoporosis)
- Improves sense of well-being, helps overcome insomnia, and decreases feelings of depression and irritability, according to anecdotal evidence from women who elect to use HRT

Risks of HRT

- Increased risk of endometrial cancer unless progestins are administered to prevent hyperplasia
- Possible increased risk of breast cancer for women who use estrogen for more than 10–20 years; however, the risk is unclear and the data are confusing (ACOG, 1996).

Contraindications for HRT

- Unexplained vaginal bleeding
- Active liver disease or chronic impaired liver function
- Recent vascular thrombosis
- Cancer of the breast (particularly if the tumor was estrogen-receptor positive)
- Cancer of the endometrium

Relative Contraindications for HRT

- Seizure disorders
- Very high levels of triglycerides and lipids
- Migraine headaches
- Current gallbladder disease (ACOG, 1996)

Alternative Medical Treatment

- Clonidine hydrochloride
- Bellergal

Nursing Considerations

Nurses are often the primary sources of information about measures to mitigate symptoms. These measures are particularly helpful when the woman cannot or chooses not to take exogenous estrogen.

- Vitamin E, ginseng, or other herbs to relieve hot flushes
- Water-soluble lubricants (Lubrin, Replens) for relief of vaginal dryness and dyspareunia
- Kegel exercises to increase tone in muscles around the vagina and urinary meatus that may atrophy without estrogen
- Drinking at least eight glasses of water a day to decrease urine concentration and reduce bacterial growth
- Wiping from front to back following urination or defecation to reduce transfer of bacteria from the anus to the urinary meatus
- Acknowledging symptoms, such as depression and irritability, that sometimes receive very little attention or sympathy

H. OSTEOPOROSIS

Osteoporosis is loss of bone density that leaves the bones porous, fragile, and susceptible to fractures. The vertebrae, wrists, and hips are the most common sites of fractures.

Risk Factors

- Slender, fair-skinned Caucasian women
- Asian women
- Family history of osteoporosis

- A sedentary lifestyle
- Early menopause (before 45 years)
- Alcoholism
- Smoking
- Frequent use of corticosteroids
- Excessive amounts of caffeine
- Inadequate lifetime intake of calcium

Signs and Symptoms

Osteoporosis is sometimes called the "silent thief" because it take place gradually without any signs or symptoms. The first noticeable signs are:

- Loss of height and back pain as vertebrae collapse.
- "Dowager's hump," which develops when vertebrae can no longer support the upper body.
- Loss of bone mass demonstrated by dual energy x-ray absorptiometry (DXA), computed tomography (CT scan), or other methods of assessing bone density.

Prevention and Management

- Weight-bearing exercise (walking, aerobics)
- Adequate daily calcium intake (1500 mg/day for adolescent and postmenopausal women, 1000 mg/day for premenopausal women)
- Vitamin D supplementation (400 to 800 mg/day for postmenopausal women or those with little exposure to direct sunlight)
- Decreasing risk factors (smoking, alcohol, caffeine)
- Estrogen replacement therapy (at least 0.625 mg/day)
- Calcitonin nasal spray (Miacalcin) for women who demonstrate low bone mass by DXA
- Alendronate (Fosamax) to inhibit bone resorption

- May cause gastrointestinal problems
- Directions for use
  - Take with 6–8 ounces of water on arising.
  - Wait at least 30 minutes before taking food, other fluids, or medications.
  - Remain upright for at least 30 minutes.

Nursing Considerations

In addition to providing information about diet, and exercise, and answering questions about medical regimen, nurses are also concerned about how to prevent falls. Teach the following important measures.

- Use ample lighting with easily available switches.
- Secure loose electrical cords.
- Area rugs should have nonskid backing.
- Install nonskid devices and grab bars by the bathtub.
- Install handrails by stairways.
- Keep loose items out of walking pathways.

I. DYSFUNCTION OF PELVIC SUPPORT

When the muscles and ligaments of the pelvic floor become weakened, pelvic organs prolapse into the vagina. The most common problems are cystocele (the bladder protrudes downward into the vagina), rectocele (the rectum protrudes into the vagina), and uterine prolapse (the uterus sags backward and downward into the vagina).

Etiology

- Genital atrophy that begins in the perimenopausal period
- Delayed result of traumatic childbirth
- Lifetime of lifting heavy objects
- Congenital defect of pelvic structures

- Coexistent medical disease (chronic respiratory disease, asthma, hay fever) that may traumatize the pelvic supports

Signs and Symptoms

- Urinary incontinence
  - Stress incontinence (loss of urine with sudden increase in intra-abdominal pressure, such as that generated by sneezing, coughing, lifting, or sudden jarring motions)
  - Urge incontinence (abrupt or strong desire to void)
  - Overflow incontinence (involuntary loss or "dribbling" of urine; associated with overdistention)
- Constipation, flatulence, or difficulty defecating
- Feelings of pelvic fullness or pelvic pressure
- Low backache
- Fatigue

Management

- Rubber barrier insert for urethra for urinary incontinence
- Anticholinergic agents for urge incontinence
- Bladder-neck support prosthesis to control stress incontinence
- Hormone replacement therapy to increase tissue elasticity and blood supply and thus reduce dyspareunia
- Surgical procedures such as anterior colporrhaphy (for cystocele), posterior colporrhaphy (for rectocele), and/or vaginal hysterectomy when other measures are unsuccessful
- Vaginal pessary if surgery is not an option (pessary must be removed, cleaned, and replaced regularly)

Nursing Considerations

- Teach methods to strengthen pubococcygeal muscles (Kegel exercises, use of incrementally weighted vaginal cones).

- Initiate bladder retraining (gradually lengthen time between voiding) that enables women to accommodate greater volumes of urine.
- Suggest voiding according to a schedule that incorporates systematic delay of voiding by using distraction and relaxation techniques, self-monitoring, and positive reinforcement.
- Recommend drinking at least 2,000 mL of fluid each day to prevent concentrated urine that can irritate the bladder.
- Advise to avoid to avoid or restrict alcohol and caffeine, which can aggravate bladder irritation.
- Provide information about practices to protect the skin and prevent odor (warm sitz baths, perineal care, thorough drying of genital area).
- Describe commercial products that trap urine and hold it away from the skin.
- Teach measures to prevent constipation.
  - Consume adequate dietary fiber and fluids.
  - Pay prompt attention to a feeling of rectal fullness.
  - Use bulk producers, stool softeners, or stimulants as indicated or as recommended by health care provider.
  - Exercise regularly.
- Instruct in measures to reduce discomfort, such as backache and pelvic pressure.
  - Lie down with legs elevated several times each day.
  - Assume knee-chest position for a few minutes as necessary.
  - Use of biofeedback.
- Advise lifestyle changes (avoiding heavy lifting, weight reduction, cessation from smoking, and treatment of respiratory diseases).

J. BENIGN DISORDERS OF THE REPRODUCTIVE TRACT

Cervical Polyps

Polyps are small tumors, usually only a few millimeters in diameter, that are generally on a pedicle. They cause intermittent vaginal bleeding. They are surgically removed in an outpatient setting and sent for cytology examination to rule out the possibility of malignancy.

Uterine Leiomyomas (Fibroids)

Fibroids develop from smooth muscle of the uterus. Growth is stimulated by estrogen and they may grow rapidly during the childbearing years. Fibroids may cause increased uterine size and excessive uterine bleeding. Treatment depends on size and may involve watchful waiting only. If abnormal bleeding is a problem, surgical intervention may be necessary and may include removal of the tumor (myomectomy), or removal of the uterus. Gonadotropin-releasing hormone agonists may reduce the size of the myoma and lessen the need for surgical removal.

Ovarian Cysts

Cysts are closed sacs filled with fluid or semifluids. They may be follicular (when the ovarian follicle fails to rupture during ovulation) or luteal (when the corpus luteum does not regress following ovulation). They are often asymptomatic, but may cause pain and some delay in the menstrual cycle. Treatment depends on differentiating a cyst from a solid tumor that may indicate cancer. Diagnosis may involve transvaginal ultrasound or laparoscopy.

If initial treatment involves watchful waiting, the woman should be instructed that

- Frequent pelvic examinations are necessary to monitor the size of the cyst.
- Oral contraceptives may be used for several months to suppress ovulation.
- Surgical removal may be necessary for large cysts or for cysts that do not shrink.

- Pain can usually be managed with analgesics and comfort measures such as application of heat to the abdomen.

K. MALIGNANT DISORDERS OF THE REPRODUCTIVE TRACT

The primary sites for cancer are the uterus, cervix, and ovaries.

Risk Factors

Risk factors vary according to the site of the cancer. See Table V-6, "Risk Factors for Cancer of the Reproductive Organs."

TABLE V-6

Risk Factors for Cancer of the Reproductive Organs

Uterus
- Obesity
- Early onset of menarche
- Late onset of menopause
- Diabetes mellitus
- Hypertension
- Infertility
- Lynch syndrome II (a familial syndrome of predisposition to endometrial, breast, ovarian, colon cancers)
- Chronic unopposed estrogen stimulation

Cervix
- Multiple sexual partners
- First coitus before 20 years of age
- Nonbarrier contraception
- History of sexually transmissible diseases (strong link with human papillomavirus)
- HIV positive
- Smoking
- Failure to obtain regular cytology screening
- Lower socioeconomic status

Ovaries
- Race (increased in Caucasian women)
- Low parity, delayed childbearing, infertility
- Family history of ovarian or uterine cancer
- Obesity and high-fat diet are possible risk factors
- Frequent use of genital powders is a possible risk factor

Signs and Symptoms

There are few signs and symptoms in the early stages of cancer of the female reproductive organs. Nurses must emphasize, however, that the following symptoms should *always* be reported.

- Irregular vaginal bleeding
- Unexplained postmenopausal bleeding
- Unusual vaginal discharge
- Dyspareunia
- Persistent vulvar or vaginal itching
- Elevated or discolored lesions on the vulva
- Persistent abdominal bloating or constipation
- Persistent anorexia or vomiting
- Blood in stools

Diagnosis

Early diagnosis is strongly associated with long-term survival. In addition to screening procedures described earlier, a variety of diagnostic procedures are useful in early detection.

- Serum tests, such as CA 125, for tumor markers
- Ultrasonography to distinguish fluid-filled cysts from solid tumors
- Endometrial biopsy to detect hyperplasia that may be associated with cancer
- Colposcopy that can identify patterns of abnormality near the cervical os where cancer often develops
- Conization (removal of a cone of tissue from the cervical canal) for diagnosis or for cure of preinvasive lesions of the cervix

Management

Treatment is based on the location and extent of the disease, as well as the age and desire of the woman to have children.

Cervical Cancer

Early treatment of cervical lesions may involve destruction of abnormal tissue.

- Cryosurgery to freeze abnormal cells, which then slough; normal tissue regenerates
- Laser surgery that allows for precise direction of a beam of light (heat) to remove diseased tissue
- Electrosurgical excision, which often uses a wire-loop electrode that can excise tissue with minimal damage to surrounding tissue

Treatment of Invasive Cancer of the Cervix

- Hysterectomy
- Radiation therapy delivered by internal radium applications to the cervix or by external radiation therapy that includes lymphatics of the pelvis
- Pelvic exenteration if treatment by radiation fails
- Chemotherapy for metastatic disease

Endometrium

Treatment of uterine cancer depends on the extent of the cancer.

- Hysterectomy with bilateral salpingo-oophorectomy (BSO)
- Radical hysterectomy, BSO, and pelvic node dissection for more advanced disease
- Radiation therapy before or after surgery (may be external or internal)
- Chemotherapy for advanced or recurrent disease

- Medroxyprogesterone (Depo-Provera) for estrogen-dependent cancers
- Anti-estrogen medications such as tamoxifen (Tamofen)

Ovarian Cancer

Because the symptoms are vague and definitive screening tests do not exist, ovarian cancer is often diagnosed at an advanced stage. Palpation of an ovary in a postmenopausal woman or palpation of a pelvic mass are usually the first signs. Prior to surgical procedures, there should be

- Evaluation of bowel, including barium enema, to detect invasion of bowel surfaces.
- Evaluation of the urinary tract by intravenous pyelogram.
- Chest x-ray, liver, bone, and brain scan to detect metastasis.
- Series of oral antibiotics to decrease pathogenic organisms in the bowel.
- Counseling regarding the possibility of temporary colostomy if tumor adheres to bowel.
- Surgical removal of as much of the tumor as possible, plus excision of the uterus, fallopian tubes, and ovaries.
- Chemotherapy plus counseling regarding the side effects and measures to control nausea, vomiting, and anorexia.
- Post-therapy monitoring, which may include serial physical examinations, serum marker determinations, and abdominal imaging.
- Second-look surgery to determine the response of the disease to chemotherapy.

Nursing Considerations

Most preoperative procedures are performed on an outpatient basis, and short hospital stays are common even for radical surgery. As a result, women need a great deal of information and support that nurses can provide and that often extends from diagnosis through home care. Common responsibilities include providing information about the following.

- Preoperative procedures (ultrasonography, biopsies, etc.)
- Postoperative events and procedures (drainage tubes, suprapubic drains, intravenous fluids, nasogastric tube to prevent distention, and frequent evaluation of vital signs, wounds, urinary output, and bowel sounds)
- Postoperative care, such as pain management and measures to prevent hypostatic pneumonia (turning, coughing, breathing deeply)
- Discharge planning and teaching
  — Monitoring appetite and diet as well as bowel function and activity
  — Explaining that temporary vaginal discharge is expected even though uterus has been removed
  — Reminding her that she will no longer have menstrual periods
  — Encouraging questions about follow-up care such as chemotherapy or radiation
  — Facilitating a discussion about common fears that many women have such as fear of death or recurrence and concern about the effects on femininity or sexuality
  — Teaching measures to overcome anorexia, nausea, and diarrhea, which are common side effects of chemotherapy (frequent small meals, high calorie snacks, protein shakes); to avoid rich fatty foods, alcohol, spicy foods, and carbonated drinks
  — Instructing about need and schedule for home follow-up appointments
  — Referring to appropriate support groups

L. SEXUALLY TRANSMISSIBLE DISEASES (STDs)

Multiple diseases can be transmitted through sexual activity. For some diseases, such as syphilis, gonorrhea, or Chlamydial infection, sexual activity is almost the only method of transmission. For other diseases, such as candidiasis or trichomoniasis, sexual activity may or may not be the mode of transmission. For information about signs and symptoms, diagnosis, and treatment, see Table V-7. See pages 86-90 for impact of STDs on pregnancy and the fetus.

TABLE V-7

Sexually Transmissible Diseases

SIGNS AND SYMPTOMS	DIAGNOSIS	MANAGEMENT
Syphilis (Spirochete *Treponema pallidum*)		
Primary stage: painless chancre of genitalia, lips, anus; Secondary stage: enlargement of spleen and liver, headache, generalized maculopapular rash; Tertiary stage: all body systems, including CNS, affected	Spirochete visible on darkfield examination; Serology (VDRL, RPR, or FTAABS) positive	Benzathine penicillin G, 2.4 million units I.M. Tetracycline 500 mg p.o. q.i.d. for 15 days is alternative for those allergic to penicillin
Gonorrhea (*Neisseria gonorrhoeae*)		
May be asymptomatic in women; dysuria, purulent discharge, and dyspareunia are most common symptoms; pelvic pain indicates PID	Identification of gonococci on culture of exudate from cervix, urethra, or other infected areas	Ceftriaxone sodium one dose I.M. followed by doxycycline hyclate p.o. for 7 days
Chlamydial Infection (*Chlamydia trachomatis*)		
May be asymptomatic in women; dysuria, purulent discharge, abnormal vaginal bleeding, pelvic pain (PID)	Culture, antigen-antibody tests, enzyme immunoassay, monoclonal antibody test	Doxycycline p.o. for 7 days
Herpes Genitalis (Herpes simplex virus I or II)		
Painful genital vesicles that ulcerate; fever, chills, muscle aches	Clinical signs and symptoms; culture of virus	No cure; acyclovir p.o. for 5–10 days for acute episodes

SECTION FIVE: Women's Health Care and Reproductive Issues **411**

Condylomata Acuminata (Genital Warts) (Human papillomavirus (HPV))

Painless anal or genital warts	Pap smear, colposcopy, or biopsy	Weekly applications of trichloroacetic acid, cryotherapy, laser therapy; podophyllin weekly for 6 weeks

Acquired Immunodeficiency Syndrome (AIDS) (Human immunodeficiency virus)

Seroconversion usually within 6 months with flu-like symptoms; asymptomatic period until there is destruction of cell-mediated immunity; opportunistic infections develop	Serology to detect antibodies (ELISA, IFA, Western Blot)	Zidovudine (AZT), Didanosine (Videx), Zalcitabine (ddC, Hivid) Protease inhibitors such as saquinavir (Invirase)

Hepatitis B (Hepatitis B virus)

Anorexia, nausea, vomiting, arthralgia, rash, jaundice, enlarged liver	HBsAg, HBcAg, HBeAg positive	Vaccine available

Candidiasis (*Candida albicans*)

Vaginal and perineal itching and inflammation; thick white vaginal discharge	Clinical signs and symptoms; visualization of organism	Vaginal applications of miconazole (Monistat), clotrimazole (GyneLotrimin), or nystatin (Mycostatin)

Trichomoniasis (*Trichomonas vaginalis*)

Thin, malodorous, greenish-yellow vaginal discharge; edema, itching, redness of the vulva	Identification of organism in a wet-mount preparation	Metronidazole (Flagyl, Protostat) if not pregnant

Bacterial Vaginosis (*Gardnerella vaginalis*)

Grayish-white vaginal discharge with "fishy" odor	Identification of clue cells in discharge	Metronidazole p.o., clindamycin cream, metronidazone gel

ELISA (Enzyme-linked immunosorbent assay)
FTAABS (fluorescent treponemal antibody absorption)
HBcAg (hepatitis B core antigen)
HBeAg (hepatitis B e antigen)
HBcAg (hepatitis B surface antigen)
IFA (immunofluorescence assay)
PID (pelvic inflammatory disease)
RPR (rapid plasma reagin)
VDRL (venereal disease research laboratory)
*Concurrent treatment of sexual partners is essential to prevent reinfection.
*Woman must be advised to complete the entire course of therapy.

American College of Obstetricians and Gynecologists (1996). Guidelines for Women's Health Care. Washington, D.C., Author.

M. PELVIC INFLAMMATORY DISEASE (PID)

Etiology

Bacteria invade the endocervical canal and cause cervicitis. The bacteria ascend to infect the endometrium, fallopian tubes, and pelvic cavity. The most common organisms are

- *Neisseria gonorrhoeae*
- *Chlamydia trachomatis*

Signs and Symptoms

Some women are asymptomatic; however, the most common signs and symptoms are

- Pelvic pain.
- Fever.
- Purulent vaginal discharge, irregular vaginal bleeding.
- Nausea, anorexia.

- Adnexal tenderness during bimanual examination.
- Leukocytosis, increased sedimentation rate.

Management

- Intravenous administration of cefoxitin, cefotetan, or clindamycin for women with fever, pain, and leukocytosis
- Oral administration of antibiotics for women who are less ill and are able to comply with recommended regimen

Nursing Considerations

Nurses play an important role in teaching women how to protect themselves from STDs. Teaching should include measures to avoid exposure.

- Limit number of sexual partners.
- Avoid intercourse with those who have multiple partners.
- Use barrier methods (latex condoms with spermicide containing nonoxynol 9, diaphragm with spermicide).
- Seek medical attention promptly after having unprotected sex with one who is suspected of having an STD or when vaginal discharge or genital lesions are apparent.
- Take medication as directed.
- Return for follow-up evaluation.

N. TOXIC SHOCK SYNDROME (TSS)

TSS is a rare but potentially fatal condition caused by toxin-producing *Staphylococcus aureus*.

Risk Factors

- Poor perineal hygiene
- Lack of hand washing before touching perineal area
- Menstruation
- Chronic vaginal infection

- Postpartum endometritis
- Use of high-absorbency tampons
- Use of diaphragm or cervical cap, which may trap and hold bacteria if left in place for a prolonged period of time

Signs and Symptoms

- Sudden spiking fever
- Flu-like symptoms (headache, sore throat, vomiting, diarrhea)
- Hypotension due to intravascular fluid leaking from blood vessels as a result of increased capillary permeability
- Generalized rash resembling sunburn

Management

- Fluid replacement
- Administration of vasopressor drugs
- Antimicrobial therapy
- Corticosteroids to treat skin changes

Nursing Considerations

Nurses are often responsible for teaching measures to prevent TSS.

- Wash hands thoroughly before inserting tampons, diaphragm, or cervical cap.
- Change tampons at least every 1–4 hours.
- Avoid superabsorbent tampons.
- Use pads rather than tampons during hours of sleep, which usually exceed 6–8 hours
- Do not use diaphragm during menstrual periods.
- Remove diaphragm within time recommended by health care provider.

SECTION SIX

Procedures and Drug Guides

CONTENTS

I. Procedures
- A. Administering Gavage Feeding 417
- B. Administering Intramuscular Injections to Newborns 419
- C. Applying a Pediatric Urine Collection Bag 420
- D. External Fetal Heart Rate and Contraction Monitoring 421
- E. Internal Fetal Heart Rate and Contraction Monitoring 423
- F. Assessing Blood Glucose in the Newborn 424
- G. Assessing Deep Tendon Reflexes 426
- H. Assessing the Perineum 427
- I. Assessing the Uterine Fundus 428
- J. Assessing Vital Signs of the Newborn 428
- K. Auscultating the Fetal Heart Rate 430
- L. Identifying Infants 431
- M. Palpating Contractions 432
- N. Performing Breast Self-Examinations 433
- O. Leopold's Maneuvers 434
- P. Performing Resuscitation in Newborns 436
- Q. Performing Vaginal Examination During Labor 438
- R. Teaching Women Fertility Awareness 440
- S. Testing for Ruptured Membranes 444
- T. Using a Bulb Syringe 445
- U. Weighing and Measuring the Newborn 445

II. Drug Guides
   A. Butorphanol 447
   C. Erythromycin Ophthalmic Ointment 450
   D. Hydralazine 451
   E. Hepatitis B Vaccine 452
   F. Magnesium Sulfate 454
   G. Medroxyprogesterone 455
   H. Methergine 456
   I. Naloxone Hydrochloride (Narcan) 458
   J. Oxytocin 459
   K. Rh$_O$(D) Immune Globulin 462
   L. Terbutaline 464
   M. Vitamin K1 (Phytonadione) 467

SECTION SIX

Procedures and Drug Guides

I. PROCEDURES

A. ADMINISTERING GAVAGE FEEDING

1. Wash hands and gather equipment: gavage tube of proper size (5–8 French, depending on the size of the infant), measured container, and 20-mL syringe. Warm breast milk or formula to room temperature. Check the chart to determine how previous feedings were tolerated. Add fortifier to breast milk if necessary.

2. Position the infant on the right side or prone if the infant regurgitates when moved.

3. Measure from the infant's mouth or nose to the earlobe and xiphoid process to determine the length of the catheter to insert. Mark the tube with a piece of tape.

4. Moisten the tip of the catheter with water. Hold the infant's head steady and gently insert the tube through the mouth or nose to the point marked. Remove the tube immediately if persistent coughing, choking, cyanosis, apnea, or bradycardia occurs.

5. Tape the tube in place.

6. Check for placement when the tube is first inserted, before beginning bolus feedings, and at least once a shift for continuous feedings.

    a. Attach a syringe to the tube and insert 0.5–1 cc of air through the tube while listening over the stomach with a stethoscope. Gently draw back on the plunger to withdraw the inserted air.

    b. Gently aspirate stomach contents. Move or rotate the tube slightly if the plunger does not withdraw easily.

7. Withdraw the stomach contents. Observe the amount, color, and consistency of the aspirate. During continuous feedings, check the gastric residual every 2–4 hours. Do not feed the infant if the aspirate is abnormal. Report abnormal appearance or amount of stomach contents.

8. Replace the aspirate before beginning the feeding. Subtract the amount of gastric residual from the amount of milk to be given.

9. Remove the plunger and attach the syringe to the feeding tube. Pour the correct amount of solution into the syringe. If it does not begin to move down the tube, insert the plunger just far enough to start the flow, then withdraw the plunger. Do not use the plunger to force the contents through the tube. Allow feeding to flow by gravity or attach to a feeding pump to regulate the flow.

10. If using gravity flow, raise or lower the syringe to increase or decrease the rate of flow so that the feeding moves slowly into stomach over 15–30 minutes.

11. For continuous feedings, place no more than a 2 to 4-hour supply of milk in a feeding bag or syringe. Set the pump to deliver the correct rate of flow. Change the equipment every 4 hours or according to hospital policy.

12. Give the infant a pactfier during the feeding to help prepare for nippling and to provide comfort.

13. When the catheter is to be withdrawn, pinch the tube and remove quickly to prevent drops of milk from entering the trachea as the tube is removed.

14. Burp the infant and position on the right side or prone, with the head of the bed elevated. If movement tends to cause regurgitation, omit burping. Allow the infant to remain on the right side or prone.

16. Record time, amount, and characteristics of gastric residual; type and amount of feeding given, and how the infant tolerated it.

SECTION SIX: Procedures and Drug Guides 419

B. ADMINISTERING INTRAMUSCULAR INJECTIONS TO NEWBORNS

1. Prepare medication for injection. Use a 1-mL syringe with a 5/8-inch 25-gauge needle. If the medication is in a glass ampule, use a filter needle to draw it up to prevent particles of glass from entering the syringe. Remove the filter needle and replace the original sterile needle to give the injection.

2. Put on gloves to protect against contamination with blood.

3. Locate the correct site (Figure VI-1). Intramuscular medication for an infant is given in the vastus lateralis muscle or, if necessary, the rectus femoris muscle. Divide the area between the greater trochanter of the femur and the knee

Figure VI-1

Correct Site for Intramuscular Injection in Infants

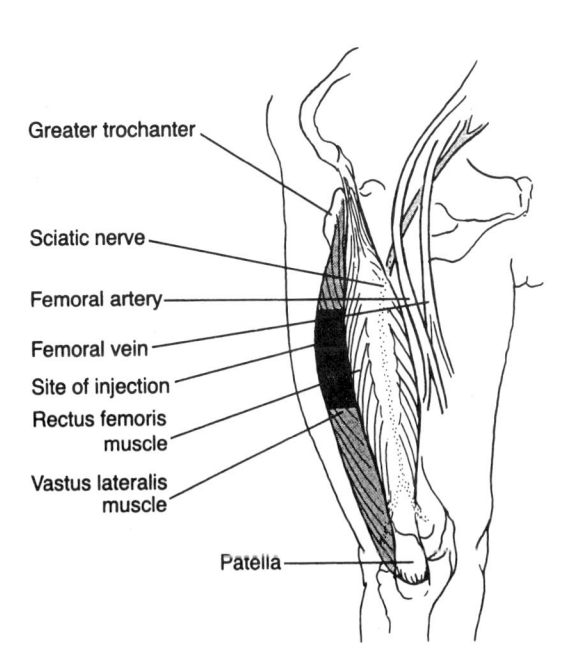

into thirds. Locate the injection site in the middle third of the muscle, lateral to the midline of the anterior thigh. (**Note:** The dorsogluteal muscle is never used until a child has been walking for at least a year. These muscles are poorly developed and dangerously near the sciatic nerve.)

4. Cleanse the area with an alcohol wipe.

5. Stabilize the leg firmly while grasping the thigh between the thumb and fingers.

6. Insert the needle at a 90° angle. Aspirate and inject the medication slowly if there is no blood return. If blood returns, withdraw the needle, discard the medication and syringe and prepare new medication.

7. Withdraw the needle quickly and wipe the site with an alcohol wipe.

C. APPLYING A PEDIATRIC URINE COLLECTION BAG

1. Wash and dry the genitalia. Apply tincture of benzoin according to hospital policy. Allow to dry until "tacky."

2. Remove the paper covering the posterior adhesive tabs first. Female infants: Fold the bag in half and apply it smoothly over the perineum, extending the tabs to the side. Male infants: Place the penis and scrotum (if small) inside the bag and apply the posterior adhesive tabs to the perineum. If the scrotum will not fit in the bag easily, apply the tabs smoothly over the scrotum.

3. Remove the paper covering the anterior adhesive tabs, and apply it to cover genitalia. Be sure that there are no wrinkles in the tabs.

4. An alternative method is to cut a small hole in a piece of transparent dressing and place it over the genitalia with hole centered over the meatus in a female and over the entire penis in a male. Attach the urine collector over the transparent dressing. This prevents trauma to the skin if the bag must be changed.

5. Place the diaper loosely over the bag or cut a slit in the diaper and gently pull the bag through the slit so urine can be seen in the bag.

6. Check the bag for urine frequently. Transfer the urine to a specimen cup by removing the tab over the hole in the bottom, cutting the lower corner, or aspirating with a syringe.

7. Clean the genitalia, and observe for irritation.

D. EXTERNAL FETAL HEART RATE AND CONTRACTION MONITORING

Purposes:

- To provide continuous or intermittent electronic fetal heart rate monitoring.
- To perform a basic evaluation of the fetal heart rate and uterine activity patterns to identify data needing further assessment by the experienced nurse, physician, or nurse-midwife.

1. Read instruction manual for equipment.

2. Perform a function test following manufacturer's instructions. Press TEST button and observe for result. Determine if result is correct for monitor model.

3. Explain the basic procedure of electronic fetal monitoring to the woman and her partner or family. Vary instructions according to equipment being used and hospital protocols.

4. Apply belts or stockinette if an adhesive ring is not used

    a. Slide both belts under the woman's back without the sensors attached. Be sure to keep belts smooth under her back.

    b. Cut a length of stockinette tubing about 15–18 inches long for the average sized woman. Cut a longer length of wide stockinette for a heavier woman. Slide the stockinette up from her feet to her abdomen.

5. Use Leopold's maneuvers to locate the fetus' back. During early labor this will usually be in the left or right lower quadrant of the woman's abdomen. During later labor, the fetal back will usually be nearer the woman's abdominal midline.

6. Apply ultrasound gel to the Doppler ultrasound transducer and place it on the woman's abdomen at the approximate location of the fetus' back. Move the transducer until a clear signal is heard. Most bedside units have a green light or flashing heart shape to indicate a good signal.

7. Place the uterine activity sensor in the fundal area, or the area where contractions feel the strongest when palpated. This will often be slightly above the umbilicus. When the woman has a contraction, observe the tracing for the bell shape. The line for uterine activity will be jagged because it also senses the rise and fall of the abdomen with breathing. Fetal or maternal movement will cause a spike in the line. Observe through several contractions.

8. Observe the strip for baseline fetal heart rate, presence of variability, periodic changes, and uterine activity (contraction duration and frequency). Palpate contractions for intensity and relaxation between contractions. Notify the physician or nurse-midwife of non-reassuring patterns.

9. Record on the properly-labeled monitor strip and the woman's chart the monitor function test, date and time of application, and the mode (external or internal).

10. Continuing documentation on the strip should include

    a. Maternal vital signs

    b. Vaginal examinations

    c. Rupture of membranes, including whether spontaneous or artificial rupture

    d. Color, quantity, and character of amniotic fluid

    e. Maternal position changes or other maternal or fetal movement that significantly affects tracing

f. Any adjustments of equipment (such as relocating sensors)

g. Medication and anesthesia and their related interventions

h. Changes of equipment, such as from external to internal monitoring mode

i. Interventions for non-reassuring patterns

j. Interruptions in the strip, such as the woman ambulating

11. Documentation in the labor record should include

a. Same information as on monitor strip

b. Periodic summary of the baseline rate, variability, periodic changes, and uterine activity

E. INTERNAL FETAL HEART RATE AND CONTRACTION MONITORING

Purpose: To provide a more accurate record of the fetal heart rate and uterine contractions during labor than with external monitoring.

Note: Women often have a combination of external and internal electronic fetal monitoring, usually external contraction monitoring and internal fetal heart rate monitoring.

1. Perform steps 1 through 3 under the external monitoring procedure. Read also the directions for insertion on the packages of the intrauterine pressure catheter (IUPC) and the fetal scalp electrode.

2. The membranes must be ruptured to allow internal electronic monitoring. The cervix must be dilated enough to identify the fetal presenting part and to allow passage of the spiral electrode or IUPC.

3. Use sterile technique for insertion of internal monitor leads. Cleanse the woman's perineum according to the facility's protocol. Avoid iodine solutions if the woman is allergic to iodine, seafood, or x-ray contrast media.

4. Insert the IUPC, following specific directions on the package. Connect to the proper port on the fetal monitor. If a fluid-filled catheter is used, the transducer that joins it to the monitor should be at the height of the tip within the uterus. Both catheters must be "zeroed" to compensate for atmospheric pressure, and some solid catheters must be zeroed before insertion.

5. Apply the internal spiral electrode to the fetal presenting part. Avoid the face, fontanelles, or genitalia. After locating the place for application (usually on the parietal bone), slide the electrode within its guide (outer) and drive (inner) tubes between the examining fingers to the presenting part. While maintaining pressure of the guide tube against the presenting part, turn the drive tube clockwise until the electrode wire catches in the skin. Release the electrode wires from the clamp on the outer part of the tube and pull the drive tube, then the guide tube, out. Connect the wires to the leg plate on the woman's thigh and the leg plate to the monitor.

6. Documentation should be the same as for external monitoring.

F. ASSESSING BLOOD GLUCOSE IN THE NEWBORN

Directions are for heel puncture using the Accu-Chek® or One Touch® glucometer or Dextrostix or Chemstrip reagent strips. Follow manufacturer's directions.

1. Wash hands and gather needed supplies: gloves, alcohol wipe, 2x2 gauze, lancet, adhesive bandage, diaper or commercial warming pack to warm the heel, glucometer and/or glucose screening reagent strips. Chemstrip and Accu-Chek®: Add a cotton ball. One Touch®: Add a pipette.

2. Calibrate or program the glucometer according to the manufacturer's guidelines.

3. If the infant's mother has a blood-borne disease such as hepatitis B or HIV, bathe the infant before puncturing the skin to avoid contamination of the puncture site with maternal blood on the infant's skin.

4. Warm the foot for a few minutes if it is cold or if blood is needed for several tests. Fasten a warm, wet, disposable diaper over the heel, or use a heel warming pack according to directions.

5. Apply gloves. Locate the site correctly to prevent permanent injury to the bone or nerves. Avoid the bone and the center areas of the heel to prevent osteomyelitis or nerve damage. Place a thumb or finger over the walking surface to shield this area (Figure VI-2).

6. Clean the lateral area of the heel with alcohol. Wipe dry with sterile gauze or allow to air dry.

7. Puncture the side of the heel with the lancet. Place the lancet in a sharps container immediately.

Figure VI-2

Correct Site for Heelstick in Infants

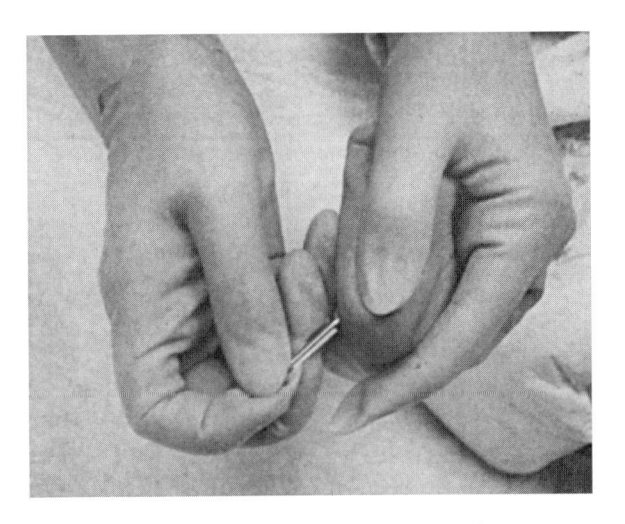

8. If an automatic puncture device is used, place it over the appropriate site and activate according to the manufacturer's directions.

9. Dextrostix and Chemstrip: Wipe away the first drop of blood with gauze because the first drop may be diluted with fluid from the area of the puncture.

10. Collect a large "stand-up" drop of blood at the puncture site. Avoid excessive squeezing of the foot that would dilute the sample with fluid from the tissues. Accu-Chek®, Dextrostix, and Chemstrip: Place a drop of blood on the treated area of the reagent strip. Cover the entire treated area of the strip and do not smear it. One Touch®: Draw blood into a pipette and place it on reagent strip that has been placed in the glucometer.

11. Remove blood at the correct time for the type of machine or reagent strip used. Use the method appropriate for the type of reagent strip used. Dextrostix: Run cold water slowly over the end of the strip to wash away the blood. Accu-Chek® and Chemstrip: Wipe blood completely away with a cotton ball. One Touch®: no removal is necessary.

12. Obtain the results. Glucometers: Read the glucometer when sound indicates the results are ready. Dextrostix and Chemstrip: Compare the reagent strips with the color chart on the bottle. Dextrostix: Read immediately. Chemstrip: Read after 60 seconds.

13. Apply an adhesive bandage.

14. Record the results. Have the laboratory draw blood for verification of abnormal results according to agency policy. Feed the infant if the screening test shows a reading below 45 mg/dL or according to agency policy.

G. ASSESSING DEEP TENDON REFLEXES

Purpose: To determine whether there are exaggerated reflexes (hyperreflexia) or diminished reflexes (hyporeflexia).

1. To assess the brachial reflex, support the woman's arm and instruct her to let it go totally limp while it is being held.

2. Place your thumb over the woman's tendon and strike the thumb with the small end of the reflex hammer. The normal response is slight flexion of the forearm.
3. The patellar reflex can be assessed in two positions, sitting or lying. When the woman is sitting, allow her lower legs to dangle freely to flex the knee and stretch the tendons. Strike the tendon with the reflex hammer just below the patella.
4. When the woman is in the supine position, the weight of her leg must be supported to flex the knee and stretch the tendons. Strike the partially stretched tendons just below the patella. Extension of the leg is the expected response.
5. Clonus should be tested, particularly when the reflexes are hyperactive. The woman's lower leg should be supported and the foot sharply dorsiflexed. Hold the stretch. With a normal response, no movement will be felt. When clonus is present, rapid rhythmic jerking motions of the foot are obvious.

H. ASSESSING THE PERINEUM

Purpose: To observe perineal trauma and state of healing.

1. Provide privacy, and explain the purpose of the procedure.
2. Put on clean gloves.
3. Ask the mother to assume a Sims position and flex her upper leg; lower the perineal pads and lift the superior buttocks; use a flashlight (if necessary) to inspect the perineal area.
4. Note the extent and location of edema or bruising.
5. Examine the episiotomy or laceration for redness, ecchymosis, edema, discharge, and approximation (REEDA).
6. Note number and size of hemorrhoids.

I. ASSESSING THE UTERINE FUNDUS

Purpose: To determine location and firmness of the uterus.

1. Explain the procedure and rationale for each step before beginning the procedure.

2. Have the mother empty her bladder if she has not voided recently.

3. Place the mother in a supine position with her knees slightly flexed.

4. Put on clean gloves; lower the perineal pads to observe lochia as the fundus is palpated.

5. Place the non-dominant hand above the symphysis pubis.

6. Use the flat part of the fingers (not the fingertips) for palpation.

7. Begin palpation at the umbilicus and palpate gently until the fundus is located. Note firmness and location of the fundus. The fundus should be firm, in midline, and approximately at the level of the umbilicus.

8. If the fundus is difficult to locate or is soft or "boggy," keep the non-dominant hand above the symphysis pubis and massage the fundus with the dominant hand until the fundus is firm.

9. Document the consistency and location of the fundus. Consistency is recorded as "fundus firm," "firm with massage," or "boggy." Fundal height is recorded in fingerbreadths above or below the umbilicus. Examples: "fundus firm, midline, U–2" (2 fingerbreaths below umbilicus); "fundus firm with light massage, U+2" (2 fingerbreadths above umbilicus), displaced to right.

J. ASSESSING VITAL SIGNS OF THE NEWBORN

Respirations

1. Assess the respirations when the infant is quiet or sleeping if possible to determine the rate at rest.

2. Assess by observing, palpating, and/or auscultating the chest and abdomen to increase accuracy.
3. Lift the infant's blanket and shirt to visualize the chest and abdomen for accuracy.
4. If desired, place a hand lightly over the infant's chest or abdomen to feel the movement.
5. Auscultate the respirations and lung sounds with a stethoscope.
6. Count for a full minute because respirations are normally irregular in the newborn.
7. If the infant is crying, allow the intant to suck on a pacifier or gloved finger.
8. Note signs of respiratory distress, including tachypnea, retractions, flaring, cyanosis, grunting, seesawing, apneic periods, or asymmetry of chest movements. Normal rate: 30–60 at rest.

Pulse

1. Listen to the apical pulse on a quiet or sleeping infant if possible.
2. Use a pediatric head on the stethoscope to listen to the apical pulse, if possible, to hear better.
3. Move the stethoscope over the entire heart area to listen to all sounds. Note arrhythmias, murmurs, or other abnormal sounds. Report abnormalities.

Temperature

Axillary

1. Place the thermometer vertically along the chest wall in the center of the axillary space with the infant's arm firmly over it.

2. Read thermometer at the proper time: glass, 5 minutes; plastic strip, 1–1.5 minutes (with a 10-second wait before reading); electronic, when the indicator sounds. Normal range: 36.5–37.5°C (97.7–99.5°F).

Rectal

1. Take a rectal temperature only when birth facility policy dictates. Use the axillary method whenever possible to avoid the risk of perforation of the rectum.

2. Lubricate the tip of the thermometer with water-soluble lubricant.

3. Place the infant in a supine position and hold the ankles firmly in one hand. Bend the infant's knees against the abdomen and raise the legs to expose the anus. Alternatively, place the infant prone or on the side and separate the buttocks.

4. Insert the thermometer gently no more than 0.5 inch into the rectum because the rectum turns to the right 1 inch from the sphincter. Inserting the thermometer farther may cause perforation. Do not force the thermometer!

5. Hold the thermometer securely throughout the time it remains in the rectum.

6. Read the thermometer at the proper time: glass, 5 minutes; electronic, when indicator sounds. Normal range: 36.5–37.6°C (97.7–99.7°F).

K. AUSCULTATING THE FETAL HEART RATE

Purpose: To evaluate the fetal condition and tolerance of labor.

1. Explain the procedure, and wash hands with warm water.

2. Use Leopold's maneuvers to identify the fetal back.

3. Assess the FHR with a fetoscope, Doppler transducer, or external fetal heart monitor.

4. *Fetoscope*: Place the bell of the fetoscope over the fetal back with the head plate pressed against your forehead. Move the fetoscope until you locate where the sound is loudest. Use your forehead to maintain pressure during auscultation.

5. *Doppler transducer*: Review manufacturer's instructions for operating the Doppler. Place water-soluble conducting gel over the transducer, and turn it on. Place the transducer over the fetal back, and move it until you clearly hear the double sounds of the fetal heart.

6. With one hand, palpate the mother's radial pulse. If her pulse is synchronized with the sounds from the fetoscope or Doppler transducer, try another location for the fetal heart.

7. Assess the FHR before, during, and after a contraction. Count the baseline FHR for 30–60 seconds between contractions. Note accelerations and slowing of the rate.

8. Note reassuring signs:

   a. Average rate of 110–120 BPM at the lower limit and 150–160 BPM at the upper limit for a term fetus. The FHR of a preterm fetus is usually higher.

   b. Accelerations of at least 15 BPM, usually with fetal movement.

   c. Presence of variability (electronic monitoring).

9. Note non-reassuring signs, and make more frequent assessments. Notify the physician or nurse-midwife.

   a. FHR outside normal limits

   b. Slowing of the FHR after the contraction ends.

L. IDENTIFYING INFANTS

1. Identify infants and mothers (or support people) with identification bands whenever reuniting them, even after a brief separation.

2. Explain the identification procedure and its purpose to the mother.

3. Expose the identification band on the infant's wrist or ankle. Do *not* rely on memory of the number.

4. Look at the number on the infant's band and ask the mother to read off the identification number on her band. Do *not* reverse the process by reading the infant's number to the mother because the mother might indicate that the numbers are correct when they are not.

5. Compare the infant's and the mother's bands visually if the mother does not speak English or might have difficulty with the process.

6. Follow the same identification procedure if the infant is to be released to a support person wearing an identification band.

M. PALPATING CONTRACTIONS

Purposes

- To determine whether a contraction pattern is typical of true labor.
- To identify abnormal contractions that may jeopardize the health of the mother or fetus.

1. Assess at least three contractions in a row. Guidelines are:

    a. Hourly during latent phase.

    b. Every 30 minutes during active phase and transition.

    c. Every 15 minutes during second stage.

    Assess more frequently if non-reassuring signs are identified.

2. Place fingertips of one hand on uterine fundus, using light pressure. Keep fingertips relatively still rather than moving them over uterus.

3. Note the time when each contraction begins and ends.

a. Determine frequency by noting average time that elapses from beginning of one contraction until beginning of the next one.

   b. Determine duration by noting average time in seconds from beginning to end of each contraction.

   c. Determine interval by noting average time between end of one contraction and beginning of the next one.

4. Estimate the average intensity of contractions by noting how easily the uterus can be indented during the peak of the contraction:

   a. Mild contractions are easily indented with the fingertips. They feel similar to the tip of the nose.

   b. Moderate contractions can be indented with more difficulty. They feel similar to the chin.

   c. Firm contractions feel "woody" and cannot be readily indented. They feel similar to the forehead.

5. Report hypertonic contractions:

   a. Durations longer than 90 seconds

   b. Intervals shorter than 60 seconds

   c. Incomplete relaxation of the uterus between contractions

N. PERFORMING BREAST SELF-EXAMINATIONS

1. Lie down. Flatten your right breast by placing a pillow under your right shoulder. If your breasts are large, use your right hand to hold your right breast while you do the exam with your left hand.

2. Use the sensitive pads of the middle three fingers on your left hand and a massaging motion to feel for lumps or changes in the breast tissue.

3. Press firmly enough to distinguish different breast textures.

4. Completely palpate or feel all parts of the breast and chest area. Be sure to examine the breast tissue that extends toward the shoulder. The amount of time required to completely palpate all the breast tissue depends on the size of the breast. Women with small breasts will need at least 2 minutes to examine each breast. Larger breasts will take longer.

5. Use the same routine or pattern to feel every part of the breast tissue. Any of three patterns will help you to make sure you have covered your entire breast—the circular pattern, the vertical strip, or the wedge. Choose the method you find easiest.

6. When you have completely examined your right breast, the left breast should be examined using the same method. Compare what you feel in one breast with the other.

7. You may also want to examine your breasts while bathing, when the skin is wet and lumps may be easily palpated.

8. You can check your breasts in a mirror by raising your arms and looking for an unusual shape, dimpling of the skin, and any changes in the nipple.

Adapted from American Cancer Society. 1992. Special touch.

O. LEOPOLD'S MANEUVERS

Purposes

- To determine presentation and position of the fetus.
- To aid in location of the fetal heart sounds.

1. Explain procedure and what is found to woman as each step is done.

2. Ask the woman to empty her bladder if she has not done so recently. Have her lie on her back with her knees flexed slightly. Place a small pillow or folded towel under one hip.

3. Wash your hands with warm water. Wear gloves if contact with secretions is likely.

4. Stand beside woman, facing her head, with your dominant hand nearest her.

First Maneuver

Determines the contents of the uterine fundus.

5. Palpate the uterine fundus. The breech (buttocks) is softer and more irregular in shape than the head. Moving the breech will also move the fetal trunk. The head is harder, with a round, uniform shape. The head can move without moving the entire fetal trunk.

Second Maneuver

Determines which side of the uterus the fetal back is on and which side the arms and legs are on.

6. Hold the left hand steady on one side of the uterus while palpating the opposite side of the uterus with the right hand. Then hold the right hand steady while palpating the opposite side of the uterus with the left hand. The fetal back is a smooth convex surface. The fetal arms and legs feel nodular and the fetus will often move them during palpation.

Third Maneuver

Determines if presenting part is engaged. Confirms presentation that was determined in first maneuver.

7. Palpate the suprapubic area. If a breech was palpated in the fundus, expect a hard, rounded head in this area. Attempt to grasp the presenting part gently between the thumb and fingers. If the presenting part is not engaged, the grasping movement of the fingers will move it upward in the uterus.

8. Omit the fourth maneuver if the fetus is in a breech presentation.

Fourth Maneuver

Determines if the fetal head is flexed (vertex) or extended (face).

9. Turn so that you face the woman's feet.

10. Place your hands on each side of the uterus with fingers pointed toward the pelvic inlet. Slide hands downward on each side of the uterus. On one side, your fingers will easily slide to the upper edge of the symphysis. On the other side, your fingers will meet an obstruction, the cephalic prominence.

P. PERFORMING RESUSCITATION IN NEWBORNS

1. If resuscitation is needed at birth, quickly dry the infant thoroughly under a preheated radiant warmer.

2. Position the infant's neck in a slightly extended, "sniffing" position to open the airway. Avoid hyperextension or flexion of the neck. Place a small blanket under the shoulders.

3. Suction the mouth and then the nose.

4. Stimulate the infant by rubbing the back or slapping the soles of the feet.

5. If there is no response after stimulating once or twice, stop and initiate immediate resuscitation. Do not delay resuscitation until the Apgar scores are given. Drying, clearing the airway, and stimulation should take no more than 20 seconds.

6. Begin positive-pressure ventilation with a bag and mask attached to 100% oxygen if there are no spontaneous respirations or if the heart rate is less than 100 BPM when respirations begin.

7. Place the mask snugly over the infant's nose and mouth. Squeeze the bag gently to force air into the infant's lungs with a pressure that will deliver 20–30 mL of air. Use a bag with a gauge measuring the pressure being used and a "pop-off" valve that releases if the pressure is too high.

SECTION SIX: Procedures and Drug Guides **437**

8. Observe the rise and fall of the chest during ventilation. If the chest does not move, suction secretions and reposition the head and the mask. Ventilate the infant at a rate of 40–60 breaths/minute until spontaneous breathing occurs and the heart rate is above 100 BPM.

9. Pause after 15–30 seconds of ventilation to take a 6-second heart rate. Use a stethoscope or feel the pulsations at the base of the cord. Multiply the rate by 10 to get the heart rate per minute. If the rate is less than 60 BPM or less than 80 BPM and not increasing, a second person should begin chest compressions while the first continues to ventilate the infant.

10. Compress the chest by placing the hands around the infant's chest with the fingers under the back for support and the thumbs over the sternum just below the nipple line. (Figure VI-3).

Figure VI-3

Performing Resuscitation in Newborns

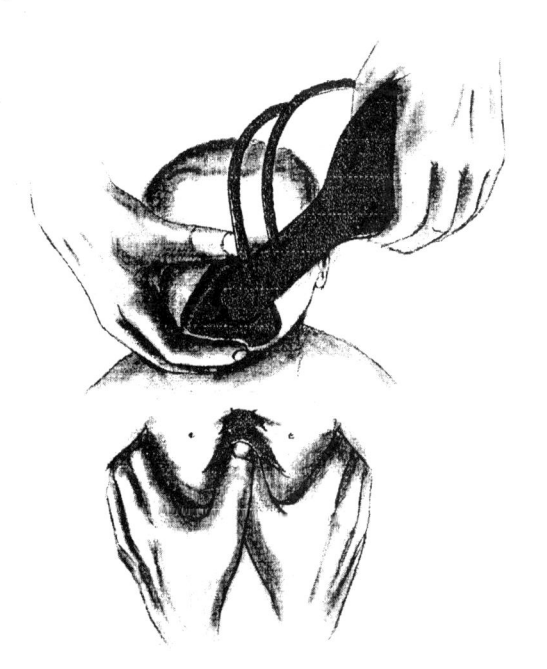

438 Clinical Manual for Foundations of Maternal Newborn Nursing

11. Compress the sternum 1/2–3/4 inch, with three compressions followed by one ventilation, for a combined rate of compressions and ventilations of 120 each minute. This is 90 compressions and 30 ventilations each minute.

12. Stop compressions after 30 seconds to check the heart rate for 6 seconds. If it is above 80 BPM, discontinue compressions but continue ventilation until spontaneous breathing begins. If the heart rate is below 80 BPM, continue compressions with rechecks of the heart rate periodically.

13. Prepare medications and fluids if the HR is below 80 after 30 seconds of compression. They may include epinephrine given through an umbilical vein catheter or through an endotracheal tube; volume expanders; naloxone; and 10% dextrose solution. Sodium bicarbonate is given only after prolonged arrest and only with effective ventilation.

Q. PERFORMING VAGINAL EXAMINATION DURING LABOR

Purposes

- To determine cervical effacement, dilation, and fetal station.
- To determine fetal presenting part, position, and station.
- To determine status of amniotic membranes.

Note: Vaginal examination should not be done if the woman is having active bleeding. Bloody show is not a contraindication.

1. Collect equipment to do examination:

    a. Sterile disposable exam gloves

    b. Sterile water-soluble lubricant

    c. Nitrazine paper if needed to check for ruptured membranes

2. Have the woman lie on her back with her head slightly elevated. Place a small pillow or wedge under one hip. Drape her to minimize exposure. Just before the examination, have her flex her thighs and abduct them, placing her heels together.

3. Open the gloves and lubricant. Eject a small amount of lubricant on an unused part of the glove wrapper.

4. If Nitrazine paper is being used to clarify if membranes have ruptured, it should be inserted into the vaginal introitus before use of lubricant.

5. Separate the inner labia with the gloved non-dominant hand to reveal the vaginal opening. Insert the lubricated and sterile-gloved index and middle fingers of the dominant hand into the vagina.

6. Gently move the fingers upward to locate the cervix. Have the woman take slow deep breaths if she tenses during the examination.

7. Determine if the amniotic sac is intact. It feels like a slippery membrane over the presenting part or a slick, fluid-filled balloon. The "balloon" has varying amounts of pressure behind it. If membranes have ruptured, manipulating the cervix often causes amniotic fluid to leak from the vagina. Note the color, odor, and amount of any fluid that leaks from the vagina during the exam.

8. Palpate the fetal presenting part to distinguish a vertex presentation from others. This is easier to do if the membranes are ruptured.

    a. Vertex presentation: The nurse feels the hard, round surface of the fetal head. The triangular posterior fontanelle is palpable if the head is well flexed. Caput (edema) may make it impossible to feel suture lines or fontanelles.

    b. Face presentation: The nurse feels an irregular surface and may elicit the fetal suck reflex as the finger is passed over the mouth.

    c. Frank breech: The nurse feels a somewhat more irregular surface than the head, although the hip area may feel quite similar to the head. Fresh meconium stool (black and thick) is often passed during a frank breech labor.

d. Footling breech: The nurse feels the small irregular surface of the fetal foot. Touching the foot often causes the fetus to curl it or draw it upward. The fetal hand will feel similar, but touching the hand may elicit the grasp reflex.

9. Palpate the cervix to identify:

   a. Dilation in centimeters. The dilation may range from closed to 10 cm (about 4 inches). A woman's index fingertip is about 1 cm.

   b. Effacement as a percentage of original length, or as actual length in centimeters. The non-effaced cervix is usually at least 2 cm long. When fully thinned (100%), it may feel like a delicate membrane that is almost indistinguishable from the fetal presenting part or amniotic sac when palpated.

   c. Fetal station in relation to the ischial spines. The ischial spines are prominences located on each side of the mid-pelvis. Station is recorded in minus numbers to signify centimeters above the ischial spines, a zero to signify that the widest part of the presenting part is at the level of the spines, and plus numbers to signify centimeters below the ischial spines.

10. Palpate the fetal head to identify fontanelles and suture lines so that position (LOA, ROP, etc.) can be determined.

11. Remove the fingers, wipe excess lubricants or secretions from the woman's genitalia, and share the results of the examination with her.

12. Record the examination on the fetal monitor strip (if being used) and on the chart.

R. TEACHING WOMEN FERTILITY AWARENESS

Purpose: To identify whether ovulation occurs and the probable time of ovulation.

Basal Body Temperature (BBT)

Detects the slight elevation in temperature that may accompany increased progesterone secretion in response to the luteinizing hormone (LH) surge and ovulation.

1. Teach the woman the relationship between her BBT and ovulation:
   a. Explain that the BBT is the lowest, or resting, temperature of the body.
   b. During the first half of the woman's menstrual cycle, her temperature is lower than during the second half of the cycle.
   c. The basal temperature often drops slightly just before ovulation. Not all women experience this fall in basal temperature.
   d. Progesterone is secreted during the second half of the cycle, rising just after ovulation. The BBT rises after the slight drop near ovulation and remains higher during the second half of the cycle.
   e. The BBT remains high if conception occurs or falls about 2–4 days before menstruation if conception does not occur.

2. Explain the occurrences that can interfere with the accuracy of her BBT: illness, restless or inadequate sleep (fewer than six hours), waking later than usual, jet lag, alcohol intake the evening before, sleeping under an electric blanket or on a heated water bed, or any activity before taking the temperature.

3. Show the woman a glass fever thermometer and a glass basal thermometer. Explain that the range of temperatures on the basal thermometer is smaller (96–100°F) and is marked in tenths of a degree. Explain how to read the marks on the thermometer. Electronic basal thermometers digitally display tenths of a degree and require less time for accurate assessment than glass ones. The woman should read the instructions that come with her specific thermometer.

4. Basal temperatures with glass thermometers can be taken orally, rectally, or vaginally. The woman should use the same site for all readings.

5. Show the woman the chart for recording her BBT and the symbols for marking relevant events, such as menstrual periods, intercourse, illness or other occurrences, which may alter her BBT.

6. Teach the woman how to take her basal temperature:

    a. If a glass thermometer is used, shake it down the night before.

    b. As soon as she awakens, but before any activity, the basal thermometer should be placed under her tongue and remain until the electronic thermometer beeps. A glass thermometer requires up to 10 minutes for an accurate reading if the oral site is used. The thermometer should remain still while it is registering the temperature.

    c. Record the reading on the chart provided.

7. Encourage the woman to demonstrate taking her temperature and recording the result. Ask her to list events other than ovulation that can alter the BBT.

8. As a method to avoid pregnancy: Explain that for greatest effectiveness, a woman should avoid intercourse from the onset of the menstrual period through the second day of elevated temperature.

9. To enhance the chances of conception, the couple should have intercourse when the temperature falls: Emphasize that the BBT primarily identifies that ovulation has already occurred and the adequacy of progesterone secretion to prepare her endometrium during the second half of her menstrual cycle. The BBT is less effective for timing intercourse to coincide with ovulation because of the short life span of the ovum after ovulation.

Cervical Mucus Assessment

The cervical mucus normally changes just before ovulation to facilitate survival of the sperm and promote their passage into the woman's uterus.

1. Teach the woman how her cervical mucus changes throughout the menstrual cycle. Spinnbarkheit describes how much the mucus can be stretched between her fingers or between a microscope slide and coverslip. Before and after ovulation, the cervical mucus is scant, thick, sticky, and opaque. It stretches less than 6 cm. Just before and for 2–3 days after ovulation, the cervical mucus is thin, slippery, and clear and is similar to raw egg white. It stretches 6 cm or more. When this ovulatory mucus is present, the woman has probably ovulated and could become pregnant.

2. Explain the factors that can interfere with the accuracy of her assessment. The mucus may be thicker if she takes antihistamines. Vaginal infections, contraceptive foams or jellies, sexual arousal, and semen can make the mucus thinner even if ovulation has not occurred. Tell her to record these factors.

3. Demonstrate how to stretch mucus between the thumb and forefinger by using raw egg white. Have the woman return demonstrate the process.

4. Teach the woman to wash her hands before and after assessing her mucus.

5. Teach the woman to obtain a small mucus sample several times a day from just inside her vagina and to note the following:

    a. The general sensation of wetness (around ovulation) or dryness (not near ovulation) on her labia.

    b. The appearance and consistency of the mucus: thick, sticky, and whitish or thin, slippery, and clear or watery.

    c. The distance the mucus will stretch between her fingers, usually at least 6 cm (2.3 inches) at the time of ovulation.

6. Have the woman record the day's typical mucus characteristics (often combined with her BBT recording).

7. As a method of contraception, the woman should avoid intercourse from the time the thin, stretchy ovulatory mucus appears until 48 to 72 hours after the mucus returns to its pre-ovulatory characteristics.

8. As a method to enhance conception, the couple should have intercourse every 2 days during the period of ovulatory mucus (approximately days 12 to 16 if the woman has a 28-day cycle).

S. TESTING FOR RUPTURED MEMBRANES

Purpose: To help clarify if membranes are ruptured, or if the woman is having episodes of urinary incontinence.

1. Equipment:
   a. Disposable gloves (sterile if a vaginal exam will immediately follow)
   b. Nitrazine tape (about 5 cm [2 inches] long)
   c. Slide and microscope if ferning will be tested.

2. Test for rupture of membranes *before* using lubricant for a vaginal examination.

3. Nitrazine tape: Touch the tape against the vaginal opening or well-soaked clothing. Compare the color with the scale on the Nitrazine tape container. A color change to blue-green or dark blue (pH >6.5) suggests that the membranes are ruptured.

4. Fern test: Spread a sample of vaginal secretions on a glass slide and allow it to dry. Examine the slide under a low-power microscope to identify the typical fern pattern of dry amniotic fluid.

T. USING A BULB SYRINGE

1. Position the infant's head to the side or pick up the infant and hold with the head lower than the rest of the body to promote drainage.

2. Compress the bulb before inserting it into the side of the infant's mouth. Do not insert it straight to the back of the throat as a vagal response could be stimulated, resulting in bradycardia or apnea.

3. Release the bulb slowly to draw secretions from the infant's mouth into the bulb. Remove and empty it by compressing it several times to prepare it for use again.

4. Gently suction the nose if necessary *after* the mouth is cleared to prevent aspiration if the infant gasps.

U. WEIGHING AND MEASURING THE NEWBORN

Weight

1. Cover the scale with a blanket and paper cover to prevent conductive heat loss and cross-contamination and to make cleaning easier.

2. Balance or adjust the scale to zero after the covering is placed. Electronic scale: push the "on" button and check to see that the digital readout is at zero. Balance scale: adjust until the balance arm is horizontal.

3. Place the infant in supine position on the scale. Keep one hand just above the infant to prevent the infant from sliding off the scale.

4. Read the weight. Electronic scales may display "stable" when ready to be read. Balance scale: Move weights slowly until the arm is level.

5. Record the weight immediately. Compare with the normal range for term infants: 2500–4000 g (5 pounds, 8 ounces–8 pounds, 13 ounces).

Length

Ruler Printed on Scale or Crib

1. Place the infant in a supine position with the head at the upper edge of the ruler on the scale.
2. Hold the infant so that the head does not move. Extend the leg along the ruler. Note the length at the bottom of the heel.

Tape Measure

1. Check that a paper tape has no partial tears so that the measurement will be accurate.
2. Place the tape beside the infant with upper end at the top of the head. Tuck it beneath the shoulder and extend it down to the feet. Keep the tape straight while extending one leg.
3. Note the measurement. Compare it with the normal range of 48–53 cm (19–21 inches).

Head and Chest Circumference

1. Measure around the fullest part of the head with the tape placed around the occiput and just over the eyebrows.
2. Measure the chest at the level of the nipples. Keep the tape even and taut.
3. Remove the tape by lifting or rolling the infant instead of pulling to avoid cutting the infant's skin.
4. Compare the measurements with the normal range. Head: 33–35.5 cm (13–14 inches). Chest: 30.5–33 cm (12–13 inches).

II. DRUG GUIDES

A. BUTORPHANOL (STADOL)

Classification

Opioid analgesic.

Action

Opioid analgesic with some agonist-antagonist effects. Exact mechanism of action is unknown. Produces respiratory depression that does not increase markedly with larger doses.

Indications

Systemic pain relief during labor.

Dosage and Route

Intravenous: 1 mg every 3 to 4 hours; range 0.5 to 2 mg. May be given undiluted.

Absorption

Onset of analgesia almost immediate with intravenous administration, peaks about 30 minutes, and lasts about 3 hours. Faster onset and shorter duration of action than meperidine or morphine.

Excretion

Excreted in urine. Crosses placental barrier. Secreted in breast milk.

Contraindications and Precautions

Contraindicated in persons who are hypersensitive. Do not use in opiate-dependent persons because antagonist activity of the drug may cause withdrawal symptoms in the woman or newborn. Use cautiously during birth of preterm infant. Drug actions are potentiated (enhanced) by barbiturates, phenothiazines, cimetidine, and other tranquilizers.

Adverse Reactions

Respiratory depression or apnea (woman or newborn), anaphylaxis. Dizziness, lightheadedness, sedation, lethargy, headache, euphoria, mental clouding, fainting, restlessness, excitement, tremors, delirium, insomnia. Nausea, vomiting, constipation, increased biliary pressure, dry mouth, anorexia. Flushing, altered heart rate and blood pressure, circulatory collapse. Urinary retention. Sensitivity to cold.

Nursing Considerations

Assess for allergies and opiate dependence. Observe vital signs and respiratory function in woman (12 per minute or more) and newborn (30 per minute or more). Have naloxone and resuscitation equipment available for respiratory depression in woman and neonate. Report nausea or vomiting to the birth attendant for a possible order for an antiemetic. Antiemetics or other central nervous system depressants may enhance the respiratory depressant effects of butorphanol.

B. CONJUGATED ESTROGENS

Classification

Hormone—estrogen

Action

Increases synthesis of DNA, RNA, and various proteins in responsive tissues. Reduces release of gonadotropin-releasing hormone, thus reducing follicle-stimulating hormone and luteinizing hormone. Promotes normal growth and maintenance of female genital organs, maintaining genitourinary function and vasomotor stability. Restores hormone balance in deficiency states, reduces blood cholesterol, and restores balance of bone resorption. Decreases serum concentration of testosterone.

Indications

Treatment of vasomotor symptoms of menopause, such as hot flashes; prevention of postmenopausal osteoporosis; management of atrophic vaginitis.

Dosage and Route

Dosage for relief of menopausal symptoms and prevention of osteoporosis, 0.6 to 1.25 mg orally. Schedule of administration depends on whether the woman has had a hysterectomy. If she has no uterus, estrogen alone may be administered daily or in a repeating cycle. If the uterus is present, both estrogen and progesterone are administered. Estrogen may be given for 21 days, with progesterone added for the final 10 days. Both medications are then stopped for 7 days. When the medication is stopped, predictable bleeding occurs. An alternative schedule involves the administration of estrogen, 0.625 mg, and progesterone, 2.5 to 5 mg daily. This schedule eliminates episodes of planned bleeding. Vaginal cream applied daily for 21 days, off for 7 days, and then repeated, may be useful for atrophic vaginitis.

Absorption

Well absorbed following oral administration; readily absorbed through skin and mucous membranes.

Excretion

Metabolized largely by the liver; as hepatic recirculation occurs, more absorption occurs from the gastrointestinal tract.

Contraindications and Precautions

Contraindicated in thromboembolic diseases, undiagnosed vaginal bleeding, pregnancy, and lactation. Used cautiously in underlying cardiovascular disease and severe hepatic or renal disease; unopposed use may increase the risk of endometrial carcinoma.

Adverse Reactions

Headache, dizziness, intolerance to contact lenses, nausea, jaundice

Nursing Considerations

Assess blood pressure, pulse, and weight gain periodically throughout therapy; assess frequency and severity of hot flashes. Instruct the woman to report skin changes and to protect skin from excessive exposure to sunlight to prevent hyperpigmentation. Assess for vaginal bleeding, amenorrhea, or changes in menstrual flow, and instruct the woman to report these signs to her health care provider. Caution the woman to avoid use of any medication that has not first been approved by her health care provider.

C. ERYTHROMYCIN OPHTHALMIC OINTMENT

Classification

Antibiotic.

Action

Inhibits cell wall replication in bacteria.

Indications

Prophylaxis against the organisms N*eisseria gonorrhoeae* and C*hlamydia trachomatis*. Prevents ophthalmia neonatorum in infants of mothers infected with gonorrhea, and conjunctivitis in infants of mothers infected with C*hlamydia*. Prophylaxis against gonorrhea is required by law for all infants whether or not the mother is known to be infected.

Neonatal Dosage and Route

A "ribbon" of 0.5% erythromycin ointment, 0.5–1 cm (0.25–0.5 inch) long, is applied to the lower conjunctival sac of each eye within an hour after birth. May also be used in drop form.

Adverse Effects

Irritation may result in chemical conjunctivitis lasting 24–48 hours. Ointment may cause temporarily blurred vision.

Nursing Considerations

Cleanse the infant's eyes before application, as needed. Hold the tube in a horizontal rather than a vertical position to prevent injury to the eye from sudden movement. Administer from the inner canthus to the outer canthus. Do not touch the tip of the tube to any part of the eye, as this may spread infectious material from one eye to the other. Do not rinse. Ointment may be wiped from outer eye after one minute. Observe for irritation. Use a new tube for each infant to prevent spread of infection. Other medications used for prevention of gonorrhea include tetracycline and silver nitrate solution.

D. HYDRALAZINE

Classification

Antihypertensive.

Action

Relaxes arterial smooth muscle to reduce blood pressure.

Indications

Used in pre-eclampsia when blood pressure is elevated to a degree that might be associated with intracranial bleeding.

Dosage and Route

For obstetric use, 10–15 mg is administered intramuscularly. Following a test dose to determine hypotensive effects, 5–10 mg may be administered by Intravenous bolus infusion as often as every 20 minutes if necessary (ACOG, 1996).

Absorption

Well absorbed from intramuscular sites. Widely distributed, crosses the placenta; enters breast milk in minimal concentrations.

Excretion

Metabolized and excreted by the liver.

Contraindications and Precautions

Contraindicated in coronary artery disease, cerebrovascular disease, and hypersensitivity to hydralazine. Used cautiously in obstetrics because safety during pregnancy and lactation has not been established.

Adverse Reactions

Headache, dizziness, drowsiness, hypotension that can interfere with uterine blood flow, epigastric pain, which may be confused with worsening pre-eclampsia.

Nursing Implications

Obstetric clients are hospitalized before initiation of hypertensive medications. Blood pressure and pulse must be monitored every 2–3 minutes for 30 minutes after initial dosage and periodically throughout the course of therapy. Therapy is repeated only when diastolic pressure exceeds limits set by physician or facility protocol (usually > 110 mm Hg).

E. HEPATITIS B VACCINE

Classification

Vaccine.

Other Names

Engerix-B, Recombivax HB.

Action

Immunization against hepatitis B infection.

Indications

Prevention of hepatitis B in exposed and unexposed infants.

Neonatal Dosage and Route

Recombivax HB: 5 mcg (0.5 mL) to infants of infected mothers, 2.5 mcg (0.25 mL) if the mother is not infected.

Engerix-B: 10 mcg (0.5 mL) (whether or not the mother is infected).

For infants of uninfected mothers, the vaccine is given at birth, 1–2 months and 6–18 months. An alternate schedule is birth to 2 months, 1–4 months, and 6–18 months.

For infants of infected mothers, the vaccine is given at birth, 1 month, and 6 months. If immune globulin is also given at birth because the mother is infected, it should be at a different site than the vaccine.

Given intramuscularly in the anterolateral thigh.

Absorption

Well absorbed from muscle.

Contraindications

Hypersensitivity to yeast.

Adverse Reactions

Pain or redness at site; fever.

Nursing Considerations

Shake solution before preparing. Give vaccine within 12 hours of birth to infants of infected mothers. Bathe infants before the injection to remove blood and prevent contamination of the injection site with maternal blood on the infant's skin. Obtain parental consent before administering.

F. MAGNESIUM SULFATE

Classification

Miscellaneous anticonvulsant.

Action

Decreases acetylcholine released by motor nerve impulses, thereby blocking neuromuscular transmission. Depresses the central nervous system to act as an anticonvulsant; also decreases frequency and intensity of uterine contractions. Produces flushing and sweating due to decreased peripheral blood pressure.

Indications

Prevention and control of seizures in severe pre-eclampsia. Prevention of uterine contractions in pre-term labor.

Dosage and Route

Magnesium sulfate is generally administered parenterally. An intravenous bolus (4 g over 20 minutes) is given and followed by continuous infusion (2–3 g/hour) via a controlled infusion device (ACOG, 1996). Therapeutic range for magnesium is generally considered to be 4–8 mg/dL (ACOG, 1996).

Absorption

Immediate onset following intravenous administration. Duration of action is 3–4 hours.

Excretion

Excreted by the kidneys.

Contraindications and Precautions

Contraindicated in persons with myocardial damage, heart block, myasthenia gravis, or impaired renal function.

Adverse Reactions

Result from magnesium overdose and include flushing, sweating, hypotension, depressed deep tendon reflexes, and central nervous system depression, including respiratory depression.

Nursing Implications

Monitor blood pressure closely during administration. Assess client for respiratory rate above 12 per minute, presence of deep tendon reflexes, and urinary output greater than 30 mL per hour before administering magnesium. Place resuscitation equipment (suction, oxygen) in the room. Keep calcium gluconate, which acts as an antidote to magnesium, in the room along with syringes and needles.

G. MEDROXYPROGESTERONE

Classification

Hormone—progestin

Action

A synthetic form of progesterone that transforms the endometrium from a proliferative to a secretory phase and promotes withdrawal bleeding when estrogen is also present. Promotes relaxation of uterine smooth muscle and growth of mammary alveolar tissue.

Indications

Used to reduce the risk of endometrial carcinoma when estrogen is administered to control postmenopausal symptoms or to prevent osteoporosis.

Dosage and Route

For induction of secretory endometrium following estrogen priming, 5 to 10 mg orally for 10 days. Or 2.5 to 5 mg daily with exogenous estrogen to prevent endometrial hyperplasia. Also used for secondary amenorrhea and abnormal uterine bleeding.

Absorption

Unknown; metabolized by the liver

Excretion

Unknown

Contraindications and Precautions

Contraindicated in pregnancy, thromboembolic disease, carcinoma of the breast, and liver disease. Used with caution with cardiovascular disease, seizure disorders, and mental depression.

Adverse Reactions

Depression, thrombophlebitis, edema, weight gain, dizziness, fatigue, headache, insomnia. Fluid retention may complicate other conditions such as asthma, heart disease, and renal disorders.

Nursing Considerations

Assess blood pressure throughout therapy. Monitor weight gain, and emphasize that steady weight gain should be reported to health care provider. Advise women to anticipate withdrawal bleeding 3 to 7 days after discontinuing medication. Emphasize the importance of reporting the following signs and symptoms: visual changes, sudden weakness, headache, leg or calf pain, shortness of breath, jaundice, depression, and skin rash.

H. METHYLERGONOVINE (METHERGINE)

Classification

Oxytocic.

Action

Directly stimulates contraction of the uterus.

Indications

Used for the prevention and treatment of postpartum or postabortion hemorrhage caused by uterine atony or subinvolution.

Dosage and Route

Usual dosage is 0.2 mg intramuscularly (IM) every 2 to 4 hours for up to five doses. Change to oral route 0.2 mg every 6 to 12 hours for 2 to 7 days.

Absorption

Well absorbed after oral or IM route.

Excretion

Metabolic fate unknown, probably metabolized by the liver.

Contraindications and Precautions

Do not use to induce labor; do not use IM if the mother is hypersensitive to phenol. Contraindicated for hypertensive women, those with severe hepatic or renal disease, and during third stage of labor.

Adverse Reactions

Dizziness, headache, dyspnea, palpitations, hypertension, nausea, and uterine and gastrointestinal cramping.

Nursing Considerations

Before administering medication, check expiration date and monitor blood pressure. Follow facility protocol if medication must be withheld (usually a reading of 136/90). Caution the mother to avoid smoking because nicotine constricts blood vessels. Remind her to report any adverse reactions.

I. NALOXONE HYDROCHLORIDE (NARCAN)

Classification

Narcotic antagonist.

Action

Reverses central nervous system and respiratory depression caused by narcotics (opiates). Competes with narcotics at receptor sites.

Indications

Severe respiratory depression when the mother has received narcotics within 4 hours of delivery.

Dosage and Route

Available in 0.4 mg/mL and 1 mg/mL. Dosage is 0.1 mg/kg. Given IV, IM, SC, or into an endotracheal tube (ET), IV and ET are preferred during resuscitation.

Absorption

Well absorbed by all routes. Onset of action is 1–2 minutes if given IV.

Excretion

Metabolized by the liver and excreted by the kidneys.

Contraindications and Precautions

Duration of effect is 1–4 hours. The dose may need to be repeated because the narcotic may have a longer half-life than naloxone. If given to an infant of a mother addicted to drugs, it will cause withdrawal and may cause seizures. Resuscitative measures should be used as necessary.

Nursing Implications

Note the strength of the medication available when calculating the dose. Prepare the syringe before birth with 1 mL of the drug. After birth, remove excess from the syringe and give the amount according to the estimate of the infant's weight. Inject rapidly. Monitor for response, and be prepared to give repeated doses if necessary.

Common Doses of Naloxone Hydrochloride

Dosage must be calculated based on weight (0.1 mg/kg). The amount for various weights is given below for two different drug concentrations.

INFANT'S WEIGHT	TOTAL DOSE	DRUG CONCENTRATION 0.4 mg/mL	DRUG CONCENTRATION 1.0 mg/mL
1 kg (2 lb, 3 oz)	0.1 mg	0.25 mL	**0.1 mL**
2 kg (4 lb, 6 oz)	0.2 mg	0.50 mL	**0.2 mL**
3 kg (6 lb, 10 oz)	0.3 mg	0.75 mL	**0.3 mL**
4 kg (8 lb, 13 oz)	0.4 mg	1.00 mL	**0.4 mL**

J. OXYTOCIN (PITOCIN)

Classification

Oxytocic.

Action

Synthetic compound identical to the natural hormone from the posterior pituitary. Stimulates uterine smooth muscle, resulting in increased strength, duration, and frequency of uterine contractions. Uterine sensitivity to oxytocin increases gradually during gestation. Has vasoactive and antidiuretic properties.

Indications

Induction or augmentation of labor at or near term. Maintenance of firm uterine contraction after birth to control postpartum bleeding. Management of inevitable or incomplete abortion.

Dosage and Route

Induction or Augmentation of Labor

1. Intravenous infusion via a secondary (piggyback) line. Dilute 10 units (1 ml) of oxytocin in 1000 ml of a balanced electrolyte solution such as lactated Ringer's solution, resulting in a concentration of 10 milliunits (mU) of oxytocin per milliliter. Other mixtures of oxytocin and solution may be used, such as 15 units of oxytocin (1.5 ml) plus 250 ml intravenous solution, resulting in a concentration of 60 mU/ml. Oxytocin infusion is controlled with a pump. The drug may also be given in 10-minute pulsed infusions rather than continuously.

2. Administration protocols vary, but guidelines from the American College of Obstetricians and Gynecologists (1995) suggest (a) starting dosages of 0.5 to 2 mU/minute, and (b) increasing dosage by 1 to 2 mU/minute increments every 30 to 60 minutes. The actual oxytocin dose is based on uterine response and absence of adverse effects. Shorter intervals between dose increases may result in uterine hyperstimulation. A lower starting dose is usually required to augment labor.

3. After an adequate contraction pattern is established and the cervix is dilated 5 to 6 cm, the oxytocin may be reduced by similar increments.

Control of Postpartum Bleeding

Intravenous infusion—Dilute 10 to 40 units in 1000 ml of intravenous solution. Rate of infusion must control uterine atony. Begin at a rate of 20 to 40 mU/minute, increasing or decreasing rate according to uterine response and rate of postpartum bleeding.

Intramuscular injection—10 units after delivery of placenta.

Inevitable or Incomplete Abortion

Dilute 10 units in 500 ml of intravenous solution, and infuse at 10 to 20 mU/minute.

Absorption

Intravenous, immediate; intramuscular, 3 to 5 minutes.

Excretion

Liver and urine.

Contraindications and Precautions

Include, but are not limited to, placenta previa, vase previa, nonreassuring fetal heart rate patterns, abnormal fetal presentation, prolapsed umbilical cord, presenting part above the pelvic inlet, previous classic uterine incision, active genital herpes infection, pelvic structural deformities, invasive cervical carcinoma.

Adverse Reactions

Most result from hypersensitivity to drug or excessive dosage. Adverse reactions include hypertonic uterine activity, impaired uterine blood flow, uterine rupture, and abruptio placentae. Uterine hypertonicity may result in fetal bradycardia, tachycardia, reduced fetal heart rate variability, and late decelerations. Fetal asphyxia may occur with diminished uterine blood flow. Fetal or maternal trauma, or both, may occur from rapid birth. Prolonged administration may cause maternal fluid retention, leading to water intoxication. Hypotension (seen with rapid intravenous injection), tachycardia, cardiac dysrhythmias, and subarachnoid hemorrhage are rare adverse reactions.

Nursing Considerations

Intrapartum

Assess fetal heart rate for at least 20 minutes before induction to identify reassuring or nonreassuring patterns. Perform Leopold's maneuvers, a vaginal examination, or both to identify fetal presentation. Do not begin induction and notify physician if nonreassuring fetal heart rate patterns are identified or if fetal presentation is other than cephalic.

Observe uterine activity for establishment of effective labor pattern: contraction frequency every 2 to 3 minutes, duration 40 to 90 seconds, intensity 50 to 80 mmHg (using intrauterine pressure catheter). Observe for hypertonic uterine activity: contractions less than 2 minutes apart, rest interval shorter than 60 seconds, duration longer than 90 seconds, or an elevated resting tone greater than 20 mmHg with an intrauterine pressure catheter. Observe fetal heart rate for nonreassuring patterns such as tachycardia, bradycardia, decreased variability, and late decelerations.

If uterine hypertonicity or a nonreassuring fetal heart rate pattern occurs, intervene to reduce uterine activity and increase fetal oxygenation: stop oxytocin infusion; increase rate of nonadditive solution; position woman in side-lying position; administer oxygen by snug face mask at 8 to 10 L/minute. Notify physician of adverse reactions, nursing interventions, and response to interventions. Record maternal blood pressure every 30 to 60 minutes or with each dosage increase. Record intake and output.

Postpartum

Observe uterus for firmness, height, and deviation. Massage until firm if uterus is soft ("boggy"). Observe lochia for color, quantity, and presence of clots. Notify birth attendant if uterus fails to remain contracted or if lochia is bright red or contains large clots. Assess for cramping. Assess vital signs every 15 minutes or according to protocol. Monitor intake and output to identify fluid retention or bladder distention.

Inevitable or Incomplete Abortion

Observe for cramping, vaginal bleeding, clots, and passage of products of conception. Observe maternal vital signs, intake, and output as noted under postpartum nursing implications.

K.   RH$_0$(D) IMMUNE GLOBULIN

Classification

Concentrated immunoglobulins directed toward the red blood cell antigen Rh$_o$(D).

Action

Prevents production of anti-Rh$_o$(D) antibodies in Rh-negative women who have been exposed to Rh-positive blood by suppressing the immune reaction of the Rh-negative woman to the antigen in Rh-positive blood. Prevents antibody response and subsequently prevents hemolytic disease of the newborn in future pregnancies of women who have conceived an Rh-positive fetus.

Indications

Administered to Rh-negative women who have been exposed to Rh-positive blood by

1. Delivering an Rh-positive infant.
2. Aborting an Rh-positive fetus.
3. Having chorionic villus sampling, amniocentesis, or intra-abdominal trauma while carrying an Rh-positive fetus.
4. Following accidental transfusion of Rh-positive blood to an Rh-negative woman.

Dosage and Route

One standard dose administered intramuscularly

1. At 28 weeks of pregnancy and within 72 hours of delivery.
2. Within 72 hours following termination of a pregnancy of 13 weeks or more of gestation.

One *microdose* within 72 hours following the termination of a pregnancy of less than 13 weeks gestation.

Dose is calculated based on the volume of blood erroneously administered in transfusion accidents.

Absorption

Well absorbed from intramuscular sites.

Excretion

Metabolism and excretion unknown.

Contraindications and Precautions

Women who are Rh-positive or women previously sensitized to Rh$_o$(D) should not receive Rh$_o$(D) immune globulin. Used cautiously for women with previous hypersensitivity reactions to immune globulins.

Adverse Reactions

Local pain at intramuscular site, fever, or both.

Nursing Implications

Type and crossmatch of mother's blood and cord blood of the newborn must be performed to determine the need for the medication. The mother must be Rh-negative and negative for Rh antibodies; the newborn must be Rh-positive. If there is doubt regarding the fetus' blood type following termination of pregnancy, the medication should be administered. The drug is administered to the mother, not the infant. The deltoid muscle is recommended for intramuscular administration.

L. TERBUTALINE

Classification

Beta-adrenergic agent

Action

Stimulates beta-adrenergic receptors of the sympathetic nervous system. Action primarily results in bronchodilation and inhibition of uterine muscle activity. Increases pulse rate and widens pulse pressure.

Indications

Stop preterm labor. Reduce or stop hypertonic labor contractions, whether natural or stimulated.

Dosage and Route

1. Intravenous (IV) infusion. Begin at 0.0025 mg/minute (2.5 µg/minute). Increase by 0.0025 mg/minute (2.5 µg/minute) at 20-minute intervals until contractions stop (maximum of 0.02 mg/minute [20 µg/minute]). Maintain this dose for at least 1 hour; then reduce the rate at 20-minute intervals to reach minimum maintenance dose. Continue maintenance dose for 12 hours after contractions stop before changing route of administration.

2. Subcutaneous (SC) (most common parenteral route). 0.25 mg (250 µg) every 1 to 3 hours

3. Oral. 2.5 to 5 mg every 2 to 4 hours

When changing from intravenous therapy to oral therapy, give oral dose 30 minutes before discontinuing intravenous infusion.

Absorption

1. Intravenous. Prompt; duration about 2 hours
2. Subcutaneous. 6 to 15 minutes; duration 1.5 to 4 hours
3. Oral. 1 to 2 hours; duration 4 to 8 hours

Excretion

Metabolized in the liver. Excreted in urine.

Contraindications

Hypersensitivity. Contraindicated before 20 weeks' gestation and if continuing the pregnancy is hazardous to the mother or fetus, as in fetal distress, hemorrhage, chorioamnionitis, and intrauterine fetal death. Contraindicated in conditions that may be adversely affected by β-adrenergic agents (uncontrolled diabetes, hyperthyroidism, bronchial asthma treated with other beta-mimetic agents or steroids, cardiac dysrhythmias, hypovolemia, and uncontrolled hypertension).

Precautions

Terbutaline is not approved by the U.S. Food and Drug Administration for inhibiting uterine activity, although it is widely used for this purpose based on extensive clinical experience. It is most effective if begun as soon as a diagnosis of preterm labor is made.

Adverse Reactions

1. Cardiovascular: Maternal and fetal tachycardia, palpitations, cardiac arrhythmias, chest pain, wide pulse pressure

2. Respiratory Dyspnea, chest discomfort

3. Central nervous system: Tremors, restlessness, weakness, dizziness, headache

4. Metabolic: Hypokalemia, hyperglycemia

5. Gastrointestinal: Nausea, vomiting, reduced bowel motility

6. Skin: Flushing, diaphoresis

Nursing Considerations

Diagnostic studies that may be ordered related to terbutaline therapy: electrocardiogram, blood glucose, electrolytes, urinalysis. Explain common side effects that are usually well tolerated, such as palpitations, tremors, restlessness, weakness, headache. Assess FHR, usually with continuous electronic fetal monitoring, recording rate and patterns every 15 minutes during IV dose increases. Assess maternal pulse, respirations, and blood pressure by same schedule as for FHR. Maintain adequate IV or oral hydration. Encourage the woman to empty her bladder every 2 hours. Notify the physician for significant or unacceptable side effects (maternal heart rate above 110/BPM, respirations above 24/minute, systolic blood pressure lower than 90 mmHg, FHR above 160/BPM, chest pain, dyspnea). Report continuing or recurrent uterine activity. Teach signs and symptoms of recurrent preterm labor and follow-up medical care after discharge.

M. VITAMIN K1 (PHYTONADIONE)

Classification

Fat-soluble vitamin.

Other Names

AquaMephyton, Konakion.

Action

Promotes the formation of factors II (prothrombin), VII, IX, and X by the liver for clotting. Provides vitamin K, which is not synthesized in the intestines for the first 5–8 days after birth because the newborn lacks intestinal flora necessary for vitamin K production.

Indication

Prevention or treatment of hemorrhagic disease of the newborn.

Neonatal Dosage and Route

0.5–1 mg (0.25–0.5 mL) given once intramuscularly within 1 hour of birth for prophylaxis. (The lower dose may be used for infants weighing less than 2500 g.) May be repeated or higher doses used if the mother took oral anticoagulants or anticonvulsants during pregnancy. May be repeated if the infant shows bleeding tendencies.

Absorption

Readily absorbed after intramuscular injection. Effective within 1–2 hours.

Adverse Reactions

Pain and edema at site of administration. Hemolysis or hyperbilirubinemia, especially in a preterm infant or when large doses are used.

Nursing Considerations

Protect the drug from light until just before administration because it decomposes and loses potency on exposure to light. Incompatible with other drugs. Observe all infants for signs of vitamin K deficiency: ecchymoses or bleeding from any site.

Appendixes

APPENDIX A

Laboratory Values in Pregnant and Nonpregnant Women

Value	Non-Pregnant	Pregnant
Blood volume, total (ml/kg)	60–80	Increases 45%
Plasma volume (ml/kg)	40–50 (average 4700 ml)	Increases 45% by 32 weeks (average 5200 ml)
Red blood cell mass (ml/kg)	20–30	Increases 20–30% (average increase of 250–450 ml)
Red blood cell count (million/mm^3)	3.8–5.1	Increases 20–30%, 4.5–6.5
Hemoglobin (g/dl)	12–16	11–12 (<11 g/dl during late pregnancy suggests anemia)
Hematocrit, packed cell volume (%)	36–48	33–46
White blood cell count	5000–10,000/mm^3	5000–12,000/mm^3 Rises during labor and post partum up to 25,000/mm^3
Platelets	150,000–400,000/mm^3	Slight decrease (values <100,000/mm^3 are considered abnormal); marked increase 3–5 days after birth

Value	Non-Pregnant	Pregnant
Prothrombin time (sec)	11–15	Slight decrease
Activated partial thromboplastin time (sec)	21–35	Slight decrease
Glucose, serum		
Fasting (mg/dl)	65–110	Decreases approximately 11 mg/dl
Postprandial (mg/dl)	1 hr: 120–170 2 hr: 70–120	Screening glucose challenge test: <140 mg/dl 1 hr: <190 mg/dl 2 hr: <165 mg/dl
Creatine, serum (mg/dl)	0.8 average	End of first trimester: 0.7 Late pregnancy: 0.5–0.6
Creatinine clearance, urine (ml/min)	85–120	150–200
Fibrinogen (mg/dl)	200–400	300–600

Data from Creasy, R.K., and Resnik, R. (1994). *Maternal-fetal medicine: Principles and practice* (3rd ed.). Philadelphia: W.B. Saunders; Cunningham, F.G., MacDonald, P.C., Gant, N.F., Leveno, K.J., Gilstrap, L.C., Hankins, G.D.V., et al. (1997). *Williams obstetrics* (20th ed.). Norwalk, Conn.: Appleton & Lange; Fischbach, F. (1996). *A manual of laboratory and diagnostic tests* (5th ed.). Philadelphia: J.B. Lippincott; and Teitz, N.W. (1995). *Clinical guide to laboratory tests* (3rd ed.). Philadelphia: W.B. Saunders.

APPENDIX B

Laboratory Values in the Newborn

TEST, SPECIMEN, AND UNIT OF MEASUREMENT	AGE	NORMAL RANGES (CONVENTIONAL UNITS)
Erythrocyte (red blood cell) count, whole blood (million/mm^3)	Cord 1–3 days 1 week 1 month	3.9–5.5 4.0–6.6 3.9–6.3 3.0–5.4
Hemoglobin, whole blood	1–3 days (capillary) 2 months	14.5–22.5 9.0–14.0
Hematocrit, whole blood	1 day (cap) 2 days 3 days 2 months	48–69% 48–75% 44–72% 28–42%
Leukocyte (white blood cell) count, whole blood (thousand/mm^3)	Birth 24 hours 1 month	9.0–30.0 9.4–34.0 5.0–19.5

White blood cell differential count, whole blood
  Myelocytes
  Neutrophils ("bands")
  Neutrophils ("segs")
  Lymphocytes
  Monocytes
  Eosinophils
  Basophils
		
		0%
		3–5%
		54–62%
		25–33%
		3–7%
		1–3%
		0–0.75%

Platelet count, whole blood (thousand/mm^3)	Newborn After 1 week	84–478 150–400
Glucose, serum (mg/dL)	Cord Newborn, 1 day Newborn, >1 day	45–96 40–60 50–90

Bilirubin, total serum (mg/dL)	Preterm	Full-term
Cord	<2.0	< 2.0
0–1 day	<8.0	< 6.0
1–2 days	< 12.0	< 8.0
2–5 days	< 16.0	< 12.0
> 5 days	< 2.0	< 0.2–1.0
Bilirubin, direct (conjugated) serum (mg/dL)	—	0–0.2

Adapted from Nicholson, J.F. & Pesce, M.A. (1996), *Laboratory medicine and reference tables*. In R.E. Behrman, R.M. Kliegman, & A.M. Arvin. Nelson Textbook of Pediatrics (15th ed.). Philadelphia: W.B. Saunders.

Appendix C

Effects of Drug Use During Pregnancy and Breastfeeding

FDA PREGNANCY RISK CATEGORIES

The U.S. Food and Drug Administration (FDA) has assigned pregnancy risk categories to many drugs on the basis of their known relative safety or danger to the fetus and on whether safer alternative drugs exist. For many drugs, little is known about the fetal risk. The categories are as follows:

A: No evidence of risk to the fetus.

B: Animal reproduction studies have not demonstrated a risk to the fetus. No adequate and well-controlled studies have been done in pregnant women.

C: Animal reproduction studies have shown an adverse effect on the fetus but no adequate, well-controlled studies have been done in humans. Potential benefits may warrant use of the drug in pregnant women despite fetal risks.

D: There is positive evidence of human fetal risk based on adverse reaction data, but potential benefits may warrant use of the drug in pregnant women despite fetal risks. Essentially, no safer alternatives to the drug are available.

X: There is positive evidence of human fetal risk based on animal or human studies and/or adverse reaction data. The risks of using the drug in pregnant women clearly outweigh potential benefits. Safer alternatives to these drugs may be available.

DRUG USE DURING LACTATION

The effects of many drugs, when used during lactation, have not been studied. In general, if a drug is safe for use in infants, it is probably safe for the lactating woman to take. Other drugs are known not to be excreted in breast milk or to be excreted in an inactive form or in very low concentrations. Modifying the time of maternal ingestion may reduce transfer of the drug to the infant. Other drugs are undesirable because they suppress lactation.

The American Academy of Pediatrics (AAP) has established classifications for safety of some drugs during lactation. The categories are as follows:

- AAP compatible: Usually compatible with breastfeeding
- AAP contraindicated: Contraindicated for use in breastfeeding mothers
- AAP reason for concern: Reports of infant side effects cause concern about use in breastfeeding mothers

DRUG	USE DURING PREGNANCY	USE DURING BREASTFEEDING
Analgesics		
Aspirin	Risk category D. May prolong pregnancy because of its antiprostaglandin effects. May cause bleeding disorders in mother or newborn if used during late pregnancy.	AAP reason for concern. Toxicity unlikely in normal doses, but higher doses could cause bleeding in infant.
Acetaminophen	Risk category B. Problems have not been documented, but drug does cross placenta. Use with caution.	AAP compatible. Very small amounts secreted into breast milk.
Narcotic analgesics (butorphanol, hydrocodone, meperidine, morphine, nalbuphine, propoxyphene)	Most are risk category C. Neonatal respiratory depression is the most significant adverse effect when narcotic analgesics are used during labor. Neonatal withdrawal may occur if the woman is addicted to the narcotic.	Most narcotics given briefly and in therapeutic doses are compatible with breastfeeding. Infant lethargy and poor feeding may be noted with large doses. Prolonged use may result in infant drug dependence and subsequent withdrawal when the mother no longer takes the drug.

Nonsteroidal anti-inflammatory drugs (NSAIDs) (fenoprofen, flurbiprofen, ibuprofen, indomethacin, ketoprofen, naproxen)	Risk category B. Not recommended after 34 weeks. May prolong pregnancy or labor because of antiprostaglandin effects. Associated with premature closure of ductus arteriosus in newborn.	Ibuprofen and indomethacin are AAP compatible. All should be used cautiously owing to potential for infant bleeding. Ketoprofen and naproxen have long half-lives and may remain in mother's blood a long time.

Antiallergic And Antiasthmatic Drugs
(See also *Hormones*, *Corticosteroids*)

Antihistamines	Risk category B: brompheniramine, chlorpheniramine, clemastine, cyproheptadine, diphenhydramine, loratadine, meclizine, triprolidine. Risk category C: astemizole, phenylephrine, phenylpropanolamine, terfenadine	All should be used with caution. Most are safe, but may cause infant drowsiness. If these adverse effects occur, a different drug may be tried. Clemastine is rated as AAP reason for concern and is contraindicated.
Cromolyn	Risk category B	Minimal oral absorption, so it is unlikely to adversely affect infant.
Epinephrine	Risk category C	Unlikely to be absorbed in infant's gastrointestinal tract after early newborn period, or if preterm.
Metaproterenol (Alupent)	Risk category C	Unknown if secreted in milk; use cautiously.

Anticoagulants

Heparin	Risk category C. Does not cross placenta; anticoagulant of choice during pregnancy	AAP compatible. Not excreted in breast milk
Warfarin (Coumadin)	Risk category D. Associated with facial abnormalities and neurologic deficit. Traumatic intracranial hemorrhage may occur in neonate if ingested near term. If used, it is typically avoided between 6 and 12 weeks' gestation and for 2 to 3 weeks before term.	AAP compatible, but should be used with caution. Very small amounts secreted in milk. No reported bleeding abnormalities in infant, but observe for bruising or petechiae.

Anticonvulsants

Carbamazepine (Tegretol)	Risk category C. Associated with craniofacial abnormalities, underdeveloped fingernails, neural tube defects, and developmental delay	AAP compatible. Small amounts secreted in breast milk; accumulation does not seem to occur. Observe infant for sedation.
Magnesium sulfate	Risk category A. Infants exposed to magnesium sulfate shortly before birth may exhibit respiratory depression, hypotonic muscle tone, depressed reflexes, hypocalcemia, or cardiac dysrhythmias.	AAP compatible. Moderate amounts secreted in milk, but most remains in infant's gastrointestinal tract. Milk levels return to normal about 24 hr after drug is stopped.

Phenobarbital	Risk category D. Fetal addiction with subsequent withdrawal is possible but rare at dose levels used for seizure control. Abnormalities similar to those seen in infants exposed to carbamazepine, phenytoin, and valproic acid have been reported.	AAP reason for concern. Significant amounts accumulate in infant's plasma. Psychomotor delay and sedation possible. Use cautiously.
Phenytoin (Dilantin)	Risk category D. The fetal hydantoin syndrome includes prenatal-onset growth deficiency, small head, mental retardation, craniofacial and other anomalies, underdeveloped nails or distal phalanges.	AAP compatible. Minimal effects if maternal dose is low. Observe for sedation and decreased sucking.
Trimethadione (Tridione)	Risk category D. Fetal risk for malformations is greater than with other anticonvulsants. Associated with developmental delay, craniofacial abnormalities, cardiovascular and other internal abnormalities.	Enters breast milk. Use cautiously.
Valproic acid (Depakene)	Risk category D. Associated with neural tube defects, craniofacial abnormalities.	AAP compatible. Secreted in small amounts. May cause drowsiness. Used for infant seizures.

Antidiabetic Agents

Insulin	Risk category B. Insulin is only appropriate drug to control diabetes during pregnancy because it does not cross placenta.	AAP compatible. Any insulin secreted would be destroyed in infant's gastrointestinal tract.
Oral hypoglycemic agents	Contraindicated; cross placenta. Insulin controls blood glucose levels without crossing placenta. May cause prolonged neonatal hypoglycemia.	Safety not established for most. Observe for infant hypoglycemia.

Antihypertensives—See also *Diuretics* because these drugs are often used to treat hypertension.

ACE inhibitors (benazepril, captopril, enalapril, fosinopril, ramipril)	Risk categories C and D. Suspected teratogenic effects. May reduce uteroplacental perfusion and cause fetal hypotension. Renal malformations with anuria, leading to oligohydramnios, lung hypoplasia, and cranial and facial deformities.	Use with caution. Captopril and enalapril are AAP compatible. Small amounts are transferred to infant. Observe for infant hypotension.

Drug	Risk	Lactation
Beta-adrenergic blockers (acebutolol, atenolol, betaxolol, labetalol, metoprolol, nadolol, penbutolol, pindolol, propranolol, timolol)	Risk category C, except acebutolol, atenolol, and pindolol, which are risk category B. Possible fetal or neonatal effects include transient bradycardia, respiratory depression, and hypoglycemia.	AAP compatible, but potentially hazardous: acebutolol, labetalol, nadolol, timolol. Observe infant for pharmacologic effects if mother is taking a beta-adrenergic blocker: hypotension, bradycardia, sedation, fatigue.
Calcium channel blockers (amlodipine, diltiazem, nicardipine, nifedipine, nimodipine, verapamil)	Risk category C. Hypotensive effects may reduce uteroplacental perfusion and may lead to fetal heart failure and atrioventricular block. Nifedipine has been used on an investigational basis to inhibit preterm labor.	Drugs excreted in breast milk. AAP compatible: diltiazem, nifedipine, and verapamil. Use with extreme caution; overdoses in young children are very dangerous. Observe for hypotension and bradycardia. Delaying nursing for 3-4 hr after the non-sustained-release form may reduce transfer to infant.
Centrally acting sympatholytics (clonidine, guanabenz, guanfacine, methyldopa)	Risk category C, except for guanfacine (risk category B).	Methyldopa is AAP compatible. Others should be used cautiously, as safety is not established. Observe for hypotension and sedation.

Vasodilators (hydralazine, minoxidil)	Risk category C. No adverse fetal effects associated with long-term use. Excessive hair has been reported.	Listed drugs are AAP compatible.

Antimicrobials

Aminoglycosides (gentamicin, kanamycin, neomycin, streptomycin)	Risk categories C and D. Associated with hearing loss and renal toxicity.	AAP compatible: kanamycin and streptomycin. Most drugs in this class are poorly absorbed orally.
Azithromycin (Zithromax)	Risk category B. Chemically related to erythromycin.	Only small amounts are likely to be ingested by infant.
Cephalosporins	Most are risk category B.	Secretion into milk is generally poor. Observe for diarrhea.
Chloramphenicol	Risk category C. Not recommended for use at term because it is associated with neonatal "gray baby syndrome" (rapid respiration, ashen and pale color, poor feeding, abdominal distention, vasomotor collapse, death).	AAP reason for concern. Generally contraindicated in breastfeeding mothers. May cause infant sensitivity.
Erythromycins	Risk category C. Little transfer to fetus across placenta, which limits the drugs' usefulness for treating syphilis.	AAP compatible. May cause alteration in gastrointestinal flora, allergies, interference with infant's cultures for infection.

Fluoroquinolones (includes ciprofloxacin, norfloxacin, ofloxacin)	Risk category C. Animal studies have shown joint abnormalities.	Contraindicated. Possible association with cartilage damage and colitis.
Metronidazole (Flagyl)	Risk category B. However, not recommended to treat Trichomonas infections during first trimester.	AAP reason for concern (primarily for oral form). Breastfeeding may be discontinued for 12-24 hr to allow mother to excrete last dose, then restarted.
Nitrofurantoin (Macrodantin)	Risk category B. Use should be avoided near term because it may cause hemolytic anemia in newborn.	AAP compatible for older infants. Should avoid if infant is younger than 1 month. Risk for hemolytic anemia if infant has an enzyme (G-6-PD) deficiency.
Penicillins (includes amoxicillin, ampicillin, penicillin G)	Risk category B. No reported adverse fetal effects. Penicillins combined with beta-lactamase inhibitors (Augmentin, Timentin, and Unasyn) have not been adequately studied, although fetal effects are unlikely.	Penicillins are AAP compatible. Observe for infant diarrhea or development of sensitivity.

Sulfonamides	Risk category B (D near term). May result in neonatal hyperbilirubinemia.	Potentially hazardous. Sulfisoxazole is considered compatible, but all should be used with great caution. Associated with jaundice, diarrhea, rash.
Tetracyclines	Risk category D. Can interfere with tooth enamel formation and cause discolored teeth. Prenatal exposure does not affect permanent teeth.	AAP compatible for short periods. Tooth discoloration, slowed bone growth, and altered bowel flora are possible.

Antineoplastics—Few cases have been studied because of the relative rarity with which these drugs are used in women of childbearing age. Therefore, their relative safety or danger cannot be accurately determined. Additionally, reported congenital defects may be more related to the mother's serious disease than to the drug itself.

Alkylating agents	Probable association with fetal anomalies. Risk category D.	Contraindicated
Antimetabolites	Risk category D. Methotrexate is contraindicated for treatment of psoriasis or rheumatoid arthritis during pregnancy (risk category X).	Contraindicated
Tamoxifen (Nolvadex)	Risk category D	Contraindicated

Antituberculosis Agents (see also Antimicrobials)

Ethambutol	Risk category B. No evidence of increased abnormalities. Fetal effects of combinations of ethambutol with other antituberculosis drugs are unknown.	AAP compatible. Concentration in breast milk is similar to that in maternal serum, so caution is indicated.
Isoniazid	Risk category C	AAP compatible, but infant should be observed for liver toxicity and neuritis.
Pyrazinamide	Risk category C. Safety is not established; try to avoid use.	Use cautiously.
Rifampin	Risk category C	AAP compatible. No reported adverse effects

Antitussives and Expectorants

Dextromethorphan	Risk category C	Safety not established
Guaifenesin	Risk category C	Unlikely to cause side effects

Antiviral Agents

Acyclovir	Risk category C	AAP compatible. Few reported toxicities. If topical drug is used on nipples, wash thoroughly before nursing.

Ribavirin (Virazole)	Risk category X. Administered by aerosol. Women who are pregnant or may become pregnant should avoid exposure.	Not known if drug is excreted in milk.
Zidovudine (formerly called AZT)	Risk category C. Given to HIV-seropositive women to reduce risk for perinatal transmission of the virus.	Contraindicated

Bronchodilators

Albuterol	Risk category C	Small amounts likely to be secreted. Observe infant for tremors and excitement.
Terbutaline (Brethine)	Risk category B. Also used in treatment of preterm labor	AAP compatible. Observe infant for tremors and nervousness.
Theophylline	Risk category C	AAP compatible. Excreted in milk. May result in infant irritability, insomnia, and fretfulness.

Cardiac Glycosides

Digoxin	Risk category C	AAP compatible

Decongestants

Ephedrine, epinephrine, oxymetazoline, phenylephrine	Risk category C. Should not be used during third trimester.	Use with caution. May cause irritability in infant.

Pseudoephedrine	Risk category C. Avoid during third trimester.	AAP compatible. Minimal amounts secreted in milk.

Diuretics

Furosemide (Lasix)	Risk category C	Effects unknown but probably minimal. May reduce milk production.
Thiazides	Risk categories B and C. Decreased intravascular volume may reduce uteroplacental perfusion. Metabolic disturbances and thrombocytopenia may occur in mother and fetus.	Probably safe. May reduce milk production.

Hormones

Corticosteroids	Risk category C. Prednisone is agent of choice for asthmatic woman who needs steroids. Betamethasone and dexamethasone are used to accelerate maturation of fetal lungs if preterm delivery is likely.	Potentially hazardous in high doses or with long-term use. Delay nursing 4 hr after dose to reduce transfer to infant. Do not apply topically to nipples.
Estrogens	Risk category X. Diethylstilbestrol (DES) is associated with development of vaginal cancer in female offspring during adolescence or adulthood.	Reduces milk volume and protein content. Try to delay drug until breastfeeding is firmly established. DES should not be used.

Oral contraceptives (estrogen-progestin combinations)	Risk category X. Doses much higher than those used in oral contraceptives are associated with masculinization of the female fetus' genitalia.	Should not be used until lactation is well established, or drugs may decrease milk quantity and quality.
Clomiphene citrate (Clomid)	Risk category X. Questionable association with neural tube defects. Drug is discontinued after pregnancy is achieved.	May suppress lactation. Unlikely to be prescribed during lactation because it is given for infertility.

Psychoactive Drugs

Benzodiazepines	Most are risk category D. The following benzodiazepines are risk category X and contraindicated during pregnancy: estazolam, quazepam, temazepam, and triazolam. Some reports of mild facial abnormalities and developmental delay, but no conclusive studies.	Potentially hazardous. Preferred drugs in this class are lorazepam or oxazepam.
Lithium	Risk category D. Slightly increased risk for cardiac abnormalities.	AAP contraindicated

Drug	Pregnancy	Lactation
Meprobamate	Contraindicated. Associated with a significant increase in malformations. Equagesic contains meprobamate.	Concentrations in milk are higher than in maternal serum. May cause sedation in infant.
Phenothiazines (chlorpromazine, perphenazine, prochlorperazine, thioridazine, trifluoperazine)	Risk category C. Risk of malformations is uncertain. Continued use during pregnancy should be carefully evaluated.	AAP reason for concern; some sources say these drugs are probably safe in usual doses. Observe infant for sedation or jerking movements.
Tricyclic antidepressants	Risk category C	Use with caution. Probably safe in usual doses. Desipramine and nortriptyline are preferred. Some sources consider these drugs contraindicated for breastfeeding mothers.

Thyroid Drugs

Drug	Pregnancy	Lactation
Antithyroids (methimazole, propylthiouracil [PTU])	Risk category D. May result in neonatal goiter or hypothyroidism, although uncommon at usual therapeutic doses. Methimazole has possible association with scalp defects.	AAP compatible. Propylthiouracil is preferred drug.
Iodine, iodides	Risk category C. Long-term exposure may produce fetal thyroid enlargement.	Use caution. May cause rash or suppress infant's thyroid function. Large quantities of iodides are contraindicated.

Thyroid replacement hormones (levothyroxine, liothyronine, liotrix)	Risk category A. Crosses placenta only to limited extent.	Small amounts secreted in milk. Observe infant for nervousness and agitation. Infant should have periodic thyroid studies.

Vitamins and Retinoids

Retinoids (etretinate [Tegison], isotretinoin [Accutane])	Risk category X. Related to vitamin A. Associated with severe fetal malformations (microcephaly, ear abnormalities, cardiac defects, central nervous system abnormalities). Etretinate has a long half-life and may have fetal effects up to 18 months after drug is stopped.	AAP contraindicated
Vitamin A	Risk category A (X at high doses). Excess intake may lead to abnormalities noted for etretinate and isotretinoin.	Breast milk usually supplies sufficient vitamin A to infant. Mother should not take more than 6000 units per day.
Vitamin B_6 (pyridoxine)	Risk category A. Large doses could produce pyridoxine deficiency in infant.	AAP compatible, but a maximum of 10 mg/day should be prescribed, and only to women having deficiencies.

Vitamin D	Risk category C (D at high doses). Excess intake associated with malformations, including aortic stenosis, facial abnormalities, and mental retardation.	AAP compatible. Should be supplemented with caution. High doses could cause high infant calcium levels.

Miscellaneous Drugs

Nicotine gum; nicotine transdermal	Risk category X	AAP contraindicated. Nicotine levels from drug may be less than those from smoking, if the mother does not smoke at all. Smoking plus use of nicotine-containing drugs could lead to high levels in infant. Observe for infant shock, vomiting, diarrhea, tachycardia, and restlessness.

Bibliography

American College of Obstetricians and Gynecologists (1996). *Guidelines for women's health care.* Washington, D.C.: Author.

American College of Obstetricians and Gynecologists (1996). *Hypertension in pregnancy.* Technical Bulletin No. 219. Washington, D.C.

Creasy, R.K., and Resnik, R. (1994). *Maternal-fetal medicine: Principles and practice* (3rd ed.). Philadelphia: W.B. Saunders.

Cunningham, F.G., MacDonald, P.C., Gant, N.F., Leveno, K.J., Gilstrap, L.C., Hankins, G.D.V., and Clark, S.L. (1997). *Williams obstetrics* (20th ed.). Norwalk, CT: Appleton & Lange.

Fischbach, F. (1996). *A manual of laboratory and diagnostic tests* (5th ed.). Philadelphia: J.B. Lippincott.

Hatcher, R.A., Trussell, J., Steward, F., et al (1994). *Contraceptive Technology* (16th ed.). New York: Irvington Publishers.

Lee, R.V. (1995). Sexually transmitted infections. In G.N. Borrow and T.F. Ferris (eds.), *Medical Complications During Pregnancy* (4th ed.), pp. 404–438. Philadelphia: W.B. Saunders.

Martens, K.A. (1994). Sexually transmitted and genital tract infections during pregnancy. *Emergency Medicine Clinics of North America,* 12(1), 91–113.

NAACOG (1990). *Fetal heart rate auscultation.* Washington, D.C.: Author.

Teitz, N.W. (1995). *Clinical guide to laboratory tests* (3rd ed.). Philadelphia: W.B. Saunders.

Trussell, J. (1990). Contraceptive failure in the United States: An update. *Studies in Family Planning,* 21(1), 52.

Youngkin, E.Q. (1995). Sexually transmitted diseases: Current and emerging concerns. *Journal of Obstetric, Gynecologic, and Neonatal Nursing,* 24(8), 743–758.

Index

A

AAP (American Academy of Pediatrics) drug safety classifications, 474
Abduction, infant, 224
Abnormal uterine bleeding, 388–389
Abortion, 54–56
　induced, 395–396
Abruptio placentae, 61–65
Accu-Check glucometer, 424–426
ACE inhibitors, 479
Acetaminophen, 475
Acquired immunodeficiency syndrome (AIDS), 87t, 273t, 411
Acyclovir, 484
Adjuvant therapy, 386
Adolescent pregnancy, 328–334
β-Adrenergics (tocolysis), Ritodrine, 177t
Affective disorders, postpartum, 326–328
Afterpains, 271, 297
Albuterol, 485
Alcohol, 336t
Alkylating agents, 483
American Academy of Pediatrics (AAP) drug safety classifications, 474
Aminoglycosides, 481
Amniotic fluid, 22
Amniotic fluid embolism, 185
Amniotomy (AROM), 149–150
Analgesics, 475–476
Anemias
　folic acid-deficiency (megaloblastic), 53
　iron deficiency, 53
　sickle cell, 53–54
Anesthesia, general, 147–148
Anomalies, infant born with congenital, 345–346
Antepartal assessment
　history, 30–32
　physical examination, 32–33
　psychosocial, 34
　scheduling, 34
　subsequent, 38
　tests and procedures, 35–38
Anterior pituitary, 2
Antiallergic drugs, 476
Antiasthmatic drugs, 476
Anticoagulants, 477
Anticonvulsants, 477–478
Antidiabetic agents, 479
Antihistamines, 476
Antihypertensives, 479–481
Antimetabolites, 483
Antimicrobials, 481–483
Antineoplastics, 483
Antithyroids, 488
Antituberculosis agents, 484
Antitussives, 484
Apgar score, 130, 131t
AROM (Amniotomy), 149–150
Asphyxia, 226–227
Aspirin, use of, during pregnancy and breastfeeding, 475
Assessment
　fetal, 125–126
　focus, 108
　intrapartum guide, 109–124
　maternal, 126
Attachment, 287, 308
Augmentation, of labor, 150–153
Autosomal dominant traits, 14–15
Autosomal recessive traits, 15
Axillary temperature, assessing, 429–430
Azithromycin, 481
AZT (Zidovudine), 485

B

Backache, 46
Bacterial vaginosis, 412t
Basal body temperature (BBT), 441–442
Bathing, during pregnancy, 42
BBT (basal body temperature), 441–442
Behavior states, 194
Benzodiazepines, 487
Beta-adrenergic blockers, 480
Bilirubin encephalopathy, 238
Birth, *see* Childbirth
Birth center, when to go to guidelines, 107–108
Birth weight, 166
Bladder, 285–286, 291t
Bleeding complications
  abortion, 54–56
  abruptio placentae, 61–65
  ectopic pregnancy, 56–58
  hydatidiform mole, 58–60
  placenta previa, 60–61
Blood glucose, *see also* Hypoglycemia
  assessing, in newborn, 424–426
  maintaining, 217–218
Blood pressure (BP), 284, 290t
Blood values, postpartum adaptations, 283
Blood volume, postpartum adaptations, 283
Bonding, 287, 308
Bowel function, 286, 291t
Bradley method, of childbirth education, 52
Breast, 11
  care of, during pregnancy, 42
  care of, for nonlactating mothers, 298
  examination, 381–382
  postpartum adaptations, 285
  postpartum assessment, 291t
Breast cancer, 384–388
Breastfeeding, 299, 302
  common problems, 302–305
  positions, 300–301t
Breast-milk jaundice, 235–236
Breast reconstruction, 387
Breast self-examination (BSE), 381, 433–434
Breathing techniques, 143
Breech presentation, 168–169
Brethine (Terbutaline), 485
Bronchodilators, 485

Bronchopulmonary dysplasia, 227
BSE (breast self-examination), 381
Bulbourethral glands, 13
Bulb syringe, using, 445
Butorphanol, 447–448

C

Calcium channel blockers, 480
Cancer
  breast, 384–388
  cervical, 405t, 407
  colorectal, 383
  ovarian, 405t, 408
  uterine, 405t
Candidiasis, 275t, 411t
Carbamazepine (Tegretol), 477
Cardiac glycosides, 485
Cardinal movements, of labor, 99–103
Cardiovascular adaptation, 188–189
Cardiovascular system, postpartum adaptations, 283
Catecholamines (stress hormones), 98
Central acting sympatholytics, 480
Cephalosporins, 481
Cervical cancer, 405t, 407
Cervical cap, 352–353
Cervical changes, 99
Cervical mucus assessment, 443–444
Cervical polyps, 404
Cesarean birth, 158–163
  common nursing diagnoses, 310
  nursing assessments, 309t
  nursing interventions, 310–311
Chemstrip reagent strips, 424–426
Chickenpox, 86t, 274t
Childbearing
  environmental influences, 17
  genetic influences, 13–17
Childbirth, *see also* Labor; Pregnancy
  before attendant arrival, 130
  nursing responsibilities during, 129
  nursing responsibilities immediately after, 130–133
  pain management, 142–148
  passage component, 91–96
  passenger component, 96–98
  powers component, 91
  psyche component, 98
Childbirth education
  methods, 52
  programs, 51

Chlamydial infections, 89t, 274t, 410t
Chloramphenicol, 481
Chromosomes, 13–14
Circulation, fetal and postnatal, 23f
Circumcision, 222–223
Cleft lip, 227–229
Cleft palate, 227–229
Clomiphene citrate, 487
Cocaine, 337t, 340
Cold stress, 189–190
Colorectal cancer, 383
Condom
  female, 354–355
  male, 353–354
Condylomata Acuminata, 90, 410t
Congenital anomalies, 345–346
Congenital heart defects, 229–231
Conjugated estrogens, 448–450
Constipation, 47
Contraception
  considerations when teaching, 349, 352
  effectiveness, failure and discontinuation rates, 350–351t
  emergency, 357
Contraceptives, oral, 363, 365–366, 487
Contraction
  monitoring external fetal heart rate, 421–423
  monitoring internal fetal heart rate, 423–424
  palpating, 432–433
Corticosteroids, 180t, 486
Cramps (primary dysmenorrhea), 389–390
Critical pathways, 213
Cromolyn, 476
Cutaneous stimulation, 142
Cysts, 404–405
Cytomegalovirus infection, 86t, 272t

D

Decongestants, 485
Deep tendon reflexes, assessing, 426–427
Deep vein thrombosis (DVT), 318–319
Delayed pregnancy, 334–335
Depakene (valproic acid), 478
Depo-Provera, *see* Hormone injections
Dextromethorphan, 484
Dextrostix reagent strips, 424–426

Diabetes mellitus, *see also* Gestational diabetes mellitus (GDM); Preexisting diabetes mellitus
  effects of, on pregnancy, 66
  effects of pregnancy on insulin production, 65–66
  fetal and neonatal risk, 66–67
  nursing considerations, 71
  types, 65
Diaphragm, 355–357
Diaphragmatic hernia, 231–232
DIC (disseminated intravascular coagulation), 64–65
Dick-Read method, of childbirth education, 52
Digoxin, 485
Dilantin (Phenytoin), 478
Dilation, 99
Diminished reflexes (hyporeflexia), 426–427
Disseminated intravascular coagulation (DIC), 64–65
Diuretics, 486
Dominant traits
  autosomal, 14–15
Douching, during pregnancy, 42
Drugs, *see also specific drugs*
  commonly used, for intrapartum pain management, 144t
  over-the-counter, during pregnancy, 45
DVT (deep vein thrombosis), 318–319
Dysfunctional labor
  abnormal duration, 171–173
  problems of the passage, 169–170
  problems of the powers, 164–166
  problems of the psyche, 170–171
  problems with the passenger, 166–169

E

Early care, 213
Ectopic pregnancy, 56–58
EDB (estimated date of birth), 24
EDC (estimated date of confinement), 24
EDD (estimated date of delivery), 24
Effacement, 99
Electronic fetal monitoring (EFM), 135
  clarifying questionable data, 140
  equipment, 135

Elimination
  postpartum adaptations, 285–286
  postpartum assessment, 291t
Emergency contraception, 357
Employment, during pregnancy, 44
Endometriosis, 390–392
Endometrium, 407–408
Engorgement, 304
Ephedrine, 485
Epididymis, 13
Epidural block, 145–146
Epinephrine, 476
Episiotomy, 157–158
Erythroblastosis fetalis, 238, *see also* Hyperbilirubinemia (jaundice)
Erythromycin ophthalmic ointment, 450–451
Erythromycins, 481
Esophageal atresia, 232–233
Estimated date of birth (EDB), 24
Estimated date of confinement (EDC), 24
Estimated date of delivery (EDD), 24
Estrogens, 486
Ethambutol, 484
Exaggerated reflexes (hyperreflexia), 426–427
Exercise, during pregnancy, 42–44
Expectorants, 484
External cephalic version, 153–154
Eye treatment, 217

F

Fallopian tubes, 6
False labor, 107
Family adaptation, 288
FDA (Food and Drug Administration), pregnancy risk categories, 473
Fecal occult blood testing (FOBT), 383
Feedings, 219
  with formulas, 298–299
Fertility, decline in, 3
Fertility awareness
  basal body temperature, 441–442
  cervical mucus assessment, 443–444
  methods, 362–363
  teaching women, 440–444
Fetal and postnatal circulation, 23f
Fetal assessment, intrapartal, 125–126

factors affecting fetal oxygenation, 134
types, 135
Fetal compromise, 126, 127
Fetal heart rate (FHR), 136–139
  auscultating, 430–431
  contraction monitoring external, 421–423
  contraction monitoring internal, 423–424
  nonreassuring patterns, 138–139t, 140–141
  reassuring patterns, 137t
Fetal membranes, 22
Fetal scalp blood sampling, 40
Fetal scalp stimulation, 139
Fibroids (uterine leiomyomas), 404
Flagyl (Metronidazole), 482
Fluoroquinolones, 482
Focus assessments, 108
Folic acid-deficiency (megaloblastic) anemia, 53
Follicle-stimulating hormone (FSH), 2
Food and Drug Administration (FDA) pregnancy risk categories, 473
Forceps, 155–156
Formula feeding, 298–299
FSH (follicle-stimulating hormone), 2
Furosemide (Lasix), 486

G

Gastrointestinal system, 191
Gastroschisis, 251–252
Gavage feeding, administering, 417–418
General anesthesia, 147–148
Genital herpes, 87t
Genital warts, 410t
Gestational age assessment, 195, 212, 214–215f
Gestational diabetes mellitus (GDM)
  assessing and managing preexisting, 69–70
  diagnosing, 67–68
  managing, 68
  nursing considerations, 71
Gonorrhea, 89t, 274t, 410t
Gravida, 24
Group B streptococcus infection, 88t, 274t
Guaifenesin, 484

H

Hand washing, 298
Headache, management of post-spinal, 147
Health maintenance
  family history, 379
  immunizations, 384
  individual history, 378–379
  physical assessment, 379–380
  screening procedures, 381–384
Heartburn, 46
Heart defects, congenital, 229–231
Heart disease
  antepartum management, 80
  functional classification, 79t
  intrapartum management, 80–81
  nursing considerations, 81–82
  postpartum management, 82
  signs and symptoms, 79
Heat loss, 189–190, 216–217
Heel puncture, 424–426
Hemorrhage
  postpartum, 312–315
  preventing postpartum, 294–296
  risk factors, 293
Hemorrhoids, 47, 296–297
Heparin, 477
Hepatic system, 191–192
Hepatitis B, 87t, 272t, 411t
Hepatitis B vaccine, 452–453
Hepatitis immunization, 225
Hernia, diaphragmatic, 231–232
Heroin, 337t, 341–342
Herpes, 273t
Herpes genitalis, 410t
High-risk pregnancy, 39
Horizontal infection, 271
Hormone implant, 357–359
Hormone injections, 361–362
Hormone replacement therapy (HRT), 397–399
Hormones, 486
HRT (hormone replacement therapy), 397–399
Human immunodeficiency virus, 273t, 411t
Hyaline membrane disease (HMD), 233, see also Respiratory distress syndrome (RDS)
Hydatidiform mole, 58–60
Hydralazine, 451–452
Hydrocephalus, 233–234
Hyperbilirubinemia (jaundice), 222, 234–239

Hyperemesis gravidarum, 82–83
Hyperreflexia (exaggerated reflexes), 426–427
Hypertensive disorders, see also Preeclampsia
  classification, 74t
  nursing considerations, 76
  nursing interventions, 77–78
  predisposing factors, 72
  signs and symptoms, 72–75
Hyperthermia, 190
Hypocalcemia, 239–240
Hypoglycemia, 191, 240–242
Hyporeflexia (diminished reflexes), 426–427
Hypothalamus, 2
Hypovolemic shock, first sign of, 132

I

Identification, infant, 219, 431–432
IDM (infant of diabetic mother), 242–243
Immune system, 192–193
Immunizations, during pregnancy, 45
Immunoglobulins, 193
Indomethacin (tocolysis), 179t
Induced abortion, 395–396
Induction, of labor, 150–153
Infant abduction, 224
Infant born with congenital anomalies, 345–348, see also Newborns
Infant care, teaching, 223
Infant communication cues, 288
Infant cues, 288
Infant identification, 219, 431–432
Infant of diabetic mother (IDM), 242–243
Infection, see also specific infections
  horizontal, 271
  preventing, 223–224
  risk factors, 293
  vertical, 271, 272–275t
Infertility
  diagnostic tests, 372–375t
  female factors, 370–371
  male factors, 370
  nursing care of couples, 377–378
  repeated pregnancy loss, 371
Infertility therapy medications, 376–377
Infiltration, local, 146
Injections, intramuscular, administering to newborns, 419–420

Insulin, 479
Insulin production, effects of pregnancy on, 65–66
Intramuscular injections, administering to newborns, 419–420
Intrapartal fetal assessment
  factors affecting fetal oxygenation, 134
  types, 135
Intrapartum period
  assessment guide, 109–124
  fetal assessments, 125–126
  nursing interventions, 126–129
Intrathecal opioid analgesics, 146
Intrauterine devices (IUDs), 359–360
Intrauterine growth restriction (IUGR), *see* Small-for-gestational-age infants
Intraventricular hemorrhage, *see* Periventricular-intraventricular hemorrhage
Involution, 281, 282t, 298, *see also* Subinvolution
Iodine, 488
Iron deficiency anemia, 53
Isoniazid, 484
IUDs (intrauterine devices), 359–360

J

Jaundice (hyperbilirubinemia), 222
  breast-milk, 235–236
  nursing considerations, 238–239
  pathologic, 236–238
  physiologic, 235

K

Kegel exercise, 306
Kernicterus, *see* Bilirubin encephalopathy
Kidneys, 285–286

L

Labor, *see also* Childbirth; Dysfunctional labor; Pregnancy; Preterm labor
  characteristics, 105–106t
  mechanisms of, 99–103
  pain management techniques, 142–148
  performing vaginal examination during, 438–440
  pharmacological techniques, 144t
  stages of, 104–106
  true *versus* false, 107
Laboratory values
  newborn, 471–472
  pregnant and nonpregnant women, 469–470
Lactation
  drug use during, 473–474
  nutrition during, 51
Lamaze method, of childbirth education, 52
Lasix (Furosemide), 486
Last menstrual period (LMP), 24
Leg cramps, 47
Leopold's maneuvers, 38, 434–436
LH (luteinizing hormone), 2
Lithium, 487
LMP (last menstrual period), 24
Local infiltration, 146
Lochia, 281–282, 289t
Luteinizing hormone (LH), 2

M

McRobert's maneuver, 167
Macrodantin (Nitrofurantoin), 482
Macrosomia, 166
Magnesium sulfate, 179t, 454–455, 477
Magnesium toxicity, 77
Mammography, 382
Marijuana, 337t
Massage, 142
Mastitis, 324–325
Maternal touch, 287–288
Meconium aspiration syndrome (MAS), 244–245
Medroxyprogesterone, 455–456, *see also* Hormone injections
Megaloblastic (folic acid-deficiency) anemia, 53
Membranes
  artificial rupture of, 149–150
  fetal, 22
  testing for ruptured, 444
Meningocele, *See* Neural tube defects
Menopause, 396–399
Menstrual cycle, 389–392
Meprobamate, 488
Metaproterenol, 476
Methergine, 456–457
Metritis, 321–323
Metronidazole (Flagyl), 482

Milk stools, 191
Multifactorial disorders, 16–17
Multifetal gestation, 169
Multigravida, 24
Mycobacterium tuberculosis (tuberculosis), 88t
Myelomeningocele, *see* Neural tube defects

N

Naloxone hydrochloride (Narcan), 458–459
Narcan (Naloxone hydrochloride), 458–459
Narcotic analgesics, use of, during pregnancy and breastfeeding, 475
Natural family planning methods, 362–363, 364t
Nausea, 45–46
Necrotizing enterocolitis (NEC), 245–246
Neonatal abstinence syndrome, 246–250
Neonatal reflexes, 220–221
Neural tube defects, 250–251
Neurological adaptation, 189–190
New Ballard Score, 195, 210–211f
Newborns, *see also* Infant born with congenital anomalies
  adaptation processes
    cardiovascular, 188–189
    gastrointestinal, 191
    hematological, 190
    hepatic system, 191–192
    immune system, 192–193
    neurological, 189–190
    psychosocial, 193–195
    respiratory system, 188
    urinary system, 192
  administering intramuscular injections, 419–420
  assessing blood glucose, 424–426
  assessing vital signs, 428–430
  common nursing diagnoses, 212–213
  continuing assessments, 218
  laboratory values, 471–472
  measuring, 446
  nursing assessments, 195–209t
  performing resuscitation in, 436–438
  positioning, 213–216
  weighing, 445
Nicotine gum, 490
Nifedipine (tocolysis), 180t
Nitrofurantoin (Macrodantin), 482
Nolvadex (Tamoxifen), 483
Nonlactating mothers, breast care and, 298
Nonreassuring patterns, of fetal heart rate, 140–141
  identifying cause of, 140
  interventions for, 141
Nonsteroidal anti-inflammatory drug (NSAIDs), 476
Nonverbal cues, infant, 288
Nonviral infections, 88t
Norplant, *see* Hormone implant
Nullipara, 24
Nutrition
  during lactation, 51
  for pregnancy, 48–49
  risk factors, 49–50
  supplementation, 50–51

O

OCs (oral contraceptives), 363, 365–366, 487
Omphalocele, 251–252
One Touch glucometer, 424–426
Oral contraceptives (OCs), 363, 365–366, 487
Oral hypoglycemic agents, 479
Osteoporosis, 399–401
Ovarian cancer, 405t, 408
Ovarian cysts, 404–405
Over-the-counter drugs, during pregnancy, 45
Oxytocin, 152, 459–462

P

Pain management, labor
  nonpharmacological techniques, 142–143
  pharmacological techniques, 144–148
  regional techniques for, 145–148
Palpating contractions, 432–433
Palpation of fundus, 32, 33f
Papanicolaou (Pap) test, 382
Para, 24
Passage, component of childbirth, 91–96, 169–170
Passenger, component of childbirth,

96–98, 166–169
Pathologic jaundice, 236–238
Pediatric urine collection bag, applying, 420–421
Pelvic inflammatory disease (PID), 412–413
Pelvic support, dysfunction of, 401–403
Pelvis, 6–9, 7f
  divisions and measurements, 91–96
  types, 169–170
Penicillins, 482
Penis, 12
Perineal trauma, 296–297
Perineum, 282–283, 290t, 427
Periodic abstinence methods, 362–363
Periventricular-intraventricular hemorrhage (PIVH), 252–253
Persistent fetal circulation, *see* Persistent pulmonary hypertension of the newborn (PPHN)
Persistent pulmonary hypertension of the newborn (PPHN), 253–254
Phenobarbital, 478
Phenothiazines, 488
Phenytoin (Dilantin), 478
Physical abuse, of women, 343–345
Physiologic jaundice, 235
Phytonadione (vitamin K1), 467–468
PID (pelvic inflammatory disease), 412–413
PIVH (periventricular-intraventricular hemorrhage), 252–253
Placenta, 22
Placenta previa, 60–61
Placental abruption, 61–65
PMS (premenstrual syndrome), 392–395
Polycythemia, 255–256
Polyps, 404
Postcoital contraception, 357
Postmaturity syndrome, 256–257
Postnatal, fetal and, circulation, 23f
Postpartum adaptation
  cardiovascular system, 283
  common nursing diagnoses, 293–294
  nursing assessments, 289–292
  reproductive system, 281–283
Postpartum blues, 326
Postpartum depression, 327
Postpartum hemorrhage, 312–315
Postpartum period
  preventing hemorrhage, 294–296
  preventing injury, 294–296
  promoting comfort, 296–297
  providing health education, 298–308
Postpartum psychosis, 328
Post-spinal headache, management of, 147
Powers, component of childbirth, 91, 164–166
PPHN (persistent pulmonary hypertension of the newborn), 253–254
PPROM (preterm premature rupture of the membranes), 173–174
Preeclampsia, *see also* Hypertensive disorders
  management of mild, 75
  management of severe, 75–76
  nursing considerations, 76
  signs and symptoms, 72–75
Preexisting diabetes mellitus, 69–70
Pregnancy, *see also* Childbirth; Labor; Preterm Labor
  danger signs, 42, 43t
  diabetes and, 66
  ectopic, 56–58
  FDA risk categories, 473
  high-risk, 39, 40–41t
  insulin production and, 65–66
  nutrition for, 48–51
  overcoming discomforts during, 45–47
  physiologic adaptations, 26–30t, 29
  psychosocial adaptations, 30, 31t
  teaching health promotion during, 42–45
Pregnancy complications
  anemias, 53–54
  bleeding, 54–64
  diabetes mellitus, 65–71
  disseminated intravascular coagulation (DIC), 64–65
  heart disease, 78–82
  hyperemesis gravidarum, 82–83
  hypertensive disorders, 71–78
  infections, 85–88t
  Rh incompatibility, 84–85
  sexually transmissible diseases, 89–90t
Pregnancy risk categories, 457
Premature infants, *see* Preterm

infants
Premature rupture of the membranes (PROM), 173–174
Premenstrual syndrome (PMS), 392–395
Prenatal development, 1
  embryonic period, 18
  fetal period, 18
  pre-embryonic period, 18
  timetable, 19–21
Preterm infants
  environmentally-caused stress, 263–264
  fluid and electrolyte balance problems, 260–261
  infection problems, 261–262
  nutrition problems, 264–266
  pain problems, 262–263
  parenting problems, 266–268
  respiratory problems, 257–258
  thermoregulatory problems, 258–269
Preterm labor, 175–181
  drugs used in, 177–180t
  maternal risk factors, 175t
Preterm premature rupture of the membranes (PPROM), 173–174
Primary dysmenorrhea (cramps), 389–390
Primigravida, 24
Primip, 24
Primipara, 24–25
Prolapsed umbilical cord, 181–182
PROM (premature rupture of the membranes), 173–174
Prophylactic medications, 217
Prostate, 13
Protozoa Toxoplasma gondii (toxoplasmosis), 88t
Pseudoephedrine, 486
Psyche, component of childbirth, 98, 170–171
Psychoactive drugs, 487
Puberty
  defined, 1–2
  female, 2–3
  male, 3
Pudendal block, 146
Puerperal infections, 321–326
  mastitis, 324–325
  metritis, 321–323
  septic pelvic thrombophlebitis, 325–326
  wounds, 323–324

Puerperal phases, 286–287
Pulmonary embolism, 319–320
Pulse, assessing, of newborn, 420
Pyrazinamide, 484

R

Reactivity, periods of, 193–194
Recessive traits
  autosomal, 15
  x-linked, 15–16
Reciprocal attachment behaviors, 288
Reconstruction, breast, 387
Rectal temperature, assessing, 430
Reflexes
  assessing deep tendon, 426–427
  neonatal, 220–221
Relaxation, assisting, 142
Reproductive anatomy
  female
    blood supply, 9
    external, 4f
    internal, 4–6, 4f
    nerve supply, 9
    support structure, 6–9
  male
    external organs, 12
    internal organs, 12–13
Reproductive cycle, female
  cervical mucus, 10–11
  endometrial, 10
  ovarian, 9–10
Reproductive system, 1, 281–283
Reproductive tract
  benign disorders, 404–405
  malignant disorders, 405–409
  risk factors for cancer, 405t
Respirations, assessing, of newborn, 428–429
Respiratory distress syndrome (RDS), 268–269
Respiratory distress syndrome, type II, *see* Transient tachypnea of the newborn (TTN)
  Respiratory system adaptation, 188
Rest, during pregnancy, 44
Resuscitation, performing, in newborns, 436–438
Retinoids, 489
Retinopathy of prematurity (ROP), 269–270
Retrolental fibroplasia (RLF), 269–

270
RH₁(D) immune globulin, 462–464
Rh incompatibility, 84–85
Ribavirin (Virazole), 485
Rifampin, 484
RLF (retrolental fibroplasia), 269–270
ROP (retinopathy of prematurity), 269–279
Rotation abnormalities, 167–168
Rubella, 86t, 273t
Ruptured membranes, testing for, 444

S

Screening tests, 225
Scrotum, 12
Secretions, suctioning, 213–216
Seminal vesicles, 13
Sepsis neonatorum, 270–277
Septic pelvic thrombophlebitis, 325–326
Sex determination, 1
Sexual activity, during pregnancy, 44–45
Sexual maturation, 1–3
Sexually transmissible diseases (STDs), 89–90t, 409–410, 410–412t
SGA (small-for-gestational-age infants), 277–278
Shoulder dystocia, 166–167
Sickle cell anemia, 53–54
Single gene inheritance, 14–16
Skincare, newborn, 219
Sleep, during pregnancy, 44
Small-for-gestational-age infants (SGA), 277–278
Spermicides, 366–367
Spina bifida occulta, *see* Neural tube defects
Spinal (subarachnoid) block, 146–147
Sterilization, 367–368
Stimulation
  cutaneous, 142
  thermal, 143
Stools, newborn, 191
Stress hormones (catecholamines), 98
Subarachnoid (spinal) block, 146–147
Subinvolution, 315–316, *see also* Involution
Substance abuse, 336–343
  effects of, 336–337
  nursing diagnoses, 339–343
Suctioning secretions, 213–216
Sulfonamides, 483
Superficial venous thrombosis, 317–318
Surfactant production, 188
Syphilis, 89t, 275t, 410t

T

Tamoxifen (Nolvadex), 483
Tegretol (Carbamazepine), 477
Temperature
  assessing axillary, 429–430
  assessing rectal, 429–430
Tendon reflexes, deep, assessing, 426–427
Teratogens, 17, 44
Terbutaline (Brethine), 178t, 464–466, 485
Testes, 12
Tetracyclines, 483
Theophylline, 485
Thermal stimulation, 143
Thermoregulation, 189–190, 216–217
Thiazides, 486
Thromboembolic disorders, 316–320
  deep vein thrombosis (DVT), 318–319
  pulmonary embolism, 319–320
  superficial venous thrombosis, 317–318
Thrombophlebitis, 317
Thrombus, 316
Thyroid drugs, 488–489
Thyroid replacement hormones, 489
Tobacco, 336t
Tocolytic drugs, 177–180t
Toxic shock syndrome (TSS), 413–414
Toxoplasmosis, 88t, 275t
Tracheoesophageal fistula (TEF), 232–233, *see also* Esophageal atresia
Transient tachypnea of the newborn (TTN), 279–280
Trauma, 185–187
Travel, during pregnancy, 45
Trichomoniasis, 90t, 411t
Tricyclic antidepressants, 488
Tridione (Trimethadione), 478
Trimester, 25
Trimethadione (Tridione), 478
True labor, 107

U

TSS (toxic shock syndrome), 413–414
TTN (transient tachypnea of the newborn), 279–280
Tubal ligation, 368–369
Tuberculosis (Mycobacterium tuberculosis), 88t

U

Umbilical cord, 22
  blood analysis, 140
  prolapsed, 181–182
Urinary frequency, 46
Urinary system, 192
Urine collection bag, pediatric, applying, 420–421
Uterine bleeding, abnormal, 388–389
Uterine cancer, 405t
Uterine fundus, assessing, 428
Uterine growth, 32, 33f
Uterine inversion, 184–185
Uterine leiomyomas (fibroids), 404
Uterine rupture, 183–184
Uterus, 5–6
  postpartum adaptations, 281
  postpartum assessment, 289t

V

Vacuum extraction, 155–156
Vagina, 5
Vaginal bleeding, 63
Vaginal examination, during labor, 438–440
Vaginal infections, 90t
Valproic acid (Depakene), 478
Varicella zoster virus (chickenpox), 86t, 274t
Varicosities, 46
Vasectomy, 368–369
Vasodilators, 481
Verbal cues, infant, 288
Verbal interaction, 287–288
Version, 153–154
Vertical infections, 271, 272–275t
Vibroacoustic stimulation, 140
Viral infections, 86–87t, 272–274t
Virazole (Ribavirin), 485
Vital signs, 290t–291t
  assessing newborn, 428–430
  postpartum adaptations, 284
Vitamin A, 489
Vitamin B_6, 489
Vitamin D, 490
Vitamin K, 217
Vitamin K1 (phytonadione), 467–468
Vitamins, 489–490
Vomiting, 45–46, 82–83
VSE (vulvar self-examination), 382
Vulvar self-examination (VSE), 382

W

Warfarin (Coumadin), 477
Weight, birth, 166
Weight gain, during pregnancy, 48
Wound infections, 323–324

X

X-linked recessive traits, 16

Z

Zidovudine (AZT), 485